Neonatology: A Clinical Approach

Neonatology: A Clinical Approach

Edited by Talia Atkins

AMERICAN
MEDICAL PUBLISHERS
www.americanmedicalpublishers.com

American Medical Publishers,
41 Flatbush Avenue,
1st Floor, New York,
NY 11217, USA

Visit us on the World Wide Web at:
www.americanmedicalpublishers.com

ISBN: 978-1-63927-422-2

Cataloging-in-Publication Data

Neonatology : a clinical approach / edited by Talia Atkins.
p. cm.
Includes bibliographical references and index.
ISBN 978-1-63927-422-2
1. Neonatology. 2. Perinatology. 3. Newborn infants. I. Atkins, Talia.
RJ251 .N46 2022
618.920 1--dc23

Table of Contents

Preface

Over the recent decade, advancements and applications have progressed exponentially. This has led to the increased interest in this field and projects are being conducted to enhance knowledge. The main objective of this book is to present some of the critical challenges and provide insights into possible solutions. This book will answer the varied questions that arise in the field and also provide an increased scope for furthering studies.

Neonatology is a field of pediatrics that is related with the medical care of newborn infants. The newborn infants who are severely ill or premature need such special medical care. Other complications which require specialized care include prematurity, low birth weight, intrauterine growth restriction, congenital malformations, sepsis, pulmonary hypoplasia and birth asphyxia. It is generally practiced in neonatal intensive care units. During this neonatal period, there are many diseases of concern. These include anemia of prematurity, atrial septal defect, brachial plexus injury, cerebral palsy, congenital heart disease, gastroschisis, lissencephaly, neonatal cholestasis, omphalocele, ventricular septal defect, etc. The development of mechanical ventilation and pulmonary surfactant replacement therapy in recent decades has improved the survival of premature infants. This book is a valuable compilation of topics, ranging from the basic to the most complex advancements in the field of neonatology. The various studies that are constantly contributing towards advancing technologies and evolution of this field are examined in detail. It will provide comprehensive knowledge to the readers.

I hope that this book, with its visionary approach, will be a valuable addition and will promote interest among readers. Each of the authors has provided their extraordinary competence in their specific fields by providing different perspectives as they come from diverse nations and regions. I thank them for their contributions.

Editor

1

Effect of combined music and touch intervention on pain response and β-endorphin and cortisol concentrations in late preterm infants

Jie Qiu[1†], Yun-fei Jiang[2†], Fang Li[1], Qian-hong Tong[1], Hui Rong[1] and Rui Cheng[1*]

Abstract

Background: Preterm neonates undergo many painful procedures as part of their standard care in the neonatal intensive care unit. However, pain treatment is inadequate in many of these routine procedures. In the present study, we investigated the impact and mechanism of combined music and touch intervention (CMT) on the pain response in premature infants.

Methods: Sixty-two preterm neonates (gestational age of <37 weeks) were randomly assigned to either the experimental or control group. Infants in the experimental group underwent painful procedures with CMT, and those in the control group underwent painful procedures without CMT. Blood samples were collected from all infants at the beginning of hospitalization and 2 weeks later to assess the cortisol and β-endorphin concentrations. Differences in the levels of cortisol and β-endorphin between two groups were examined using analysis of covariance (ANCOVA).

Results: In total, 3707 painful procedures were performed on 62 neonates during their hospitalization. The average number of painful procedures in the control group ($n = 35.5$) was higher than that in the experimental group ($n = 29.0$) during hospitalization, although no significant difference was reached ($P > 0.05$). After 2 weeks, the Premature Infant Pain Profile scores were significantly higher in the control group than experimental group (13.000 ± 0.461 *vs* 10.500 ± 0.850, respectively; $P < 0.05$). The cortisol concentration was not significantly different between the control and experimental groups either at the beginning of hospitalization (131.000 ± 18.190 *vs* 237.200 ± 43.860, respectively; $P > 0.05$) or 2 weeks later (162.400 ± 23.580 *vs* 184.600 ± 21.170, respectively; $P > 0.05$). However, the serum β-endorphin concentration was higher in the experimental group than in the control group both at the beginning of hospitalization (1.640 ± 0.390 *vs* 1.179 ± 0.090, respectively; $P < 0.05$) and 2 weeks later (2.290 ± 0.740 *vs* 1.390 ± 0.410, respectively; $P < 0.05$).

Conclusions: CMT might decrease the pain response of preterm neonates by significantly improving the β-endorphin concentration, but not the blood cortisol concentration.

Keywords: Preterm infant, Pain, Cortisol, β-Endorphin, Music, Touch

* Correspondence: chengrui350@163.com
Equal contributors
Department of Newborn Infants, Children's Hospital of Nanjing Medical University, Nanjing 210008, China
Full list of author information is available at the end of the article

Background

Preterm neonates undergo many painful procedures as part of their standard care in the neonatal intensive care unit (NICU) [1, 2]. Accumulating evidence shows that preterm infants are able to experience pain [3, 4] and are highly sensitive to pain because of their immature and vulnerable nervous systems [5]. Repetitive, prolonged, and poorly treated pain has many deleterious consequences. Short-term effects include excessive crying, choking, gagging, vomiting, and long-term effects include altered pain sensitivity as well as permanent neuroanatomical and behavioral abnormalities [6]. Therefore, there is an urgent need to establish safe and effective treatments for pain relief in infants.

However, pain treatment for routine procedures in the NICU is inadequate. In fact, many doctors are reluctant to use analgesic medications such as nonsteroidal anti-inflammatories or acetaminophen in the NICU because the effectiveness of these medications has not been proven or because of potential adverse effects in the short term (e.g., opioid-induced ileus or apnea) or long term (e.g., ketamine-induced neuroapoptosis). Various nonpharmacological treatments, including non-nutritive sucking both with and without sucrose, swaddling or kangaroo care, music therapy, and multisensorial stimulation, reportedly exert a pain-modulating effect on preterm neonates because they activate the neonates' attention, distract them from the pain, and thus modify pain perception [7–14]. Music therapy may help to relieve procedural pain in both full-term and preterm infants because it can provide an auditory stimulus that modulates pain perception, obviating or decreasing the need for pharmacological agents [10, 12, 13, 15, 16]. Another nonpharmacological intervention, touching, also helps to reduce pain in preterm and term neonates. Prasopkittikun and Tilokskulchai [17] reported that touching, swaddling, maternal holding, and repositioning were effective nonpharmacological interventions that reduced pain using validated pain assessment measures in preterm and term infants. However, a combination of these nonpharmacological interventions may be more useful because their effectiveness may vary across infants. Furthermore, few data specifically address premature infants, who are exposed to the most procedural pain and are the most vulnerable to altered developmental trajectories in childhood. Especially in China, no study has addressed the effects of combined music and touch intervention (CMT) on the pain response in late preterm infants. Therefore, in the present study, we investigated the impact of CMT on the premature infant pain response. We also studied the levels of cortisol and β-endorphin after the intervention because these parameters may provide evidence of the effectiveness of CMT in alleviating pain in premature infants. Pain may activate the hypothalamic-pituitary-adrenal (HPA) axis, inducing an endocrine response in premature infants that increases cortisol levels [18]. Cortisol affects the metabolism, cardiovascular system, and central nervous system [19]. In various studies, cortisol has been used to assess the effects of nonpharmacological interventions against pain in newborn infants, including sucrose, the kangaroo position, and developmental care [20–22]. β-Endorphin is an endogenous opioid that is released in response to pain and increases the inhibition of pain at several sites within the β-endorphin inhibitory pathway. It is released when an organism is exposed to stress or painful stimuli. During acute stress and pain, the HPA system increases the blood β-endorphin concentration. This circulatory release of β-endorphin can be reduced by systemic analgesia [23–25]; thus, plasma β-endorphin concentrations have frequently been used to determine analgesic efficacy.

The purpose of this study was to examine whether CMT is an effective pain management method for premature infants during the painful procedures performed on a daily basis in the NICU. We compared the Premature Infant Pain Profile (PIPP) scores and cortisol and β-endorphin concentrations between infants who did and did not receive CMT. To the best of our knowledge, this is the first study to examine the relationship between CMT and the pain response in premature infants.

Methods

Participants

This randomized controlled trial was conducted in the NICU of Children's Hospital of Nanjing Medical University from June 2011 to March 2012. The inclusion criteria were as follows: (1) admission within 72 h after birth and (2) a gestational age of <37 weeks. The exclusion criteria were one or any combination of the following: (1) serious birth injuries, (2) serious malformations (especially in the oral cavity or external ear), (3) significant parenchymal brain injury (grade IV intraventricular hemorrhage or periventricular leukomalacia), (4) treatment with analgesics or sedatives within 72 h of the assessment, or (5) failed hearing screening.

Procedures

The research team comprised a neonatologist, three research nurses, a child health care expert, and three assistants with extensive research and clinical experience. A list of daily painful procedures was designed [26–28]; this list also included other procedures that the clinicians or nurses considered painful, such as tracheal aspiration, nasal aspiration, removal of intravenous lines, and removal of adhesives (Table 2). After consent was obtained from the infants' parents, the infants were randomly assigned to either the experimental or control group using a random numbers table. Infants in the control group underwent daily painful procedures without intervention. Infants in the experimental group underwent painful procedures with CMT. Only nurses on the research team administered the CMT to ensure consistency. A compact disc player (AZ-1103; Philips, Amsterdam, Netherlands) was used for the music intervention. Audio stimulation was provided by "Smart Baby Lullaby" compact discs. The music included lullabies and nursery rhymes, which are musically simple songs with a lower pitch and slower tempo. The most appropriate decibel level for the disc player was determined to be 55 to 65 decibels (dB) using an A-weighted scale, measured using a TES-1351B Sound Level Meter (TES Electrical Electronic Corp., Taipei, Taiwan). This volume level was implemented to meet criteria consistent with current knowledge of infant auditory development in relationship to the ambient NICU sound environment. Music applications of 55 to 65 dB for short-timed interventions met the recommendations for infants and supported a variance of 10 dB between the ambient sound floor and sound interventions to ensure audibility [29]. Although environmental sound was not within the scope of this investigation, the staff members in our NICU were cognizant of the noise and ambient sounds. The disc player was placed approximately 15 to 20 cm above the infants' heads, which allowed for continuous play of the music from 5 min before the experimental procedure until 30 min after the procedure. The touch intervention protocol (Gentle Human Touch, GHT), started from the beginning of each procedure until 10 min after the procedure and was performed as previously described [30]. Briefly, the nurse gently placed her left hand on the infant's head with her fingertips resting immediately above the eyebrow line and her palm touching the infant's crown. Her right hand was placed with the right thumb on the infant's right shoulder (midline position) with the rest of her hand and fingers on the infant's arm, above the elbow. The video camera was positioned for a close-up of the face. The signals were fed directly to a VCR before, during, and after each painful procedure. These procedures were repeated for every painful procedure during the 2-week data collection period.

PIPP

The PIPP is a pain measure for premature infants and comprises seven indicators: two contextual (gestational age and behavioral state), two physiologic (heart rate and oxygen saturation), and three behavioral (brow bulge, eye squeeze, and nasolabial furrow). Each indicator is scored on a 4-point scale (0–3) for a maximum total score of 21 [31, 32]. The internal consistency and inter- and intra-rater reliability were summarized with good face validity and content validity in a review article on pain assessment in children [32]. Video sequences were assessed by three different nurses. The three nurses were supervised to ensure that they did not consult one another, and all were blinded to the intervention *vs* control group.

Cortisol and β-endorphin concentrations

The β-endorphin concentration is known to exhibit a circadian rhythm that repeats once in a 24-h period. Therefore, a 2-ml blood sample was collected from each infant between 6 and 7 AM to minimize any circadian rhythm effects. The cortisol and β-endorphin concentrations were quantitatively assessed using a highly sensitive electrochemiluminescence immunoassay (Roche Diagnostics, Mannheim, Germany) and a modular analytics analyzer (Elecsys Modular Analytics E170; Roche Diagnostics, Tokyo, Japan).

Statistical analysis

Unless otherwise stated, numerical results are presented as the mean ± standard error of the mean. Statistical analyses were performed using the SPSS 19.0 statistical package (IBM Corp., Armonk, NY, USA). Demographic data and pain experience were compared between the two groups using the unpaired *t*-test (normally distributed data), the Mann–Whitney U test (non-normally distributed data), or Fisher's exact test (categorical data). Gestational ages were compared using one-way analysis of variance and the least significant difference test. Wilcoxon signed-rank tests were carried out to examine PIPP scores. ANCOVA was used to evaluate the difference in the levels of cortisol and β-endorphin between two groups. Statistical significance was defined as $P < 0.05$.

Results

Demographic variables

During the study period (June 2011 to March 2012), 74 of 141 eligible infants were enrolled in this study (flow diagram, Fig. 1). We excluded seven neonates in the experimental group and five neonates in the control group who were discharged within 2 weeks. Thus, 62 neonates were finally included in the analysis. The primary purpose of the pilot study was to refine the study methodology and obtain adequate data with which to conduct an analysis for an expanded study. Based on the advice of a biostatistician, a sample size of 30 was determined to be adequate for this purpose. In addition, the severity of illness was assessed using the Score for Neonatal Acute Physiology II [33]. Table 1 shows the demographic characteristics of the neonates. There were no differences in the demographic characteristics between the experimental and control groups.

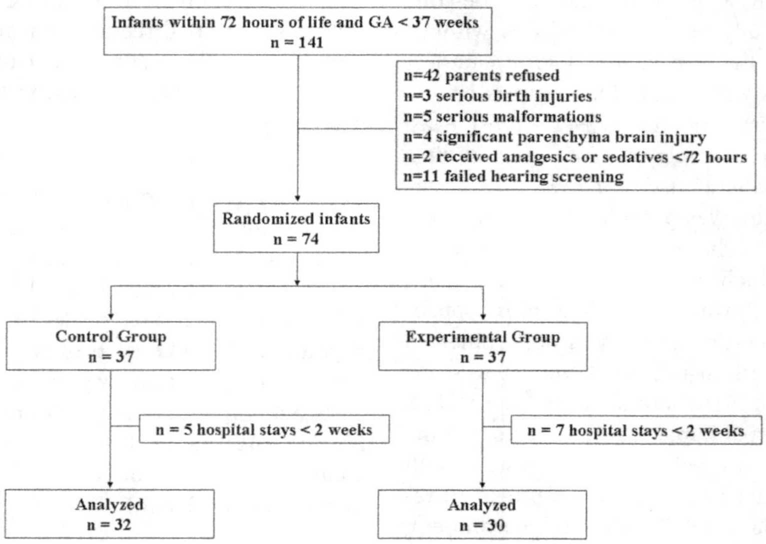

Fig. 1 Study profile and patient flow

Numbers and types of pain experiences

In total, 3707 painful procedures were performed on 62 neonates during their hospitalization. Among these procedures, 1913 were performed in the control group and 1794 were performed in the experimental group. The median number of painful procedures for each preterm neonate in the control group was 35.5 (range, 18–325). The median number in the experimental group was 29 (range, 14–316). The average number of painful procedures in the control group was higher than that in the experimental group during hospitalization, although no statistical difference was reached ($P > 0.05$). The types of painful procedures performed on the neonates are listed in Table 2.

PIPP

The mean PIPP scores were 11.17 ± 0.91 and 12.14 ± 0.46 (control *vs.* experimental), respectively, at the beginning of the hospitalization. After 2 weeks, the PIPP score in the control group had significantly increased ($t = 2.573$; $P < 0.05$) and that in the experimental group had significantly decreased ($t = 2.216$; $P < 0.05$). There was no significant difference between the two groups at the beginning. Two weeks later, however, the experimental group had a significantly lower score than the control group (10.50 ± 0.85 *vs* 13.00 ± 0.46, respectively; $P < 0.05$) (Fig. 2).

Table 1 Clinical and demographic characteristics of neonates

	Control group $n = 32$	Experimental group $n = 30$	*P*
Gestational age (weeks)	33.33 ± 0.54	34.30 ± 0.67	0.10
Birth weight (kg)	2.00 ± 0.07	1.93 ± 0.13	0.64
Sex (male/female)	15/17	13/17	0.80
1-min APGAR	8.67 ± 0.24	9.37 ± 0.32	0.96
5-min APGAR	9.40 ± 0.22	9.64 ± 0.15	0.47
Severity (SNAP-II)	8 (0–57)	8 (0–33)	0.69

Data are presented as mean ± SD or median (range)
APGAR indicates appearance, pulse, grimace, activity, respiration

Cortisol concentration

In the control group, the cortisol concentration significantly decreased after 2 weeks of hospitalization (131.00 ± 18.19 *vs* 237.20 ± 43.86, respectively; $P < 0.05$). Additionally, no significant changes occurred in the experimental group from the beginning of hospitalization to 2 weeks later (184.60 ± 21.17 *vs* 162.40 ± 23.58, respectively; $P > 0.05$). No significant differences were noted between the two groups either at the beginning of hospitalization or 2 weeks later (Fig. 3).

β-Endorphin

The β-endorphin concentration increased significantly in the experimental group, but not in the control group, after 2 weeks ($P < 0.05$). Neonates in the experimental group had higher β-endorphin levels than those in the control group both at the beginning of hospitalization (1.64 ± 0.39 *vs* 1.18 ± 0.09, respectively; $P < 0.05$) and 2 weeks later (2.29 ± 0.74 *vs* 1.39 ± 0.41, respectively; $P < 0.05$) (Fig. 4).

Discussion

In this study, we randomly assigned 62 preterm neonates to either an experimental or control group to demonstrate whether CMT can relieve pain such patients in the

Table 2 Types of painful procedures on neonates

Procedure Types	Procedure no. (%) on control group	Procedure no. (%) on experimanetal group
Tracheal aspiration	183 (9.57)	165 (9.20)
Nasal aspiration	283 (14.79)	241 (13.43)
Intravenous cannulation	256 (13.38)	231 (12.88)
Removal of intravenous lines	229 (11.97)	206 (11.48)
Adhesive removal	229 (11.97)	206 (11.48)
Fingerstick	89 (4.65)	95 (5.30)
Heelstick	69 (3.61)	85 (4.74)
Femoral venous puncture	108 (5.65)	107 (5.96)
Arterial puncture	53 (2.77)	49 (2.73)
Laxative or enema	48 (2.51)	43 (2.40)
Gastric tube insertion	34 (1.78)	30 (1.67)
Tracheal intubation	7 (0.37)	6 (0.33)
Tracheal extubation	7 (0.37)	6 (0.33)
Chest physiotherapy	285 (14.90)	295 (16.44)
Lumbar puncture	9 (0.47)	8 (0.45)
Intradermal injection	24 (1.25)	21 (1.17)
Total	1913 (100.01)	1794 (99.99)

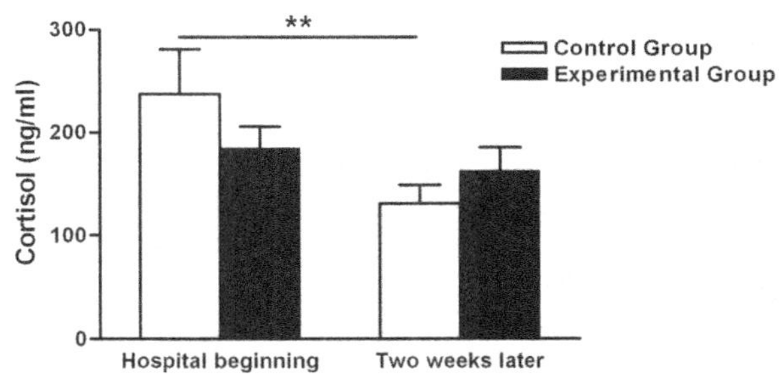

Fig. 3 Effects of CMT on cortisol concentration. In the control group, the cortisol concentration had significantly decreased after 2 weeks of hospitalization *vs* the beginning (131.00 ± 18.19 *vs* 237.20 ± 43.86, respectively; $^{**}P < 0.05$), while there was no significant change in the experimental group after 2 weeks *vs* the beginning (162.40 ± 23.58 *vs* 184.60 ± 21.17, respectively; $^{**}P > 0.05$). No significant difference was noted between the two groups either at the beginning of hospitalization or 2 weeks later

NICU. Infants in the experimental group underwent daily painful procedures with CMT, while those in the control group underwent daily painful procedures without interference. Details on the daily painful procedures, PIPP scores, and circulatory cortisol and β-endorphin concentrations were analyzed at the beginning of hospitalization and 2 weeks later.

The hospitalized preterm neonates in this study underwent an average of 29.0 to 35.5 painful procedures during 2 weeks of hospitalization. Among these procedures, those related to tracheal aspiration (e.g., tracheal aspiration, nasal aspiration, and chest physiotherapy) and intravenous cannulation (e.g., intravenous cannulation, removal of intravenous lines, and adhesive removal) are the most frequent types of painful procedures performed among preterm infants. This might be because preterm infants commonly have complications such as breathing difficulties and nutrient defects. These complications lead most preterm neonates to require ventilation, support, and prolonged infusion of parenteral nutrition. Thus, the numbers of related procedures are significantly increased.

The PIPP was chosen as the pain measurement tool for this study because it is a composite of seven multidimensional indicators of pain. These pain indicators include physiological, behavioral, and contextual measures that adjust for the influence of gestational age at the time of treatment and the infant's state of awareness [34–37]. As shown in Fig. 2, after 2 weeks, the PIPP score in the control group had significantly increased and that in the experimental group had significantly

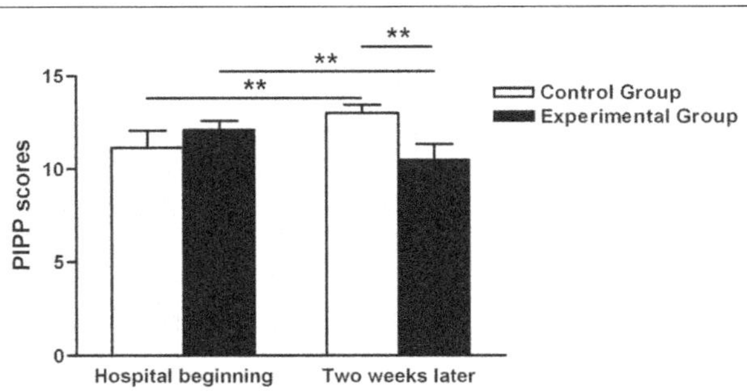

Fig. 2 Effects of CMT on PIPP. The mean PIPP scores were 11.17 ± 0.91 and 12.14 ± 0.46 (control vs. experimental) at the beginning of the hospitalization, respectively. There was no significant difference between the two groups at the beginning of hospitalization ($^{**}P > 0.05$). Two weeks later, the experimental group had significantly lower scores than the control group (10.50 ± 0.85 *vs* 13.00 ± 0.46, $^{**}P < 0.05$)

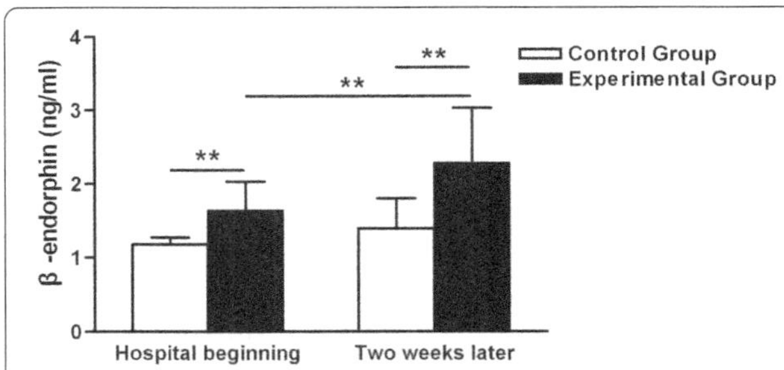

Fig. 4 Effects of CMT on β-endorphin concentration. Neonates in the experimental group had higher serum β-endorphin levels than those in the control group both at the beginning of hospitalization (1.64 ± 0.39 *vs* 1.18 ± 0.09, respectively; $^{**}P < 0.05$) and 2 weeks later (2.29 ± 0.74 *vs* 1.39 ± 0.41, respectively; $^{**}P < 0.05$). The β-endorphin concentration increased significantly in the experimental group after 2 weeks, but not in the control group

decreased; the PIPP score in the experimental group was significantly lower than that in the control group. Therefore, we presume that CMT can reduce the pain response in premature infants.

Cortisol, the steroid end product of the HPA axis, increases with painful procedures [38] and decreases with comforting procedures such as massage [39] and skin-to-skin care [40] in preterm infants. Thus, we supposed that the cortisol concentration would not differ between the two groups at the beginning of hospitalization and would significantly increase in the control group but not in the experimental group after 2 weeks of hospitalization. However, although there was no significant difference in the cortisol concentration between the two groups in this study, the cortisol concentration in the experimental group was slightly lower than that in the control group after a single blood collection at the beginning of hospitalization. After 2 weeks, the cortisol concentration had decreased in both groups, especially in the control group, in which the cortisol concentration had significantly decreased against the beginning of hospitalization. Two meaningful hypotheses can be offered to explain this phenomenon. First, at the beginning of hospitalization, the cortisol level in the control group increased because of a single painful procedure while that in the experimental group decreased because of a single CMT procedure. Measurement of the salivary cortisol concentration may be more accurate because there is no painful procedure at first. This would allow comparison of the baseline concentration and subsequent concentrations after single or repeated pain exposures. Second, after 2 weeks of hospitalization, the lower cortisol concentration may have occurred because repeated exposure to procedural pain was associated with downregulation of the HPA axis, such that the cortisol responses were dampened while the infants were still in the hospital [41]. Overall, the HPA axis responsiveness, cortisol regulation, and normal cortisol concentrations in preterm infants are very complex, and continued research is needed.

In this study, at the beginning of hospitalization, we found that the β-endorphin concentration significantly increased in the preterm infants of the experimental group after a single CMT; this prompted the β-endorphin concentration to change immediately after the intervention. However, no significant differences in the PIPP scores were detected at the beginning. After 2 weeks, the β-endorphin concentration in the experimental group had significantly increased while that in the experimental group had significantly decreased. These data suggest that in preterm infants, although the β-endorphin concentration increased, the increase was not adequate to reduce the pain response after a single intervention; repeating CMT might decrease the pain response by improving the β-endorphin concentration.

This study has shown that CMT is effective in comforting late preterm infants when they undergo painful procedures. As advocates for premature infants, neonatal nurses must continually explore treatment modalities to provide these infants with quality care and hope for a bright future. CMT plays a potential role in this field. A limitation of this study is that it was a pilot study with a small sample size; it would be advantageous to enlarge the sample size. Furthermore, it was a single-center case series that may not represent the situation in China as a whole. Thus, future studies involving other NICUs are needed to map the epidemiology of neonatal pain in China.

Conclusions

CMT might decrease the pain response of preterm neonates by improving the β-endorphin concentration, but not the blood cortisol concentration.

Abbreviations

CMT: Combined music and touch intervention; HPA axis: Hypothalamic-pituitary-adrenal axis; NICU: Neonatal intensive care unit; PIPP: Premature Infant Pain Profile

Acknowledgements

Not applicable.

Funding

This project was supported by grants from Nanjing Health bureau (YKK12108).

Authors' contributions

JQ was an assistant of the research team, measured the cortisol concentration, and performed the statistical analysis. YFJ was an assistant of the research team and measured the β-endorphin concentration. FL, QHT, and HR were research nurses of the research team. RC was a neonatologist of the research team and participated in the study's design and coordination. All authors read and approved the final manuscript.

Competing interests

The authors declare that they have no competing interests.

Author details

[1]Department of Newborn Infants, Children's Hospital of Nanjing Medical University, Nanjing 210008, China. [2]Department of Pediatrics, Yixing People's Hospital Affiliated to Jiangsu University, Yixing 214200, China.

References

1. Johnston CC, Collinge JM, Henderson SJ, Anand KJ. A cross-sectional survey of pain and pharmacological analgesia in Canadian neonatal intensive care units. Clin J Pain. 1997;13:308–12.
2. Simons SH, van Dijk M, Anand KS, Roofthooft D, van Lingen RA, Tibboel D. Do we still hurt newborn babies? A prospective study of procedural pain and analgesia in neonates. Arch Pediatr Adolesc Med. 2003;157:1058–64.
3. Giannakoulopoulos X, Teixeira J, Fisk N, Glover V. Human fetal and maternal noradrenaline responses to invasive procedures. Pediatr Res. 1999;45:494–9.
4. Anand KJ, Carr DB. The neuroanatomy, neurophysiology, and neurochemistry of pain, stress, and analgesia in newborns and children. Pediatr Clin North Am. 1989;36:795–822.
5. Andrews K, Fitzgerald M. The cutaneous withdrawal reflex in human neonates: sensitization, receptive fields, and the effects of contralateral stimulation. Pain. 1994;56:95–101.
6. Batton DG, Barrington KJ, Wallman C. Prevention and management of pain in the neonate: an update. Pediatrics. 2006;118:2231–41.
7. Stevens B, Gibbins S, Franck LS. Treatment of pain in the neonatal intensive care unit. Pediatr Clin North Am. 2000;47:633–50.
8. Cignacco E, Hamers JP, Stoffel L, van Lingen RA, Gessler P, McDougall J, et al. The efficacy of non-pharmacological interventions in the management of procedural pain in preterm and term neonates. A systematic literature review. Eur J Pain. 2007;11:139–52.
9. Pillai Riddell RR, Racine NM, Turcotte K, Uman LS, Horton RE, Din Osmun L, et al. Non-pharmacological management of infant and young child procedural pain. Cochrane Database Syst Rev. 2011;10:CD006275.
10. Joyce BA, Keck JF, Gerkensmeyer J. Evaluation of pain management interventions for neonatal circumcision pain. J Pediatr Health Care. 2001;15:105–14.
11. Johnston CC, Filion F, Nuyt AM. Recorded maternal voice for preterm neonates undergoing heel lance. Adv Neonatal Care. 2007;7:258–66.
12. Bo LK, Callaghan P. Soothing pain-elicited distress in Chinese neonates. Pediatrics. 2000;105:E49.
13. Lai HL, Chen CJ, Peng TC, Chang FM, Hsieh ML, Huang HY, et al. Randomized controlled trial of music during kangaroo care on maternal state anxiety and preterm infants' responses. Int J Nurs Stud. 2006;43: 139–46.
14. Johnston CC, Filion F, Campbell-Yeo M, Goulet C, Bell L, McNaughton K, et al. Enhanced kangaroo mother care for heel lance in preterm neonates: a crossover trial. J Perinatol. 2009;29:51–6.
15. Hartling L, Shaik MS, Tjosvold L, Leicht R, Liang Y, Kumar M. Music for medical indications in the neonatal period: a systematic review of randomised controlled trials. Arch Dis Child Fetal Neonatal Ed. 2009;94: F349–54.
16. Robb SL, Burns DS, Carpenter JS. Reporting guidelines for music-based interventions. Music Med. 2011;3:271–9.
17. Prasopkittikun T, Tilokskulchai F. Management of pain from heel stick in neonates: An analysis of research conducted in Thailand. J Perinat Neonatal Nurs. 2003;17:304–12.
18. Grabska J, Walden P, Lerer T, Kelly C, Hussain N, Donovan T, et al. Can oral sucrose reduce the pain and distress associated with screening for retinopathy of prematurity? J Perinatol. 2005;25:33–5.
19. Dedovic K, Duchesne A, Andrews J, Engert V, Pruessner JC. The brain and the stress axis: the neural correlates of cortisol regulation in response to stress. Neuroimage. 2009;47:864–71.
20. Cignacco E, Denhaerynck K, Nelle M, Bührer C, Engberg S. Variability in pain response to a non-pharmacological intervention across repeated routine pain exposure in preterm infants: a feasibility study. Acta Paediatr. 2009;98: 842–6.
21. Cong X, Ludington-Hoe SM, Walsh S. Randomized crossover trial of kangaroo care to reduce biobehavioral pain responses in preterm infants: a pilot study. Biol Res Nurs. 2011;13:204–16.
22. Kleberg A, Warren I, Norman E, Mörelius E, Berg AC, Mat-Ali E, et al. Lower stress responses after Newborn Individualized Developmental Care and Assessment Program care during eye screening examinations for retinopathy of prematurity: a randomized study. Pediatrics. 2008;121: e1267–78.
23. Matejec R, Ruwoldt R, Bödeker RH, Hempelmann G, Teschemacher H. Release of beta-endorphin immunoreactive material under perioperative conditions into blood or cerebrospinal fluid: significance for postoperative pain? Anesth Analg. 2003;96:481–6.
24. Anand KJ, Sippell WG, Aynsley-Green A. Randomised trial of fentanyl anaesthesia in preterm babies undergoing surgery: effects on the stress response. Lancet. 1987;1:62–6.
25. Fisk NM, Gitau R, Teixeira JM, Giannakoulopoulos X, Cameron AD, Glover VA. Effect of direct fetal opioid analgesia on fetal hormonal and hemodynamic stress response to intrauterine needling. Anesthesiology. 2001;95:828–35.
26. Carbajal R, Rousset A, Danan C, Coquery S, Nolent P, Ducrocq S, et al. Epidemiology and treatment of painful procedures in neonates in intensive care units. JAMA. 2008;300:60–70.
27. Anand KJ. Consensus statement for the prevention and management of pain in the newborn. Arch Pediatr Adolesc Med. 2001;155:173–80.
28. Lehr VT, Taddio A. Topical anesthesia in neonates: clinical practices and practical considerations. Semin Perinatol. 2007;31:323–9.
29. Standley JM. A meta-analysis of the efficacy of music therapy for premature infants. J Pediatr Nurs. 2002;17:107–13.
30. Modrcin-Talbott MA, Harrison LL, Groer MW, Younger MS. The biobehavioral effects of gentle human touch on preterm infants. Nurs Sci Q. 2003;16:60–7.
31. Stevens B, Johnston C, Petryshen P, Taddio A. Premature Infant Pain Profile: development and initial validation. Clin J Pain. 1996;12:13–22.
32. Stevens B, Gibbins S. Clinical utility and clinical significance in the assessment and management of pain in vulnerable infants. Clin Perinatol. 2002;29:459–68.
33. Richardson DK, Corcoran JD, Escobar GJ, Lee SK. SNAP-II and SNAPPE-II: Simplified newborn illness severity and mortality risk scores. J Pediatr. 2001; 138:92–100.
34. Craig KD, Whitfield MF, Grunau RV, Linton J, Hadjistavropoulos HD. Pain in the preterm neonate: behavioural and physiological indices. Pain. 1993;52: 287–99.
35. Johnston CC, Stevens B, Yang F, Horton L. Developmental changes in response to heelstick in preterm infants: a prospective cohort study. Dev Med Child Neurol. 1996;38:438–45.
36. Johnston CC, Stevens BJ, Yang F, Horton L. Differential response to pain by very premature neonates. Pain. 1995;61:471–9.
37. Stevens BJ, Johnston CC. Physiological responses of premature infants to a painful stimulus. Nurs Res. 1994;43:226–31.
38. Herrington CJ, Olomu IN, Geller SM. Salivary cortisol as indicators of pain in preterm infants: a pilot study. Clin Nurs Res. 2004;13:53–68.
39. Acolet D, Modi N, Giannakoulopoulos X, Bond C, Weg W, Clow A, et al. Changes in plasma cortisol and catecholamine concentrations in response to massagein preterm infants. Arch Dis Child. 1993;68:29–31.
40. Mörelius E, Theodorsson E, Nelson N. Salivary cortisol and mood and pain profiles during skin-to-skin care for an unselected group of mothers and infants in neonatal intensive care. Pediatrics. 2005;116:1105–13.
41. White-Traut RC, Schwertz D, McFarlin B, Kogan J. Salivary cortisol and behavioral state responses of healthy newborn infants to tactile-only and multisensory interventions. J Obstet Gynecol Neonatal Nurs. 2009;38:22–34.

2

Population-based study of the incidence of congenital hip dysplasia in preterm infants from the Survey of Neonates in Pomerania (SNiP)

A. E. Lange[1,6*], J. Lange[2], Till Ittermann[3], M. Napp[2], Paul-Christian Krueger[4], H. Bahlmann[1], R. Kasch[5] and M. Heckmann[1]

Abstract

Background: Some etiological factors involved in developmental dysplasia of the hip (DDH) occur in the last trimester of pregnancy, which could result in a decreased incidence of DDH in preterm infants. The aim of this study was to compare the incidence of DDH between preterm and term infants.

Methods: Ultrasound of the hip joint was performed in 2,534 term infants and 376 preterm infants within the population-based Survey of Neonates in Pomerania (SNiP) study.

Results: A total of 42 (1.66%) term infants had DDH (Graf type II c, 0.8%; type D, 0.3% left and 0.4% right; type III a, 0.2% left). Eighteen infants had bilateral findings. Hip dysplasia occurred more frequently in female neonates (32/1,182 vs. 10/1,302, $p < 0.023$; 95% CI 0.012–0.022, χ^2 test). A familial disposition for DDH was found in 169 (6.7%) term infants and 181 (7.1%) infants in the overall population. In preterm infants, dysplasia of the hip was found in only three late preterm infants with gestational age between 36 and 37 weeks ($n = 97$) and not in preterm infants <36 weeks gestational age ($n = 279$). Regression analysis revealed a narrowly significant association between gestational week of birth and DDH (relative risk = 1.17; 95% confidence interval 0.99–1.37; $p = 0.065$).

Conclusion: Our study suggests that preterm infants <36 weeks gestational age have a decreased risk of DDH.

Keywords: Preterm neonate, Ultrasound of the hip, Hip dysplasia, Screening of neonates

Background

Developmental dysplasia of the hip (DDH) is one of the most common congenital malformations with a regionally varying incidence of 1.5–4.9% [1–5]. The diagnostic standard for DDH is ultrasound imaging using the Graf classification [6–8]. In 1996, as part of the guidelines for early detection of childhood disease, Germany implemented screening for hip dysplasia in the form of a routine hip ultrasound for all neonates at 4–6 weeks of life. Many hospitals deviate from this by performing the hip ultrasound at 3–10 days of life as part of the routine examination (U2) given at this time. Schilt et al. screened nearly 15,000 babies immediately after birth over 15 years and showed that earlier treatment may lead to a shorter duration [1, 2]. Preterm infants are generally screened at a corrected age of more than 36 weeks [9].

Hip development is based on the interaction between genetically determined maturation of the cartilage and bone elements of the acetabulum and the pressure applied by the muscular forces of the centered femur head [10]. Regarding etiology, there are endogenous, exogenous, and genetic factors that cause malposition of the femur, which in turn causes malformation of the acetabulum or too shallow of an acetabulum to form with primary malpositioning of the femur head [10]. Known

* Correspondence: anja.lange@uni-greifswald.de
[1]Departments of Paediatrics and Neonatology & Paediatric Intensive Care Medicine, University of Greifswald, Greifswald, Germany
[6]Klinik und Poliklinik für Kinder- und Jugendmedizin, F.-Sauerbruch-Str., 17487 Greifswald, Germany

risk factors for DDH are breech presentation, oligohydramnion, or multiparous pregnancies, resulting in less intrauterine space. In addition, skeletal malformations and neuromuscular disease due to teratogenic agents can also cause types of hip luxation [11]. Furthermore, gender plays a role, with a two- to three-times higher incidence of DDH in females compared to males [12].

Only a few studies have reported the incidence of hip dysplasia in preterm infants, which has been reported to be 0.2–2.8 [11–13] compared to 1.5–4.9 in term infants [1–3].

Intrauterine risk factors for DDH with respect to less intrauterine space occur in the last trimester and are partially or completely absent in the case of preterm birth. The objective was to test the hypothesis that the incidence of DDH is lower in preterm infants than term infants by comparing the incidence of hip dysplasia between these groups. For this purpose, the population-based cohort study Survey of Neonates in Pomerania (SNiP) served as the database [14].

Methods

Survey of Neonates in Pomerania

The SNiP study is a prospective, population-based survey that collected comprehensive data on pregnancies, mothers, and their offspring in eastern Pomerania. Details were reported elsewhere [14]. All neonates whose place of residence was in eastern Pomerania were eligible for this survey. Infants were excluded from the survey if communication was impaired due to language barriers or a consent form was missing.

Trained physicians participating in the survey according to a standardized protocol collected the data. The questionnaires were pseudonymized and entered into the study database by a medical archivist.

In the study, data for 95% of all pregnant women in the Ostvorpommern region were recorded and >80% of mothers actively participated over the years. For the non-participants, risk factors during pregnancy, birth mode, and outcome of the child were recorded.

SNiP received a positive vote from the Ethics Committee of the University Medicine Greifswald and written informed consent was obtained from the parents.

Gestational age

Gestational age was defined as the time elapsed during the pregnancy from the first day of the woman's last menstrual cycle to the current date. A normal pregnancy ranges from 37 to 42 weeks. To investigate the influence of gestational age on hip development, preterm infants were categorized as late preterm (34 weeks and 0 days–36 weeks and 6 days gestation), very preterm (28 weeks and 0 days–33 weeks and 6 days gestation), or extremely preterm (less than 28 weeks gestation). To investigate the influence of birth weight, preterm infants were categorized as having normal birth weight (>2,500 g), low birth weight (1,500 g–2,500 g), very low birth weight (1,000 g–1,500 g), or extremely low birth weight (<1,000 g).

Ultrasound examination

Ultrasound of the hip was established for preterm infants not before January 2004. Therefore, only data on hip ultrasound in term and preterm infants born between January 2004 and November 2008 ($n = 2,910$) were included in this subgroup-analysis of the SNiP-cohort. The subgroup represented 42.6% of all live births and 45.4% of all infants included in SNiP between January 2002 and November 2008 (Fig. 1). During this period, 80% of all preterm infants and 70% of term infants underwent a hip ultrasound. Neonates with major congenital malformations, muscular or skeletal disease, or chromosomal anomalies were excluded.

For term infants, ultrasound screening of the hip was performed at the time of the regular second health check (3–10 days of age, called U2 in Germany) in the maternity ward. Briefly, the U2 comprises a physical exam, medical history, and counseling the mother on preventive measures, such as Vitamin D and K prophylaxis and vaccination. Preterm infants were screened at the corrected age of more than 36 weeks. Ultrasound scans, documentation, and classification were performed according to Graf [6–8]. The standard protocol was described previously by Graf [7].

A familial disposition for DDH was defined as dysplasia of the hip in first degree family members (siblings, parents, grandparents), or family members with hip replacement before 50 years of age.

All examiners passed their specialist's examination as a pediatrician. The structured training comprised a minimum number ($n = 200$) of performed hip ultrasounds. The final board certification implied an assessment of the candidate's ability to perform an ultrasound. In addition, a DEGUM II certified examiner supervised all pathological results (DEGUM: Deutsche Gesellschaft für Ultraschall in der Medizin). All research was conducted in a Graf storage tray [7] and an ultrasonic instrument with a 7.5 MHz linear transducer (Logia TM 200, Pro Serius, 7, 5-MHz linear transducer, Wi Pro GE Medical Systems, Bangalore, India).

Statistical analysis

Continuous data were expressed as mean and standard deviation according to their normal distribution and categorical data as absolute numbers and percentages. Differences in mature hip prevalence across groups of gestational age and birth weight were tested

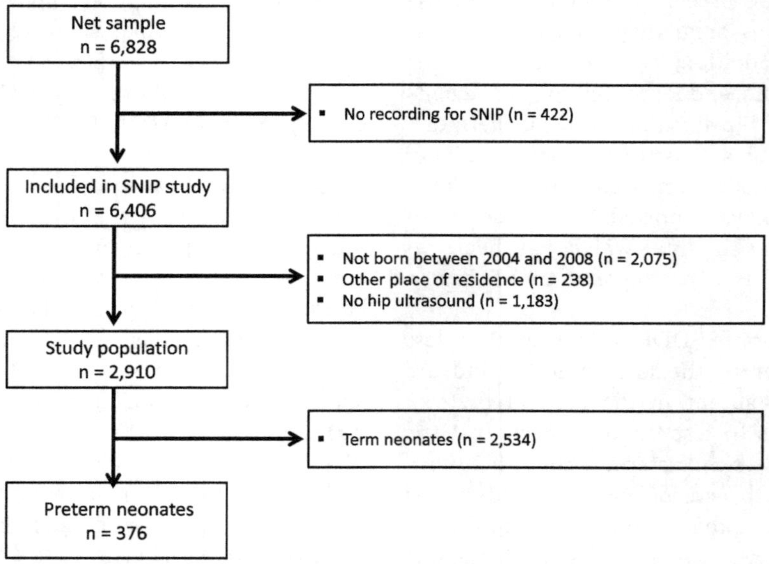

Fig. 1 Effect of gestational age and birth weight on Graf classification in preterm infants of the SNiP cohort. For the left ($p < 0.001$) and right hip ($p < 0.001$), extremely preterm and very preterm neonates had a significantly higher incidence of mature hips than late preterm babies. χ^2 95% confidence interval 0.99–1.37

by Fisher's exact test. We also performed a Poisson regression to test whether gestational week of birth was significantly associated with the prevalence of hip dysplasia. A p-value < 0.05 was considered significant. A medical statistician (T.I.) carried out all analyses using Stata 13.1 (Stata Corporation, College Station, TX, USA).

Results

Hip ultrasound was documented in 2,534 term neonates and 376 preterm neonates born between January 2004 and November 2008 (Fig. 2). The perinatal characteristics of the study population are shown in Table 1. Preterm infants were more often twins ($p < 0.001$) and more often born in breech presentation than term infants ($p < 0.001$).

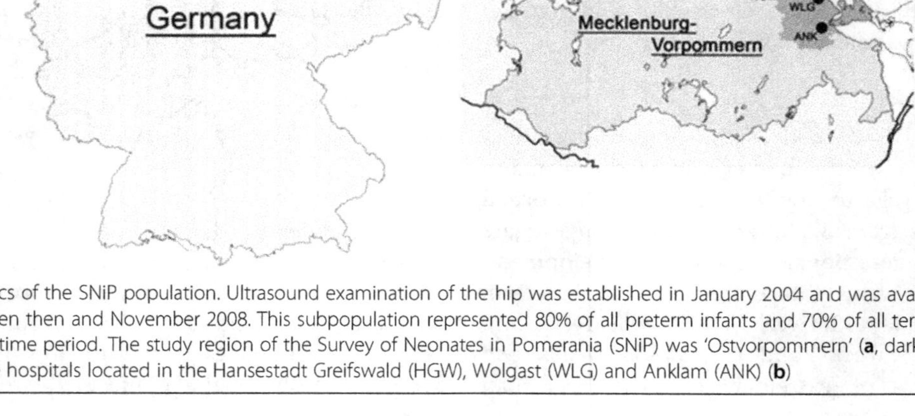

Fig. 2 Characteristics of the SNiP population. Ultrasound examination of the hip was established in January 2004 and was available in 2,910 infants born between then and November 2008. This subpopulation represented 80% of all preterm infants and 70% of all term infants included in SNiP during the time period. The study region of the Survey of Neonates in Pomerania (SNiP) was 'Ostvorpommern' (**a**, dark grey). SNiP was carried out in three hospitals located in the Hansestadt Greifswald (HGW), Wolgast (WLG) and Anklam (ANK) (**b**)

Table 1 Characteristics of the study population

	Term neonates N = 2534	Preterm neonates N = 376
Gestational age (w)	39.4 (1.2)	33.0 (3.4)
- Late Preterm (34 weeks–36 weeks and 6 days)	-	223 (59.2%)
- Very preterm (28 weeks–33 weeks and 6 days)	-	115 (30.7%)
- Extremely Preterm (<28 weeks)	-	38 (10.1%)
Birth weight (g)	3,463 (480)	2,067 (724)
- Normal birth weight (≥2,500 g)	2,473 (97.6%)	121 (32.1%)
- Low birth weight (<2,500 g)	63 (2.5%)	168 (44.8%)
- Very low birth weight (<1,500 g)	0 (0.0%)	41 (10.9%)
- Extremely low birth weight (<1,000 g)	0 (0.0%)	47 (12.5%)
- SGA	33 (1,5%)	78 (21,4%)
- IUGR	1 (0.03%)	5 (1.3%)
Gender		
- Female	1,211 (47.8%)	183 (48.4%)
- Male	1,320 (52.1%)	193 (51.1%)
Parity		
- Twin	28 (1.1%)	67 (17.7%)
- Triplet	0 (0.0%)	4 (1.1%)
Delivery presentation		
- Cephalic	2,299 (90.7%)	285 (75.8%)
- Breech	152 (6.1%)	78 (20.7%)
Familiary Disposition for developmental dysplasia of the hip	169 (6.7%)	12 (3.1%)

Data are presented as mean (standard deviation) or absolute numbers (percentage). *SGA* small for gestational age (defined as birthweight < 3th.percentile *
IUGR intrauterine growth retardation (defined as birthweight, birth length, <3th percentile)
*[New percentile values for the anthropometric dimensions of singleton neonates: analysis of perinatal survey data of 2007–2011 from all 16 states of Germany]
Voigt M, Rochow N, Schneider KT, Hagenah HP, Scholz R, Hesse V, Wittwer-Backofen U, Straube S, Olbertz D
Z Geburtshilfe Neonatol. 2014 Oct;218 (5):210–7. doi:10.1055/s-0034-1385857. German. PMID:25353215

A familial disposition for hip disease did not differ between term and preterm neonates. Table 2 shows the Graf classification of the hips in term and preterm infants.

For the left ($p < 0.001$) and right hip ($p < 0.001$), preterm infants had a significantly higher incidence of mature hips than term infants. The incidence of Graf II was twice as high in term infants as in preterm infants. Overall, the incidence of Graf II c or higher dysplasia of the hip was greater in term infants (left hip: 1.3%, right hip: 1.2%) than in preterm infants (left hip: 0.53%, right hip: 0.53%). By individual years, the incidence of hip dysplasia in term infants was 2.10% in 2004, 2.23% in 2005, 2.2% in 2006, 0.9% in 2007, and 1.5% in 2008. A familial disposition for

Table 2 Graf classification in term and preterm infants of the birth cohort

	Term ($n = 2{,}534$)		Preterm ($n = 376$)	
Type	Left hip	Right hip	Left hip	Right hip
I a	1,449 (57.2%)	1,462 (57.7%)	296 (78.7%)	302 (80.3%)
II a	1,052 (41.5%)	1,041 (41.1%)	78 (20.5%)	72 (18.9%)
II c	21 (0.8%)	20 (0.8%)	1 (0.3%)	0 (0.0%)
D	8 (0.3%)	9 (0.4%)	1 (0.3%)	2 (0.5%)
III a	2 (0.2%)	0 (0.0%)	0 (0.0%)	0 (0.0%)
IV	0 (0.0%)	0 (0.0%)	0 (0.0%)	0 (0.0%)

Data are presented as absolute numbers (percentage)
Survey of Neonates in Pomerania (SNiP)

dysplasia of the hip was found in 169 (6.7%) term infants and 181 (7.1%) infants in the overall population.

Figure 1 shows the influence of gestational age and birth weight on Graf classification in preterm infants. For the left ($p < 0.001$) and right hip ($p < 0.001$), extremely preterm and very preterm neonates had a significantly higher incidence of mature hips than late preterm babies (χ^2 test). The incidence of Graf II a was 10-times higher in late preterm infants than in extremely preterm infants, and three-times higher than in very preterm neonates. Only three late preterm infants with a gestational age of more than 36 weeks had dysplasia of the hip: two female preterm neonates (the first born 36 weeks and 4 days, 2,520 g, transverse position, right and left hip type D; the second one was born 36 weeks, 2,480 g, breech position, right hip type II a, left hip type II c) and one male preterm neonate (born 36 weeks and 1 day, 2,700 g, cephalic position, right hip type D, left hip type II a). Preterm infants with extremely low or very low birth weight had a higher incidence of mature hips than preterm babies with low or normal birth weight for the left ($p < 0.001$) and right hip ($p = 0.004$). The incidence of type II a was six-times higher in preterm infants of normal birth weight than preterm infants with extremely low birth weight. In the Poisson regression, we found no significant differences between term infants (1.75%) and preterm infants (0.53%) with respect to the prevalence of hip dysplasia (relative risk = 2.14, 95% CI 0.66–6.92, $p = 204$). Therefore, we added analyses based on the continuous gestational week of birth variable, which revealed a barely significant association between gestational week of birth and dysplasia of the hip (relative risk = 1.17, 95% CI 0.99–1.37, $p = 0.065$). One week of gestation was associated with a 16% increased risk of hip dysplasia (Fig. 3).

Discussion

Intrauterine risk factors for DDH in the last trimester are partially or completely absent in the case of preterm birth. In our large cohort of preterm infants, hip dysplasia was not found at less than 36 weeks gestational age. Our

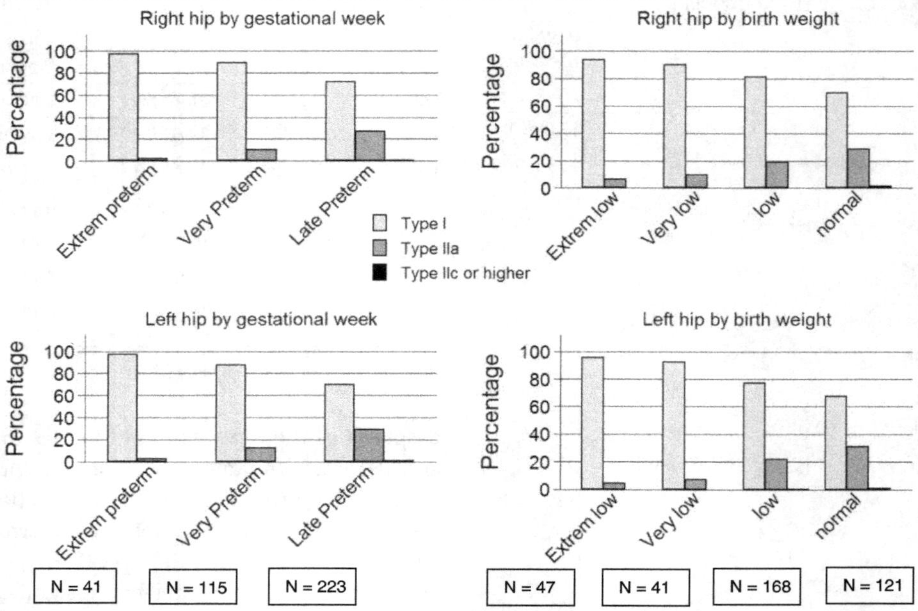

Fig. 3 Gestational age and risk of developmental dysplasia of the hip (DDH). Regression analysis of the association between gestational week of birth and risk of DDH (relative risk = 1.17, 95% confidence interval 0.99–1.37, $p = 0.065$). One week of gestation was associated with a 16% increased risk of hip dysplasia. Dotted line: 95% confidence interval 1.08–1.63

findings are consistent with recently published long-term studies conducted in infants during the neonatal period to evaluate multiple risk factors for DDH. In our preterm cohort, the incidence of dysplasia of the hip defined as type II c or greater was 0.53%. Compared to unselected newborns, preterm babies exhibited a significantly higher incidence of types I a and II a.

In contrast, the incidence of DDH in our term group corresponds to the findings in the literature [1–3]. Further findings in our term group are in accordance with the literature, including female neonates being affected two- to three-times more often than their male counterparts [11]. In our study, 32 female and 10 male neonates had hip dysplasia. Moreover, the left hip is more often affected because of the high prevalence of cephalic vertex presentation at birth [15]. In over 94% of neonates who are born from the cephalic presentation the fetal lie is the left occipito anterior position. In this position, the back of the fetus is left and the left hip lies narrowed to the mother's spine. Therefore, it could be speculated that the left hip joint is more likely to be restricted in mobility than the right one [16].

In our cohort, the incidence of fully mature hip joints was distinctly higher in preterm neonates than in term neonates (Table 2). At the time of ultrasound screening, 80% of preterm neonates had a Graf I a hip classification and approximately 20% still had a physiological maturation deficit (Graf II a), whereas 41% of term neonates were classified as type II a. Bick et al. examined the hips of 92 preterm neonates by ultrasound over the period of 1 year. Using the Graf classification, only 7% had an angle alpha between 50 and 60°, which is characteristic of type II a hips. In all other examinations, the angle alpha was > 60° (type I). Sonographically there were no pathological findings [15]. Timmler et al. showed in a large cohort study comprising 143 preterm infants that preterm delivery was not a risk factor for the development hip dysplasia [5].

Sezar et al. showed that prematurity regardless of maternal risk factors did not have an effect on the incidence of DDH [17]. Preterm infants are no longer subject to maternal hormones or lack of intrauterine space after their birth and have complete freedom to move their lower extremities. Due to better cardiorespiratory stability, the prone position is preferred in preterm infants [18]. If these infants are placed on their backs, thick diapers encourage correct positioning of the femur head in the acetabulum. All of these factors should be discussed as stimuli for development of the hip joint. These preterm infants are not subject to intrauterine restrictions; therefore, muscular, cartilaginous, and bone development can occur unhindered. In addition, maternal steroid hormones lead not only to the relaxation of maternal ligaments, but also similar effects on the ligaments of the fetal hip joint [19, 20]. These suggestions are supported by our finding that the proportion of mature hips was greater in the group of the most immature infants (Fig. 1).

Strengths and limitations

Our study has several limitations. First, we report on data from a birth cohort study that was not designed to exclusively investigate hip ultrasound data. Second, the examiners were not particularly trained or re-evaluated for the study; therefore, intra- and inter-observer variability could not be reported. Nevertheless, high quality standards for qualification of the examiners were applied. Third, our study did not report on outcome data (re-examination of the immature hips and details of therapy), which may have influenced the results due to the low incidence of DDH. However, the strengths of this study were the large number of newborns, particularly preterm infants, investigated and that the cohort was population-based.

Conclusion

Our study suggests that preterm infants (<36 weeks gestational age) have a decreased risk of DDH. Furthermore, the incidence of fully mature hip joints was twice as high in preterm infants as in term infants and the proportion of mature hips was highest in the group with the most immature infants. These findings suggest that the absence of intra-uterine factors, such as lack of space, atypical positioning (e.g., breech presentation), and maternal steroid hormones, promotes maturation of the hip in preterm infants.

Acknowledgment

This work is part of the Research Cooperation Community Medicine (RCC) of the University of Greifswald, Germany, which is funded by the Federal Ministry of Education and Research (grant no. ZZ96030). The RCC encompasses several research projects, which are sharing data of population-based studies (http://www.community-medicine.de). SNiP was supported by (a) the German Federal Ministry for Education and Research (NBL3 program, grant 01 ZZ 0103), (b) the Excellence Support Programme of the Federal State of Mecklenburg-Western-Pomerania (UG 07 034) "Genetics of frequent variants in INSIG2, their role in the pathogenesis of obesity and other disorders particularly in children" and, (c) the Epidemiological Study on Childhood Cancer and Malformations in the Vicinity of Nuclear Power Plants (Stsch 4493). AL received a training grant from the Medical Faculty of the Ernst Moritz Arndt University of Greifswald.

Funding

SNiP was supported by (a) the German Federal Ministry for Education and Research (NBL3 program, grant 01 ZZ 0103), (b) the Excellence Support Programme of the Federal State of Mecklenburg-Vorpommern (UG 07 034) 'Genetics of frequent variants in INSIG2, their role in the pathogenesis of obesity and other disorders particularly in children' awarded to D. Rosskopf and J. P. Haas, (c) the Epidemiological Study on Childhood Cancer and Malformations in the Vicinity of Nuclear Power Plants (StSCH 4493).

Availability of data and materials

The data of the SNIP-study is publicly available via https://www.fvcm.med.uni-greifswald.de/dd_service/data_use_intro.php?lang=ger. This is a data repository where any researcher can register and find data dictionary as well as an online application tool for getting access to data. Upon an application by registered users, the Research Cooperation Community Medicine (RCC) of the University of Greifswald, Germany, which is funded by the Federal Ministry of Education and Research (grant no. ZZ 96030) decides on granting access to the data based on scientific guidelines.

Authors' contributions

AEL was responsible for data collection and writing of the manuscript, JL, PCK, and HB were responsible for data collection, quality assessment and classification and revising the manuscript, TI was responsible for the statical analysis, MN and RK contributed to scientific interpretation of the results and manuscript revision, MH contributed to scientific interpretations and manuscript revision. All authors read and approved the final manuscript.

Competing interests

The authors declare that they have no competing interests.

Ethics approval and consent to participate

Research based on patient-related data and human DNA is strictly regulated by German law. The collection of detailed personal data combined with sampling of biomaterials demands strict confidentiality. Our study complies with international guidelines of ethical research based on the Declaration of Helsinki. The study design was reviewed and approved by the Ethics Committee of the Board of Physicians Mecklenburg-Western Pomerania at the University of Greifswald. Eligible women were asked for written informed consent; in cases of legally minor mothers, i.e. aged <18 years, the additional signature of the newborn's legal care-giver was required. Written informed consent included data assessment in face-to-face interviews, self-administered questionnaires and patient records. It also covered bio samples of blood. Furthermore, data storage of pseudonymized data was given informed consent to, as well as their analyses and publication.

Author details

[1]Departments of Paediatrics and Neonatology & Paediatric Intensive Care Medicine, University of Greifswald, Greifswald, Germany. [2]Department of Trauma Surgery, University of Greifswald, Greifswald, Germany. [3]Institute for Community Medicine, Div. SHIP – Clinical Epidemiological Research, University Medicine Greifswald, Greifswald, Germany. [4]Department of Radiology, University of Greifswald, Greifswald, Germany. [5]Department of Orthopaedics and Orthopaedic Surgery, University of Greifswald, Greifswald, Germany. [6]Klinik und Poliklinik für Kinder- und Jugendmedizin, F.-Sauerbruch-Str., 17487 Greifswald, Germany.

References

1. Partenheimer A, Scheler-Hofmann M, Lange J, et al. Correlation between sex, intrauterine position and familial predisposition and neonatal hip ultrasound results. Ultraschall Med. 2006;27(4):364–7.
2. Schilt M. Optimal age for hip sonography screening. Ultraschall Med. 2001;22(1):39–47.
3. Exner GU, Mieth D. Sonographic screening for hip dysplasia in newborn infants. Schweiz Med Wochenschr. 1987;117(27–28):1015–20.
4. Treiber M, et al. Ultrasound screening for developmental dysplasia of the hip in the newborn: a population-based study in the Maribor region, 1997–2005. Wien Klin Wochenschr. 2008;120(1–2):31–6.
5. Timmler T, et al. The hip joints of preterm neonates in sonographic evaluation. Chir Narzadow Ruchu Ortop Pol. 2005;70(4):301–5.
6. Graf R. Fundamentals of sonographic diagnosis of infant hip dysplasia. J Pediatr Orthop. 1984;4(6):735–40.
7. Graf R. Hip sonography in infancy. Procedure and clinical significance. Fortschr Med. 1985;103(4):62–6.
8. Graf R. The anatomical structures of the infantile hip and its sonographic representation. Morphol Med. 1982;2(1):29–38.
9. Tuncay IC, et al. Is prematurity important in ultrasonographic hip typing? J Pediatr Orthop B. 2005;14(3):168–71.
10. Dezateux C, Rosendahl K. Developmental dysplasia of the hip. Lancet. 2007;369(9572):1541–52.
11. Stevenson DA, et al. Familial predisposition to developmental dysplasia of the hip. J Pediatr Orthop. 2009;29(5):463–6.
12. Fox AE, Patron RW. The relationchip between mode of delivery and developmental dysplasia of the hip in breech infants: a 4-year prospective cohort study. J Bone Joint Surg (Br). 2010;92(12):1695–9.
13. Yau CH, et al. Frequency of developmental dysplasia of the hip in breech-presented Chinese neonates in Hong Kong. Hong Kong Med J. 2012;18(5):407–11.

14. Ebner A, Thyrian JR, Lange A, Lingnau ML, Scheler-Hofmann M, Rosskopf D, et al. Survey of Neonates in Pomerania (SNiP): a population-based birth study–objectives, design and population coverage. Paediatr Perinat Epidemiol. 2010;24(2):190–9.
15. Bick U, Muller-Leisse C, Troger J. Ultrasonography of the hip in preterm neonates. Pediatr Radiol. 1990;20(5):331–3.
16. Quan T, Kent AL, Carlisle H. Breech preterm infants are at risk of developmental dysplasia of the hip. J Paediatr Child Health. 2013;49(8):658–63.
17. Sezer C, Unlu S, Demirkale I, et al. Prevalence of developmental dysplasia of the hip in preterm infants with maternal risk factors. J Child Orthop. 2013;7:257–61.
18. van der Burg PS, Miedema M, DeJongh FH, Frerichs I, Van Kaam AH. Changes in lung volume and ventilation following transition from invasive to noninvasive respiratory support and prone positioning in preterm infants. Pediatr Res. 2015;77:484–8. doi:10.1038/pr.2014.201.
19. Ishikawa N. The relationship between neonatal developmental dysplasia of the hip and maternal hyperthyroidism. J Pediatr Orthop. 2008;28(4):432–4.
20. Trotter A, et al. Effects of postnatal estradiol and progesterone replacement in extremely preterm infants. J Clin Endocrinol Metab. 1999;84(12):4531–50.

3

Evaluation of Helping Babies Breathe Quality Improvement Cycle (HBB-QIC) on retention of neonatal resuscitation skills six months after training in Nepal

Ashish KC[1,2*], Johan Wrammert[1], Viktoria Nelin[1], Robert B. Clark[3], Uwe Ewald[1], Stefan Peterson[1,4,5,6] and Mats Målqvist[1]

Abstract

Background: Each year 700,000 infants die due to intrapartum-related complications. Implementation of Helping Babies Breathe (HBB)-a simplified neonatal resuscitation protocol in low-resource clinical settings has shown to reduce intrapartum stillbirths and first-day neonatal mortality. However, there is a lack of evidence on the effect of different HBB implementation strategies to improve and sustain the clinical competency of health workers on bag-and-mask ventilation. This study was conducted to evaluate the impact of multi-faceted implementation strategy for HBB, as a quality improvement cycle (HBB-QIC), on the retention of neonatal resuscitation skills in a tertiary hospital of Nepal.

Methods: A time-series design was applied. The multi-faceted intervention for HBB-QIC included training, daily bag-and-mask skill checks, preparation for resuscitation before every birth, self-evaluation and peer review on neonatal resuscitation skills, and weekly review meetings. Knowledge and skills were assessed through questionnaires, skill checklists, and Objective Structured Clinical Examinations (OSCE) before implementation of the HBB-QIC, immediately after HBB training, and again at 6 months. Means were compared using paired t-tests, and associations between skill retention and HBB-QIC components were analyzed using logistic regression analysis.

Results: One hundred thirty seven health workers were enrolled in the study. Knowledge scores were higher immediately following the HBB training, 16.4 ± 1.4 compared to 12.8 ± 1.6 before (out of 17), and the knowledge was retained 6 months after the training (16.5 ± 1.1). Bag-and-mask skills improved immediately after the training and were retained 6 months after the training. The retention of bag-and-mask skills was associated with daily bag-and-mask skill checks, preparation for resuscitation before every birth, use of a self-evaluation checklist, and attendance at weekly review meetings. The implementation strategies with the highest association to skill retention were daily bag-and-mask skill checks (RR-5.1, 95% CI 1.9–13.5) and use of self-evaluation checklists after every delivery (RR-3.8, 95% CI 1.4–9.7).

(Continued on next page)

* Correspondence: aaashis7@yahoo.com; http://www.kbh.uu.se/imch
[1]International Maternal and Child Health, Department of Women's and Children's Health, Uppsala University, Uppsala, Sweden
[2]United Nation's Children's Fund (UNICEF), Nepal Country Officer, UN House, Lalitpur, Nepal

(Continued from previous page)

Conclusions: Health workers who practiced bag-and-mask skills, prepared for resuscitation before every birth, used self-evaluation checklists, and attended weekly review meetings were more likely to retain their neonatal resuscitation skills. Further studies are required to evaluate HBB-QIC in primary care settings, where the number of deliveries is gradually increasing.

Keywords: Neonatal resuscitation, Helping babies breathe, Retention of skills, Multi-faceted implementation strategy, Quality improvement cycle, Nepal

Background

Globally, 2.9 million neonates die every year, of which 700,000 die due to intrapartum-related complications [1]. The first minute after a baby is born—the "Golden minute™"—is the crucial window for the initiation of neonatal resuscitation among the 10 million non-breathing babies born annually [2]. Neonatal resuscitation competency among health workers is therefore critical in every delivery room to ensure the safety and health of newborn infants. Resuscitation training in facilities has been shown to reduce the number of intrapartum-related neonatal deaths by 30% [3]. Although health workers are the key personnel in the provision of neonatal resuscitation, it has been revealed that in low-resource settings staff usually have inadequate training and knowledge, and that additional formal guidance and support are needed [4, 5].

Nepal has a neonatal mortality rate of 23 per thousand live births and intrapartum-related complications account for 23% of neonatal deaths [1, 6]. In Nepal, more than half of all deliveries take place at health institutions, but the quality of resuscitation provided at the time of birth has been found to be inadequate [7]. Identifying the implementation strategies that could improve and sustain neonatal resuscitation competency will be key to improve the quality of resuscitation care provided.

There are a number of intervention strategies that have been identified to improve the performance and competencies of health workers for a number of other clinical guidelines [8]. However, strategies to improve and sustain competency on neonatal resuscitation have not been evaluated.

Helping Babies Breathe® (HBB), developed by the American Academy of Pediatrics, is designed to train birth attendants in developing countries on the essential skills of neonatal resuscitation [9]. It is based on evidence from a neonatal evaluation study done by ILCOR (International Liaison Committee on Resuscitation), and recognizes that in many countries only one birth attendant is present to provide care to both the mother and the newborn [10, 11].

The educational material of HBB consists of a well-tested pictorial representation of the resuscitation protocol, learner workbooks, facilitator flip charts, neonatal simulators and the required equipment – i.e., reusable ventilation bag-and-mask devices and bulb suction devices [9]. An evaluation of the HBB program in Tanzania showed that intrapartum-related stillbirth and early neonatal mortality was reduced by 24% and 47%, respectively [12]. The Tanzanian study showed that the HBB program is a low-cost intervention, with the estimated cost per life saved at USD 233 and USD 4.21 per life year gained [13]. However, implementation strategies for HBB in the Tanzania study were not evaluated in relation to the retention of neonatal resuscitation competencies among health workers.

An evaluation study conducted in Ethiopia found that HBB training improved the neonatal resuscitation knowledge of health workers immediately after training and also eliminated the knowledge difference that was present prior to training among health workers [14]. A study from Rwanda revealed that neonatal resuscitation competency dropped to an unsatisfactory level 3 months after the training, indicating that training alone was not adequate to retain the health worker's neonatal resuscitation knowledge and skills [15]. The proportion of providers at a rural hospital in Tanzania who were competent in simulated routine care and neonatal resuscitation scenarios increased after HBB training, and their knowledge remained at 7 months after training; however, the improvement did not transfer into clinical competency [16]. There is thus a need to further evaluate multi-faceted interventions to promote retention of resuscitation skills, as well as to make sure that knowledge is translated into clinical practice.

We therefore conducted this study to evaluate the impact of a multi-faceted implementation strategy for HBB as a Quality Improvement Cycle (HBB-QIC), on change and retention of health workers' knowledge and skills of neonatal resuscitation.

Methods

We conducted this study in a tertiary hospital in Kathmandu, Nepal. In 2011, the hospital had around 22,000 deliveries, and an early neonatal mortality of nine per thousand live births [17]. The hospital provides level III obstetric and gynecological services and is publicly funded.

Labor and delivery services are provided in the admission unit, antenatal care unit, labor unit, maternal and newborn service center (MNSC), and the operation theatre. The hospital also has a system that rotates the staff of these units on a periodic basis.

This was a sub-set of a larger study conducted to evaluate the change in perinatal mortality before and after the implementation of a simplified neonatal resuscitation protocol, the HBB-QIC, in the hospital [18]. The duration of the larger study was 18 months, from July 2012 to September 2013. As part of the larger study evaluating the impact of neonatal resuscitation protocol implementation, the study received approval from the Hospital's Institutional Review Committee, the Nepal Health Research Council (Reg. No. 37/2012) and the Ethical Review Board of Uppsala University (dnr 2012/267). The study was registered as clinical trial, ISRCTN 97846009 [18].

All 137 nurses working in the admission unit, antenatal care unit, labor unit, MNSC, operation theatre and postnatal ward were included in the study. Informed written consent was obtained from each health worker participating in the study.

Study design

This was a time-series design where a series of periodic measurements were completed to evaluate our multi-faceted implementation strategy for the HBB-QIC, at three different time points (Table 1).

The knowledge and skills of health workers were assessed using the standard tools included in the HBB package, which were validated and used in other settings where HBB knowledge and skill evaluations have been conducted [9]. A questionnaire with 17 multiple-choice questions was used to assess the knowledge of health workers on the HBB protocol. The following tools were used to evaluate the skills of health workers in using the HBB protocol: a 7-step checklist for bag-and-mask skill checks, a 5-step checklist for preparation for resuscitation before every birth skill checks, a 13-step checklist with simulation for the first Objective Structured Clinical Examination (OSCE A), and a 18-step checklist with simulation for OSCE B. Two OSCEs tested healthcare worker's ability to prepare for, assess, and act in a scenario of routine newborn care (OSCE A) and a scenario requiring bag-and-mask ventilation (OSCE B) [9]. Successful completion of each OSCE required correct overall performance (≥80%), as well as the completion of key assessments and interventions such as "recognizes baby not breathing/crying" and "provides bag-and-mask ventilation" [9]. Assessment using these tools was completed before the HBB training was provided, immediately after the training, and again at 6 months after completion of the training (Table 1).

Information on each health worker's daily routines, including daily bag-and-mask skill checks, preparation for resuscitation before every birth, self-evaluation checklist usage, completion of the peer evaluation process, and attendance at the weekly review meetings was assessed using a direct observation checklist (Table 1).

Table 1 Evaluation of HBB QIC

	Thematic area	Tools	Evaluation design
Knowledge and skill competency	Knowledge assessment	17 multiple choice questions	Before training, immediately after training and 6 months after training
	Bag-and-mask skill	7 step skill observation checklist	Before training, immediately after training and 6 months after training
	Preparation at birth	5 step skill observation checklist	Before training, immediately after training and 6 months after training
	OSCE A	13 step observation checklist	Before training, immediately after training and 6 months after training
	OSCE B	18 step observation checklist	Before training, immediately after training and 6 months after training
Clinical practice	Daily skill check	7 step skill observation checklist	Observation on a daily basis using a checklist
	Preparation for resuscitation before every birth	5 step skill observation checklist	Observation on a daily basis using a checklist
	Self-evaluation checklist	21 step checklist	Observation on a daily basis using a checklist
	Peer evaluation process	HBB schematic protocol	Observation on a daily basis using a checklist
	Weekly review meetings	Notes of the meeting	Observation on a daily basis using a checklist

HBB QIC intervention

The HBB-QIC was implemented from January until September 2013. The HBB-QIC included multi-faceted implementation strategy including: HBB training, daily bag-and-mask skill checks, preparation for resuscitation before every birth, self-evaluation and peer review on neonatal resuscitation skills and weekly review meetings (Table 2).

First, a two-day training package on the HBB-QIC was provided to all hospital staff working in the three delivery units. There were 6 trainers who trained all the staff in each of the delivery units in a cascade manner. During the study period, there was no rotation of staff among the delivery units. Following the training, bag-and-mask kits and penguin (bulb) suctions™ were provided to each delivery unit. Additionally, HBB mannequins were placed at the entry of each delivery unit for daily skill checks; self-evaluation checklists were also attached to each clinical record form; and HBB schematic posters were placed in front of each resuscitation table for peer review. Weekly review meetings were conducted by each unit in-charge to discuss progress on the implementation of HBB-QIC standards.

Data management

In order to complete sampling and data collection, an independent surveillance team was formed. The team consisted of eight female surveillance officers with an academic background in nurse-midwifery and sufficient experience in clinical research. A research manager supervised the activities of this surveillance team. The surveillance team was trained to collect information using an observation checklist. Surveillance officers who conducted the HBB trainings collected information from the study participants, including demographic characteristics, academic qualifications and clinical experience.

After the surveillance officers collected this information, it was given to the data entry officer for dataset creation and management. The information was reviewed for completeness and then entered into an electronic database that was developed in the Census and Survey Processing System (CS Pro) software (US Census Bureau, ICF Macro). The data was then cleaned and transferred into the Statistical Package for the Social Sciences (SPSS) software (IBM Corporation) for data analysis.

Data analysis

The background characteristics of the health workers that were analyzed included age, professional experience, number of deliveries attended per month, number of neonatal resuscitations conducted per month and academic qualifications. The mean ± SD and median (IQR) for age of the health worker were calculated; mean and median years of professional experience in midwifery were calculated; the mean and median number of deliveries and resuscitations attended per month were also calculated. Academic qualifications were categorized into two groups, those who had completed an intermediate level of education in nursing or who were axillary nurse midwives compared to those who had completed a bachelor in nursing or higher.

Table 2 Description of the multi-faceted implementation strategy for Helping Babies Breathe (HBB) Quality Improvement Cycle (QIC)

Component	Activity	Facilitators and participants
HBB training	Two-day training: First day on HBB knowledge and skills as per standard package and second day on components of HBB QIC standards, training of trainers on how to conduct weekly review meeting, how to fill self-evaluation checklists and conduct peer evaluations.	Facilitators: HBB trainers Participants: Staff of the delivery units
Setting up HBB QIC standards	At each unit: Development of QIC goals and objectives, development of a place for daily bag-and-mask skill checks, QIC weekly review meetings, use of self-evaluation checklists and peer reviews after each resuscitation.	Facilitators: Study team Participants: Staff of the delivery units
QIC Weekly review meeting	At each unit, the unit in-charge facilitates the weekly review meetings on the progress of implementation of HBB QIC standards.	Facilitators: HBB trainers Participants: Staff of the delivery units
Daily bag-and-mask skill check	At each unit, each staff does a bag-and-mask skill check on a mannequin before starting duty.	Facilitators: Unit in-charge Participants: Staff of the delivery units
Self-evaluation checklist after each delivery	A self-evaluation checklist, which consists of a list of steps for immediate newborn care and neonatal resuscitation as per HBB protocol with checkboxes. After completing care of each newborn, the nurse midwife will fill up the self-evaluation checklist based on the steps completed as per the HBB protocol.	Facilitators: Unit in-charge Participants: Staff of the delivery units
Peer review after each resuscitation	A mounted poster with the steps of the HBB protocol will be attached at each resuscitation table, so that peers can review with the colleague completing resuscitation on whether the steps were followed.	Facilitators: Unit in-charge Participants: Staff of the delivery units

The mean numeric scores obtained on the knowledge questionnaire, preparation for resuscitation before every birth checklist, bag-and-mask skill check, and OSCEs A and B at baseline, immediately after the training, and at 6 months after the training were compared using paired t-tests. The proportion of health workers who scored ≥80% on the bag-and-mask skill checks before the training, immediately after the training, and at 6 months after the training was compared using paired t-tests.

The retention of bag-and-mask skills was calculated based on the change in bag-and-mask skill scores immediately after the training compared to 6 months after the training. The health workers who scored the same or better at 6 months after the training, as compared to immediately after training, were categorized as having retained their skills.

We then analyzed the association ($p < 0.01$) between retention of skills and health worker's completion of HBB-QIC components – i.e., daily bag-and-mask skill checks, preparation for resuscitation before every birth, use of self-evaluation checklists, peer evaluation following each resuscitation occurrence, attendance at weekly meetings – as well as with the completion of at least one neonatal resuscitation per month using the Fischer's exact test.

We also conducted logistic regression analysis to assess the level of association between the completion of each implementation strategy included in the HBB-QIC and the retention of bag-and-mask skills at 6 months.

Missing data that occurred randomly was adjusted for using the multiple imputation method [19].

Results

All 137 health workers included in this study participated in knowledge and skill evaluation before the HBB training, immediately after training and at 6 months after the training. The mean age of the health workers was 31.8 ± 10.2 years and the median age was 27.0 (IQR 24.0–39.0) years. Among the health workers, the mean number of professional years of experience was 10.5 ± 3.3 years and the median was 9 (IQR 6.0–15.0) years. The mean number of deliveries attended by each health worker was 8.0 ± 5.5 and the median was 7.0 (5.0–9.0). The mean number of resuscitations conducted by each health worker per month was 3.0 ± 1.5 and median was 3.0 (2.0–4.0). More than half, 65%, of health workers had intermediate level nursing qualifications or were axillary nurse-midwives, and the remaining health workers had bachelor degrees in nursing or higher (Table 3).

There was a significant change (<0.001) in the mean knowledge score after the HBB training, 16.4 ± 1.4 compared to 12.8 ± 1.6, and the knowledge was retained 6 months after the training (16.5 ± 1.1) ($p = 0.6$). There was a significant change (<0.001) from baseline in the mean skills scores for preparation for resuscitation before every birth, bag-and-mask skills, OSCE A, and OSCE B after the training, which was retained 6 months after the training (Table 4).

Table 3 Background characteristics of the Health workers-nurse

Background Characteristics	Mean ± SD	Median (IQR)
Age in complete years	31.8 ± 10.2	27.0 (24.0–39.0)
Professional experience in midwifery in complete years	10.5 ± 3.3	9.0 (6.0–15.0)
Number of deliveries attended per month	8.0 ± 5.5	7.0 (5.0–9.0)
Number of resuscitation	3.0 ± 1.5	3.0 (2.0–4.0)
Academic Qualifications	Frequency *N* = 137 (%)	
Axillary nurse midwives/ intermediate in nursing	90 (65.7)	
Bachelor in nursing	47 (34.3)	

There were no health workers who were competent in bag-and-mask skills before the training; 93% of health workers were competent immediately after the training ($p < 0.001$); and 99% of the health workers were competent 6 months after the training ($p = 0.8$) (Fig. 1).

More than half of the health workers practiced their bag-and-mask skills daily, 61% of them prepared for resuscitation before every birth, 82% of them used self-evaluation checklists after every birth, 43% of them completed peer evaluation after each resuscitation and 85% of them attended weekly review meetings (Table 5).

There was a positive association ($p < 0.01$) between retention of bag-and-mask skills and health worker's completion of daily bag-and-mask skill checks, preparation for resuscitation before every birth, use of self-evaluation checklists and attendance at weekly review meetings (Table 6).

The regression analysis showed that health workers who conducted daily bag-and-mask skill checks were five times more likely to retain neonatal resuscitation skills than those who did not (RR-5.1, 95% CI 1.9–13.5). Health workers who prepared for resuscitation before every birth had a two-fold increased likelihood of retaining the skills than those who did not (RR-2.4, 95% CI 1.0–5.6). Health workers who used self-evaluation checklists after each delivery were four times more likely to retain their skills than those who did not (RR-3.8, 95% CI 1.4–9.7). Health workers that attended weekly meetings had a 2.6 times increased likelihood of retaining their skills than those who did not attend (RR-2.6, 95% CI 1.0–7.4) (Table 7).

Discussion

We applied different implementation strategies as part of a HBB-QIC to improve the knowledge and

Table 4 Changes in knowledge and completion of preparation at birth, bag-and-mask skill checks, and OSCEs before, immediately after and 6 months after HBB training

	Before the training (N = 137)	Immediately after training (N = 137)		Follow up after 6 months (N = 137)	
	Mean ± SD	Mean ± SD	p-value	Mean ± SD	p-value
Knowledge (out of 17)	12.8 ± 1.6	16.4 ± 1.4	<0.001	16.5 ± 1.1	0.6
Preparation for resuscitation before every birth (out of 5)	2.2 ± 0.5	4.7 ± 0.1	<0.001	4.8 ± 0.03	0.1
Bag and Mask (out of 7)	2.3 ± 0.5	6.7 ± 0.6	<0.001	6.7 ± 0.5	0.815
OSCE A (out of 13)	3.9 ± 2.6	12.3 ± 0.9	<0.001	12.2 ± 0.8	0.07
OSCE B (out of 18)	3.7 ± 1.6	16.5 ± 1.2	<0.001	16.8 ± 1.1	p = 0.1

competency at different time points during the intervention period. Our study showed health workers who conducted bag-and-mask skill checks daily, who were prepared for resuscitation before every birth, who used self-evaluation checklists after each delivery, and those who attended weekly review meetings were more likely to retain their neonatal resuscitation skills, even at 6 months after the completion of training.

There are, however, certain limitations to our study. First, this study had a time-series design, thus the effectiveness of each individual component within the HBB-QIC cannot be evaluated, and we can only derive the association between the implementation strategy as a whole and the retention of neonatal resuscitation skills. Second, the use of self-evaluation checklists was evaluated based on whether these forms were completed correctly by the participants along with the other forms that had to be completed following every delivery. Therefore, there may be some discrepancy between actual practice and what was recorded. The final limitation was the presence of surveillance officers to observe the implementation of the HBB QIC, especially the bag-and-mask skill checks and weekly review meetings, which might have a Hawthorne effect (observer's bias) in changing health worker's behaviors. The strength of our study was that we used a

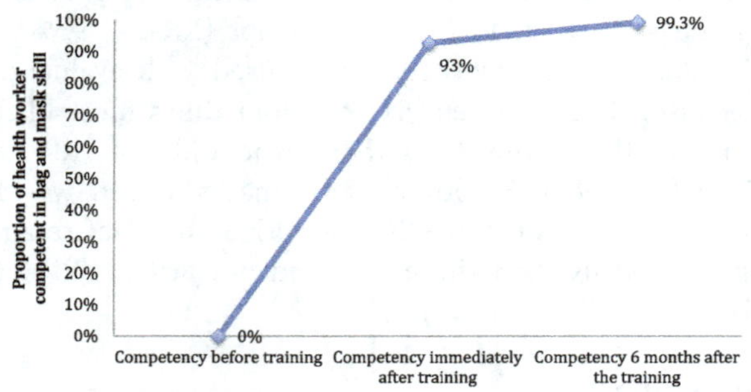

Fig. 1 Change in the proportion of the health worker who were competent (≥80%) in bag and mask skill

tested tool to evaluate the neonatal resuscitation knowledge and skills of the health worker [9].

Several studies in high-income and low-income countries have shown that resuscitation knowledge and skills improve immediately following training, however, these resuscitation skills tend to deteriorate over a period of time [15, 20–25]. Therefore, neonatal resuscitation training in itself is not an effective implementation strategy to retain resuscitation skills. Similar to our findings from this study, a study done in Canada has shown that the review of schematic posters on neonatal resuscitation before or after resuscitation of babies is not an effective strategy for retention of neonatal resuscitation skills [26].

Several systematic reviews have shown that the review of clinical performance among health workers on a periodic basis provides an opportunity to share the challenges faced in the clinical setting and to improve the

Table 5 Level of participation in the Helping Babies Breathe (HBB) Quality Improvement Cycle (QIC)

	Frequency (N = 137)	Percent
Frequency of bag-and-mask skill checks		
Every day	71	51.8
2 times a week	46	33.6
Weekly	20	14.6
Frequency of preparation for resuscitation before every birth		
At every birth	84	61.3
Occasionally	30	38.7
Frequency of practicing self-evaluation		
For every birth	112	81.8
Occasionally	25	18.2
Frequency of practicing peer evaluation		
For every resuscitation	59	43.0
Occasionally	78	57.0
Attendance of weekly review meeting		
Yes	117	85.4
No	20	14.6

Table 6 Association between the different implementation strategies of the Helping Babies Breathe (HBB) Quality Improvement Cycle (QIC) and the retention of bag-and-mask skills

		Non-retention (*N* = 27)	Retention (*N* = 110)	*p*-value
Daily bag-and-mask skill checks	Yes	6 (22.2%)	65(40.9%)	$p = 0.001$
	No	21 (77.8%)	45 (59.1%)	
Preparation for resuscitation before every birth	Yes	12(44.4%)	72(65.5%)	$p = 0.038$
	No	15 (55.6%)	38 (34.5%)	
Use of self-evaluation checklist	Yes	17 (63.0%)	95(86.4%)	$p = 0.008$
	No	10 (37.0%)	15 (13.6%)	
Peer evaluation after each resuscitation	Yes	12 (44.4%)	47 (42.7%)	$p = 0.5$
	No	15 (55.6%)	63 (57.3%)	
Attendance of weekly review meetings	Yes	20 (74.1%)	97 (88.2%)	$p = 0.065$
	No	7 (25.9%)	13 (11.8%)	

clinical skills and performance as a team, especially if the baseline performance on the clinical protocol is poor [27–30]. We showed that weekly review meetings among the nursing staff on the clinical performance of resuscitation helped to improve resuscitation skills to a moderate extent, as the baseline neonatal resuscitation competency was poor in this setting. Systematic reviews have also shown that a combination of implementation strategies (such as weekly review meetings, periodic simulated skill checks, checklists, and self-evaluation) is a more effective strategy to improve clinical performance as compared to the use of a singular strategy [31–36]. However, these implementation strategies were never implemented in combination to improve and increase the retention of neonatal resuscitation skills.

In the context of Nepal, the current number of neonatal deaths due to intrapartum-related complications needs to be reduced by at least three quarters in order to reach the pledged Every Newborn Action Plan target of a neonatal mortality of 10 or less per 1000 live birth by 2035 [37]. Further, the quality of neonatal resuscitation needs to be improved from that of the current state by improving health worker performance of neonatal resuscitation [7, 38]. Health workers need to be fully competent in neonatal resuscitation skills, and further need to be able to retain this competency such that knowledge is translated into clinical practice to reduce the burden of intrapartum-related death and morbidity. Nepal's current national strategy to provide skilled attendance at birth through neonatal resuscitation training programs is not adequate to sustain clinical competency of neonatal resuscitation as shown by several previous studies [38–41]. A combination of strategies should be considered for implementation in health facilities across the country.

Table 7 Logistic regression analysis on the level of association between different implementation strategies of the Helping Babies Breathe (HBB) Quality Improvement Cycle (QIC) and bag-and-mask skill retention

HBB QIC	Relative Risk	95% CI
Bag and mask skill check daily	5.1	1.9–13.5
Preparation for resuscitation before every birth	2.4	1.0–5.6
Use of self-evaluation checklist	3.8	1.4–9.7
Attendance of weekly review meeting	2.6	1.0–7.4

Conclusion

To our knowledge this is the first study done to evaluate the impact of a multi-faceted implementation strategy of HBB on the retention of neonatal resuscitation skills in low-income settings. We demonstrate that health workers, who conduct bag-and-mask skill checks daily, make preparation for resuscitation at every birth, use self-evaluation checklists after each delivery, and attend weekly review meetings have a higher likelihood for retention of neonatal resuscitation skills, even at 6 months post-training. Since, the HBB-QIC was implemented in a setting with a high number of deliveries, with a large team of nursing staff in each delivery unit, the implementation strategy such as weekly review meetings can be suitable in similar settings, but may not be suitable in primary care settings where there are fewer nursing staff. The other effective implementation strategies of daily bag-and-mask skill checks, preparation for resuscitation at every birth, and use of self-evaluation checklists can be applied in primary care settings to improve retention of resuscitation skills. However, the combination of different strategies needs to be evaluated in primary care settings, the point of access for delivery services among most women in rural areas. The innovative aspect of HBB-QIC is the multi-faceted implementation strategy approach. Future research should focus on further determining and refining those components that improve retention of neonatal resuscitation skills and clinical performance.

Abbreviations

HBB: Helping Babies Breathe; QIC: Quality Improvement Cycle; MNSC: Maternal Newborn Service Center; OSCE: Objective structured clinical evaluation; IQR: Inter quartile range; SD: Standard deviation; RR: Relative risk

Acknowledgement

Laerdal Foundation for Acute Medicine (Stavanger, Norway) provided financial support this study as part of the larger study to evaluate the impact of a simplified neonatal resuscitation protocol on birth outcomes and health workers performance. Part of this study was supported through a grant from the Swedish Society of Medicine. MM, JW, UE and VN were supported through a grant from Uppsala University (Uppsala, Sweden). The study group would like to thank Professor Gehanath Baral, Dr. Sheela Verma and Dr. Dhan Raj Aryal who reviewed and provided input for the design and data collection components of the study. The group is very grateful to the health workers who participated in the study.

Funding

Funding for the study was provided through grants from the Swedish Society of Medicine, Sweden and Laerdal Foundation for Acute Medicine (Stavanger, Norway). The views expressed in the publication is that of the authors and do not reflect the funding agency.

Authors' contributions

AK, MM, JW and UE conceptualized and designed the study. AK was the principal applicant for funding. AK was responsible for the data collection and data management. AK and VN were responsible for the data analysis and drafting of the manuscript. MM, JW, RC, UE, and SP contributed to the development of the manuscript. All authors read and approved the final manuscript.

Competing interests

The authors declare that they have no competing interests.

Author details

[1]International Maternal and Child Health, Department of Women's and Children's Health, Uppsala University, Uppsala, Sweden. [2]United Nation's Children's Fund (UNICEF), Nepal Country Officer, UN House, Lalitpur, Nepal. [3]Latter-day Saint Charities, Salt Lake City, UT, USA. [4]Global Health, Public Health Services, Karolinska Institute, Stockholm, Sweden. [5]School of Public Health, Makerere University, Kamala, Uganda. [6]Health Section, Programme Division, United Nations Children Fund (UNICEF), United Nations Plaza, New York, NY 10017, USA.

References

1. Lawn JE, Blencowe H, Oza S, You D, Lee AC, Waiswa P, Lalli M, Bhutta Z, Barros AJ, Christian P, Mathers C, Cousens SN, Lancet every newborn study group. Every newborn: progress, priorities, and potential beyond survival. Lancet. 2014;384(9938):189–205.
2. Lee AC, Kozuki N, Blencowe H, Vos T, Bahalim A, Darmstadt GL, Niermeyer S, Ellis M, Robertson NJ, Cousens S, Lawn JE. Intrapartum-related neonatal encephalopathy incidence and impairment at regional and global levels for 2010 with trends from 1990. Pediatr Res. 2013;74(Suppl 1):50–72.
3. Lee AC, Cousens S, Wall SN, Niermeyer S, Darmstadt GL, Carlo WA, Keenan WJ, Bhutta ZA, Gill C, Lawn JE. Neonatal resuscitation and immediate newborn assessment and stimulation for the prevention of neonatal deaths: a systematic review, meta-analysis and Delphi estimation of mortality effect. BMC Public Health. 2011;11(Suppl 3):S12.
4. Murila F, Obimbo MM, Musoke R. Assessment of knowledge on neonatal resuscitation amongst health care providers in Kenya. Pan Afr Med J. 2012; 11:78.
5. Harvey SA, Blandon YC, McCaw-Binns A, Sandino I, Urbina L, Rodriguez C, Gomez I, Ayabaca P, Djibrina S. Are skilled birth attendants really skilled? A measurement method, some disturbing results and a potential way forward. Bull World Health Organ. 2007;85(10):783–90.
6. UNICEF, Government of Nepal. Multiple indicator cluster survey (MICS). Kathmandu: UNICEF; 2015.
7. Lindback C, KC A, Wrammert J, Vitrakoti R, Ewald U, Malqvist M. Poor adherence to neonatal resuscitation guidelines exposed; an observational study using camera surveillance at a tertiary hospital in Nepal. BMC Pediatr 2014, 14:233.
8. Grimshaw JM, Shirran L, Thomas R, Mowatt G, Fraser C, Bero L, Grilli R, Harvey E, Oxman A, O'Brien MA. Changing provider behavior: an overview of systematic reviews of interventions. Med Care. 2001;39(8 Suppl 2):II2–45.
9. Singhal N, Lockyer J, Fidler H, Keenan W, Little G, Bucher S, Qadir M, Niermeyer S. Helping babies breathe: global neonatal resuscitation program development and formative educational evaluation. Resuscitation. 2012; 83(1):90–6.
10. Kattwinkel J. Neonatal resuscitation guidelines for ILCOR and NRP: evaluating the evidence and developing a consensus. J Perinatol. 2008; 28(Suppl 3):S27–9.
11. Roehr CC, Hansmann G, Hoehn T, Buhrer C. The 2010 guidelines on neonatal resuscitation (AHA, ERC, ILCOR): similarities and differences–what progress has been made since 2005? Klin Padiatr. 2011;223(5):299–307.
12. Msemo G, Massawe A, Mmbando D, Rusibamayila N, Manji K, Kidanto HL, Mwizamuholya D, Ringia P, Ersdal HL, Perlman J. Newborn mortality and fresh stillbirth rates in Tanzania after helping babies breathe training. Pediatrics. 2013;131(2):e353–60.
13. Vossius C, Lotto E, Lyanga S, Mduma E, Msemo G, Perlman J, Ersdal HL. Cost-effectiveness of the "helping babies breathe" program in a missionary hospital in rural Tanzania. PLoS One. 2014;9(7):e102080.
14. Hoban R, Bucher S, Neuman I, Chen M, Tesfaye N, Spector JM. 'Helping babies breathe' training in sub-saharan Africa: educational impact and learner impressions. J Trop Pediatr. 2013;59(3):180–6.
15. Musafili A, Essen B, Baribwira C, Rukundo A, Persson LA. Evaluating helping babies breathe: training for healthcare workers at hospitals in Rwanda. Acta Paediatr. 2013;102(1):e34–8.
16. Ersdal HL, Vossius C, Bayo E, Mduma E, Perlman J, Lippert A, Soreide E. A one-day "helping babies breathe" course improves simulated performance but not clinical management of neonates. Resuscitation. 2013;84(10):1422–7.
17. Ministry of Health and Population, GoN. Annual Report "Smarika" 2068/69. Kathmandu: Paropakar Maternity and Women's Hospital; 2011.
18. Ashish KC, Malqvist M, Wrammert J, Verma S, Aryal DR, Clark R, Naresh PK, Vitrakoti R, Baral K, Ewald U. Implementing a simplified neonatal resuscitation protocol-helping babies breathe at birth (HBB) - at a tertiary level hospital in Nepal for an increased perinatal survival. BMC Pediatr. 2012; 12:159.
19. Barnard J, Meng XL. Applications of multiple imputation in medical studies: from AIDS to NHANES. Stat Methods Med Res. 1999;8(1):17–36.
20. Smith KK, Gilcreast D, Pierce K. Evaluation of staff's retention of ACLS and BLS skills. Resuscitation. 2008;78(1):59–65.
21. Hamilton R. Nurses' knowledge and skill retention following cardiopulmonary resuscitation training: a review of the literature. J Adv Nurs. 2005;51(3):288–97.
22. Skidmore MB, Urquhart H. Retention of skills in neonatal resuscitation. Paediatr Child Health. 2001;6(1):31–5.
23. Kaczorowski J, Levitt C, Hammond M, Outerbridge E, Grad R, Rothman A, Graves L. Retention of neonatal resuscitation skills and knowledge: a randomized controlled trial. Fam Med. 1998;30(10):705–11.
24. Carlo WA, Wright LL, Chomba E, McClure EM, Carlo ME, Bann CM, Collins M, Harris H. Educational impact of the neonatal resuscitation program in low-risk delivery centers in a developing country. J Pediatr. 2009;154(4):504–8. e505
25. Enweronu-Laryea C, Engmann C, Osafo A, Bose C. Evaluating the effectiveness of a strategy for teaching neonatal resuscitation in West Africa. Resuscitation. 2009;80(11):1308–11.
26. Bould MD, Hayter MA, Campbell DM, Chandra DB, Joo HS, Naik VN. Cognitive aid for neonatal resuscitation: a prospective single-blinded randomized controlled trial. Br J Anaesth. 2009;103(4):570–5.
27. Reeves S, Zwarenstein M, Goldman J, Barr H, Freeth D, Hammick M, Koppel I. Interprofessional education: effects on professional practice and health care outcomes. Cochrane Database Syst Rev. 2008;1:CD002213.
28. Jamtvedt G, Young JM, Kristoffersen DT, Thomson O'Brien MA, Oxman AD. Audit and feedback: effects on professional practice and health care outcomes. Cochrane Database Syst Rev. 2003;3:CD000259.
29. Jamtvedt G, Young JM, Kristoffersen DT, O'Brien MA, Oxman AD. Audit and feedback: effects on professional practice and health care outcomes. Cochrane Database Syst Rev. 2006;2:CD000259.
30. Ivers N, Jamtvedt G, Flottorp S, Young JM, Odgaard-Jensen J, French SD, O'Brien MA, Johansen M, Grimshaw J, Oxman AD. Audit and feedback: effects on professional practice and healthcare outcomes. Cochrane Database Syst Rev. 2012;6:CD000259.
31. Peters DH, SE S, Siadat B, Janovsky K, Vujicic M. Improving health service delivery in developing countries : from evidence to action. Washington: World Bank; 2009.

32. Forsetlund L, Bjorndal A, Rashidian A, Jamtvedt G, O'Brien MA, Wolf F, Davis D, Odgaard-Jensen J, Oxman AD. Continuing education meetings and workshops: effects on professional practice and health care outcomes. Cochrane Database Syst Rev. 2009;2:CD003030.
33. Pageler NM, Longhurst CA, Wood M, Cornfield DN, Suermondt J, Sharek PJ, Franzon D. Use of electronic medical record-enhanced checklist and electronic dashboard to decrease CLABSIs. Pediatrics. 2014;133(3):e738–46.
34. Davis DA, Taylor-Vaisey A. Translating guidelines into practice. A systematic review of theoretic concepts, practical experience and research evidence in the adoption of clinical practice guidelines. CMAJ. 1997;157(4):408–16.
35. Lion KC, Ebel BE, Rafton S, Zhou C, Hencz P, Mangione-Smith R. Evaluation of a quality improvement intervention to increase use of telephonic interpretation. Pediatrics. 2015;135(3):e709–16.
36. Ambroggio L, Thomson J, Murtagh Kurowski E, Courter J, Statile A, Graham C, Sheehan B, Iyer S, Shah SS, White CM. Quality improvement methods increase appropriate antibiotic prescribing for childhood pneumonia. Pediatrics. 2013;131(5):e1623–31.
37. WHO, UNICEF. Every newborn: an action plan to end preventable deaths. Geneva: World Health Organization; 2014.
38. UNICEF, Ministry of Health and Population. Assessment of readiness, availability and quality of neonatal services in 12 hospitals of Nepal. Kathmandu: UNICEF; 2014.
39. Ministry of Health and Population, GoN. National Neonatal Health Strategy-2004. Kathmandu: Family Health Division; 2004.
40. Ministry of Health & Population. National in-service training strategy for skilled birth attendant. Kathmandu: Ministry of Health & Population; 2007.
41. Dickson, KE, Simen-Kapeu A, Kinney MV, Huicho L, Vesel L, Lackritz E, de Graft Johnson J, Von Xylander S, Rafique N, Sylla M, Mwansambo C, Daelmans B, Lawn JE The Lancet Every Newborn Study Group. Every Newborn: health-systems bottlenecks and strategies to accelerate scale-up in countries. Lancet. 2014;384(9941):438–54.

4

Comparison of three different methods for risk adjustment in neonatal medicine

Mark Adams[1,2*], Julia Braun[2], Hans Ulrich Bucher[1], Milo Alan Puhan[2], Dirk Bassler[1], Viktor Von Wyl[2] and The Swiss Neonatal Network

Abstract

Background: Quality improvement in health care requires identification of areas in need of improvement by comparing processes and patient outcomes within and between health care providers. It is critical to adjust for different case-mix and outcome risks of patient populations but it is currently unclear which approach has higher validity and how limitations need to be dealt with. Our aim was to compare 3 approaches towards risk adjustment for 7 different major quality indicators in neonatal intensive care (21 models).

Methods: We compared an indirect standardization, logistic regression and multilevel approach. Parameters for risk adjustment were chosen according to literature and the condition that they may not depend on processes performed by treating clinics. Predictive validity was tested using the mean Brier Score and by comparing area under curve (AUC) using high quality population based data separated into training and validation sets. Changes in attributional validity were analysed by comparing the effect of the models on the observed-to-expected ratios of the clinics in standardized mortality/morbidity ratio charts.

Results: Risk adjustment based on indirect standardization revealed inferior c-statistics but superior Brier scores for 3 of 7 outcomes. Logistic regression and multilevel modelling were equivalent to one another. C-statistics revealed that predictive validity was high for 8 and acceptable for 11 of the 21 models. Yet, the effect of all forms of risk adjustment on any clinic's comparison with the standard was small, even though there was clear risk heterogeneity between clinics.

Conclusions: All three approaches to risk adjustment revealed comparable results. The limited effect of risk adjustment on clinic comparisons indicates a small case-mix influence on observed outcomes, but also a limited ability to isolate quality improvement potential based on risk-adjustment models. Rather than relying on methodological approaches, we instead recommend that clinics build small collaboratives and compare their indicators both in risk-adjusted and unadjusted form together. This allows qualitatively investigating and discussing the residual risk-differences within networks. The predictive validity should be quantified and reported and stratification into risk groups should be more widely used to correct for confounding.

Keywords: Risk adjustment, Quality improvement, Neonatology, Effectiveness, Indirect standardization, Logistic regression, Multilevel, Mean brier score, and ROC area under curve

* Correspondence: mark.adams@usz.ch
[1]Division of Neonatology, University Hospital Zurich and University of Zurich, Wagistrasse 14, 8952 Schlieren, Switzerland
[2]Epidemiology, Biostatistics and Prevention Institute, University of Zurich, Zurich, Switzerland

Background

Risk adjustment is ubiquitously used to compare health care providers for the identification of quality improvement potential. Its effectivity is usually accepted as given. Literature reports an abundance of variations in vital patient outcome measures between clinics, regions and even networks, as shown, for instance, in neonatology [1–3]. Could these clinics, regions or networks all achieve the same potentially best standard, the resulting effect would dwarf many successful introductions of new drugs or methods. Over the last 20 years, several neonatal networks have shown beneficial developments for patients that were associated with quality improvement efforts [4–7].

A number of publications have addressed the need for risk adjustment in quality improvement [8–10]. Several of the introduced models rely on processes or diagnostics performed by the site under observation, thereby inadvertently adjusting for factors that may well be in need of improvement [11].

The use of risk-adjustment thereby assumes that the discrepancy between predicted and observed outcome is at least partially attributable to the quality of care provided. If the observed outcome exceeds the predicted outcome, then this discrepancy is assumed to be due to poor care. To which degree this assumption is valid is an important but often neglected aspect of the validation of risk-adjustment methods [12, 13]. Literature therefore recommends observing predictive and attributional validity to assess the validity of the risk adjustment approaches. The predictive validity is the extent to which the method accurately predicts the probability of outcome whereas the attributional validity allows attributing differences in outcome to the quality of care [12].

As a national neonatal network, our aim was to setup a reliable, clinic-independent, achievable quality improvement concept for several vital outcome measures and test its validity. For this, we compared 3 approaches for adjusting our 7 most important outcome measures for very preterm born children and analysed their effect on the differences that the clinics show for these outcomes.

Methods

Study population

The study includes data on all children born alive between 22 0/7 and 31 6/7 weeks gestational age during the years 2006 to 2014 that were prospectively collected in our national, population based registry (SwissNeoNet). Data are collected electronically from birth until death or first discharge home by all nine Level III and three of six Level IIB neonatal units using immediate plausibility and completeness checks and subsequent repeated challenge until corrected. All items are defined in a publicly available manual [14]. They cover typical aspects of perinatal care, demographics, common diagnoses and treatments, growth and hospitalization duration. In this study we include all infants born between 2006 and 2014. Population coverage was assessed by comparison with the birth registry of the Swiss Federal Statistical Office yielding 94% completeness when including births of non-resident mothers living outside Switzerland.

Outcome definitions

We selected outcomes that were strictly defined and whose incidence was alterable by variations in process or structure [9, 15]. Overall mortality was calculated for all infants born alive. The following proportions of newborns with the respective outcome (i.e. cumulative incidence proportion over a 9-year time span) were based on infants admitted to a NICU: in-hospital mortality; late onset sepsis with clear clinical evidence of infection as well as at least one microbiologically relevant positive blood culture occurring after day 3 of life (with day of birth as day 1); necrotizing enterocolitis (NEC) was defined as clinical signs (abdominal distension, bilious aspirates and/or bloody stools) confirmed by radiographically visible intramural gas or at laparotomy (Bell stages 2 and 3); [16] severe intraventricular haemorrhage (sIVH) was based on the most severe ultrasound result during hospital stay using stages 3 to 4 of the classifications defined by Papile et al. [17]. The remaining outcome incidence proportions were based on infants discharged home alive: severe retinopathy of prematurity (sROP) using the international classification published by the committee for the classification of ROP grades 3–4; [18] and bronchopulmonary dysplasia (BPD) defined as an oxygen requirement at 36 weeks gestational age according to the NICHD consensus conference paper [19].

Risk adjustment parameter definitions (risk adjustors)

We selected risk adjustors that were first and foremost predictive, i.e. known to vary with changes in severity in outcomes. Beyond this, they were easily available to restrict bias due to missing data, measurable, frequent, reliable, and accurately recorded with limited interpretation margins to minimize definition bias [9]. Another selection criterion was that they were consistent with literature, i.e. that their validity has already been documented for the listed outcomes [10, 11, 20]. Our risk adjusters also hold the ability to be updated periodically, based on an ongoing research commitment and investment [8].

The following risk adjusters were included in the model: Gestational age (GA), GA squared (GA^2), birth-weight z-score (BW z-score), male sex, multiples, Apgar at 1 min, major malformation, outborn and parent socio economic status (SES). GA was calculated based on ultrasound examinations during the first trimester of pregnancy and defined as postmenstrual age in weeks and days. Major congenital malformation was defined as any type of malformation severely impacting prognosis (e.g. complex congenital heart disease, malformation syndromes). SES was estimated by a validated 12-point socioeconomic score based on maternal education and current paternal occupation whereas the value 2 designates the combination of highest education and occupation versus the value 12 which represents no education and no occupation [21]. Outborn designates an infant transferred to any one of the 12 participating units after birth.

Statistical methods

Based on the risk-adjustment methodology published in literature, three approaches were compared: indirect standardization based on the units' individual distribution of children into gestational age weeks, the most commonly used multivariable logistic regression to account for multiple confounding variables, and multivariable multilevel modelling [5, 22, 23]. The latter was added in case clustering of data into neonatal units should be of importance. A previous publication revealed that the survival of Swiss infants with very low gestational age without severe neonatal morbidity was strongly influenced by the medical centre that treated them [24]. Data of infants born from 2006 to 2012 were used for model building (training set) whereas data from 2013 to 2014 were used for goodness-of-fit analysis (validation set). This split was performed to avoid overfitting, to be able to use the best acquired model on our own data and to accurately describe what effect each model has on the observed-to-expected ratios of the clinics.

In order to avoid collinearity between GA and birthweight, birthweight entered the model as z-scores relative to GA based on the growth curves published by Voigt et al. [25]. To better model the non-linear dependency of most neonatal outcomes on gestational age, its quadratic value (GA^2) was included into the latter 2 models. As several of the examined outcomes are known to have improved over the years, [26] year was added as a covariate as a continuous variable assigning the value 0 to the last year (2012) and subtracting 1 for each previous year (value range [−6, 0]); this covariate adjusts the remaining predictors for a linear effect of time. It was omitted in validation.

As one of the predictors, i.e. SES, yielded 20% missing values in the entire dataset, equally distributed over the years but with higher concentration on datasets of infants that died in the delivery room, we first calculated the models using fivefold imputation with chained equations [27]. The results were compared to those resulting from models without imputation and without SES as predictor. Models with imputation and SES were used only if SES yielded a significant adjusted odds ratio (i.e. 95% confidence interval outside 1). All other predictors yielded less than 2% missing data and were therefore not treated separately. No other model selection process was undertaken.

In the multilevel models, centre was included as a random intercept to adjust for centre differences while providing parameter estimates to permit centre-free predictions [20]. As the compared units were all of the same standard (swiss perinatal units are legally required to fulfil the same structural qualifications on staffing and equipment), we did not add any cluster level covariates. All statistical analyses were performed using R [28]. *P*-values below 0.05 were considered significant.

Validity assessments

To compare predictive validity of the different adjustment approaches, we compared the mean Brier score and the area under receiver operating characteristics curve (AUC). The Brier score measures the accuracy of probabilistic predictions as the mean squared difference between the predicted probability assigned to the possible outcome and the actual outcome. The closer the score is to 0, the better the sharpness and calibration of the prediction. A poor Brier score of 0.25 is reached by assigning each patient with a constant probability of 0.5 for the outcome [29]. AUC values between 0.7–0.8 were considered to represent moderate predictive validity whereas and >0.8 to represent high predictive validity. As no goodness-of-fit can be calculated for indirect standardization, comparison was approximated using a logistic regression model based on gestational weeks alone. The difference in prediction between both was less than 0.5% (Additional file 1: Table S1).

As we were not able to measure attributional validity, we instead measured changes to attributional validity by assessing what the effect of a specific risk adjustment model was on the differences seen in the risk-adjusted outcome measures. Standardized mortality / morbidity ratios were calculated as observed over expected ratios for each clinic. Expected outcome per clinic was calculated as sum of standardized outcome ratio per gestational age week in the case of indirect standardization and per each clinic's sum of individual patient probabilities ($0 < p < 1$) to acquire a specific outcome in the case of logistic regression or multilevel modelling, respectively. Individual patient probability was calculated as $P(Y = 1 | X_i = x_i) = \exp(\beta_0 + \beta_1 X_1 + \ldots + \beta_n X_n)/1 + \exp(\beta_0 + \beta_1 X_1 + \ldots + \beta_n X_n)$.

Results

Table 1 lists the 6 outcome variables and the proportion of new-borns presenting the respective outcome (i.e. cumulative incidence proportion) for which risk adjustment was performed. It also reveals the available data for prediction modelling and sensitivity

Table 1 Outcomes observed, collective used, study population size (N), valid responses per outcome (valid N) and cumulative incidence proportions (%) for prediction modelling and sensitivity analysis

Variable	Collective	2006–2012			2013–2014		
		Training set			Validation set		
		N[a]	valid	%	N	valid	%
Mortality	All Live-born	5212	5212	14.6	1572	1572	14.0
In hospital mortality	Admitted to ward	4876	4874	8.8	1465	1465	7.7
Late onset sepsis			4874	9.5		1465	8.1
NEC[b]			4874	2.4		1465	2.4
sIVH[c]			4865	6.5		1459	5.7
BPD[d]	Discharged home alive	4449	4439	9.3	1352	1349	11.2
sROP[e]			3990	1.9		1200	1.6

[a]*N* Sample size for analysis
[b]*NEC* Necrotizing enterocolitis
[c]*sIVH* intra-/periventricular haemorrhage grade 3–4
[d]*BPD* bronchopulmonary dysplasia
[e]*sROP* retinopathy of prematurity grade 3 and above

analysis and the number of valid responses per outcome. Proportions are relative to the number of valid responses. There were sufficient data available for model building and testing. Other than severe ROP, for which 11% of data were estimated using data imputation, the outcomes had a maximum of ten missing valid responses.

Table 2 compares the predictive validity of the three approaches for risk adjustment: indirect standardization based on GA stratification, logistic regression and multilevel modelling. Model parameters were calculated using the training set while prediction was tested using the validation set. For mortality, in hospital mortality and BPD, the indirect standardization had an inferior AUC but a superior Brier score. All other outcomes revealed close to identical Brier scores and a very similar AUC, whereas the values for logistic regression and multilevel modelling overall were almost identical. The variances of the random effect intercepts were all below 1.5 (not shown).

The 3 risk adjustment approaches over 7 outcomes yielded 21 risk adjustment models. Nineteen of these models reached a Brier Score below 0.1. Equally 19 reached at least an acceptable predictive validity (AUC > 0.7) of which 11 even reached a high predictive validity (AUC > 0.8) (Table 2).

Next we looked at the effect each risk adjustment approach had on the distribution of the individual clinic's outcomes in the standardized mortality / morbidity ratio (SMR) charts in order to ascertain if the differences in case-mix were effectively adjusted for and the remaining differences can be attributed to differences in care. SMR charts are ubiquitously used to analyse a clinic's performance by comparing the risk adjusted ratio of observed to expected mortality / morbidity cases to a standard population as shown in Fig. 1. For this we first determined for each model the number of clinics in the validation set whose observed to expected ratio were above 1, i.e. worse than expected, the value that usually interests the clinicians most (Table 3a). Mortality, in-hospital mortality

Table 2 Predictive validity for indirect standardization, logistic regression and multilevel random intercept approach respectively using the mean Brier score and AUC for assessing the predictive abilities of the respective model using the validation set

	Indirect Standardization		Logistic regression		Multilevel	
Variable	Brier Score	AUC	Brier Score	AUC	Brier Score	AUC
Mortality	0.070	0.896	0.113	0.935	0.109	0.936
In hosp. mortality	0.060	0.831	0.095	0.892	0.093	0.893
Late onset sepsis	0.068	0.788	0.067	0.804	0.067	0.803
NEC[a]	0.023	0.716	0.024	0.694	0.024	0.694
sIVH[b]	0.050	0.765	0.049	0.786	0.049	0.786
BPD[c]	0.084	0.807	0.195	0.843	0.195	0.843
sROP[d]	0.015	0.765	0.016	0.773	0.016	0.773

[a]*NEC* Necrotizing enterocolitis. Values based on imputed data
[b]*sIVH* intra-/periventricular haemorrhage grade 3–4
[c]*BPD* bronchopulmonary dysplasia
[d]*sROP* retinopathy of prematurity grade 3 and above. Values based on imputed data

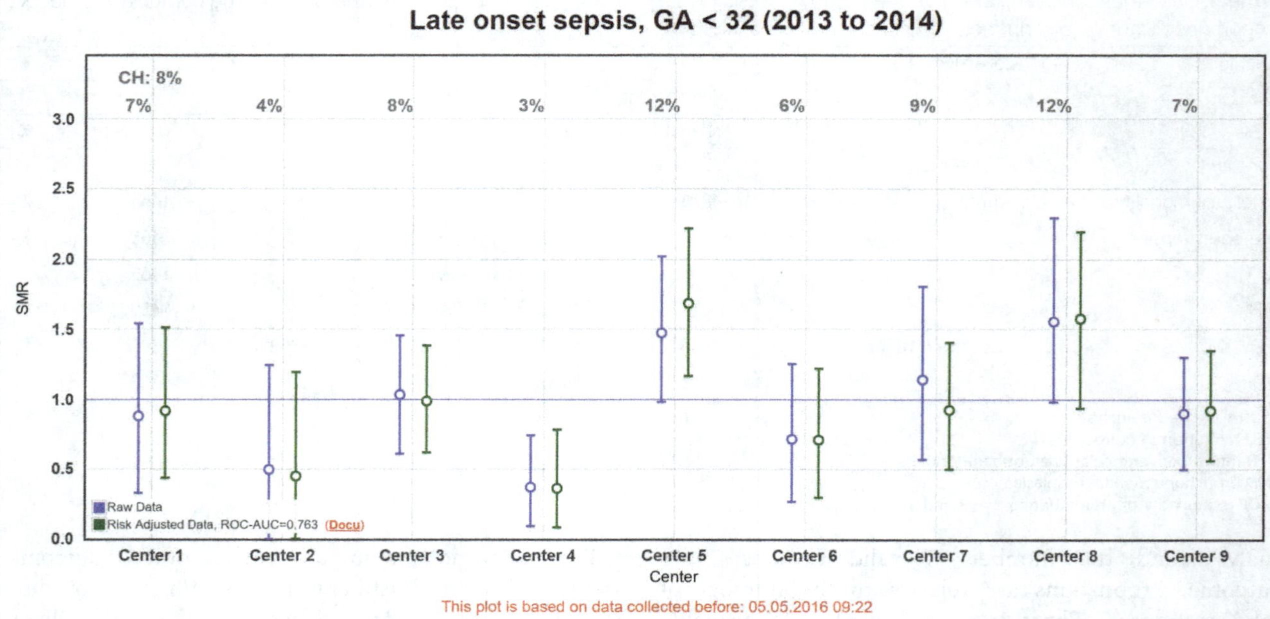

Fig. 1 Standardized morbidity ratio chart displaying late onset sepsis prediction for 9 Swiss NICUs with 95% confidence intervals (screenshot from SwissNeoNet member platform). *Blue*: crude observed over expected data, *green*: risk adjusted relation of observed to expected deaths in hospital (including delivery room). Expected deaths were calculated as sum of each child's probability to die depending upon the predictor values listed in Table 4

Table 3 Effect of risk-adjustment approach on standardized mortality/morbidity ratio chart. a) Number of clinics with observed-expected ratio > 1. b) Cumulative absolute distances of observed-expected ratio of all clinics to the standard value 1

	Raw values	Indirect standardization	Logistic regression	Multilevel
Outcome	a) SMR values above 1			
Mortality	3	3	3	3
In hosp. Mortality	3	3	3	3
Late onset sepsis	4	2	2	2
NEC[a]	3	4	3	3
sIVH[b]	5	5	6	6
BPD[c]	4	4	4	4
sROP[d]	2	2	1	2
	b) Cumulative absolute distances to 1			
Mortality	2.8	2.7	3.0	3.0
In hosp. Mortality	3.0	3.2	3.1	3.0
Late onset sepsis	2.7	3.0	3.0	3.1
NEC	3.4	3.4	3.6	3.6
sIVH	2.2	2.3	2.4	2.4
BPD	4.1	3.2	3.8	3.8
sROP	5.7	5.4	5.4	5.5
Total	23.9	23.2	24.3	24.4

[a] *NEC* Necrotizing enterocolitis
[b] *sIVH* intra-/periventricular haemorrhage grade 3–4
[c] *BPD* bronchopulmonary dysplasia
[d] *sROP* retinopathy of prematurity grade 3 and above

and BPD listed the same amount of SMR values above 1. The values for the other outcomes remained largely untouched. To determine if these values above 1 represent the same clinics, we analysed all of the 252 possible SMR changes generated out of the total of 7 (outcomes) × 9 (clinics) × 4 (approaches) (not shown). Of 252 possible changes of orientation between all approaches, a total of 14 changes were observed, 7 of which were between raw values and all other risk adjustment models, and 7 between indirect standardization and unadjusted as well as adjusted models. These changes of orientation concern clinics with observed to expected ratios close to one. There was no other fluctuation of clinics from above to below one due to risk adjustment. Our second analysis concerned the cumulative absolute distance of the observed to expected ratio from 1 for each approach in order to determine if the approaches lead to larger or smaller overall differences between clinics (Table 3b). Absolute here means that the distances of all clinics above and below one are summarized. The higher the value, the more the clinics seem to differ from each other. Again, the differences between the approaches per outcome are marginal but somewhat higher when using a logistic regression or multilevel approach. In order to exclude that the lack of effect of risk adjustment is based on a lack of difference between the clinics' risk potential, we calculated the expected mortality for the clinic with the lowest risk in the validation set as 11.2% versus 15.9% for the clinic with the highest risk according to the logistic regression model (AUC 0.935). Thus, the risk heterogeneity between the two clinics lies at 40%.

Table 4 summarizes the adjusted odds ratios of the risk adjustors per approach (indirect standardization, logistic regression and multilevel). Our indirect standardization approach relies on gestational age stratification alone which explains the difference between the odds ratios per outcome in comparison with the other approaches. The risk adjustor's odds ratios for the logistic regression and the multilevel approach are however largely congruent with only marginal differences, explaining the close comparability in the analyses above. The cumulatively strongest effect, i.e. the largest difference in relation to 1, is attributable to gestational age. A relatively high impact on some of the models is observable in major malformation. SES score only had an effect for the outcome NEC [OR 1.13, 95% CI 1.04–1.22] (note that the highest SES score (12) stands for lowest socio economic *status* whereas the lowest score (2) stands for the highest SES collected).

Discussion

In our study we analyse prospectively collected population based data with high population coverage. The aim was to develop and compare risk adjustment models for quality improvement purposes within a network of 12 Swiss neonatal units. The selected outcomes for risk adjustment represent some of the most important outcome measures in the field of neonatology [30]. We selected the two well-known and most often implemented approaches for risk adjustment, indirect standardization and logistic regression modelling and added a multilevel approach due to the nested data structure in which patients were associated with a particular clinic and its ability to provide clinic-independent predictions. Both prediction and outcome parameters fulfil multiple requirements for risk adjustment. Over half of the 21 risk adjustment models (three risk adjustment approaches for 7 outcomes each) yielded high predictive validity in the validation set with a majority of the remaining models being at least moderately predictive. In summary, the three risk adjustment approaches are similar to each other and lead to results that differ marginally when compared with the unadjusted raw outcome comparisons.

The simplest approach, indirect standardization based on GA, performed surprisingly well in comparison and may be more useful for quality assessments than previously thought. This may be due to the high impact of gestational age on outcome in very preterm infants and may not be generalizable into other areas of medicine. Nevertheless, reduction to one reliably available risk parameter may have removed bias that lead to an inferior accordance between predicted and true values in the multivariable approach. New medical registries without available previous data could profit from the observation that a non-model based approach achieves comparable if not better calibrated results to model based approaches. The lack of differences between the logistic regression and the multilevel approach and the small variances of the random effect intercepts of the multilevel model revealed that the effect of a nested data structure is lower than expected for a neonatal setting [20].

In summary, the three approaches reveal very little difference in predictive or attributional validity between each other. Nevertheless, their ability to isolate quality improvement potentials of the units is limited. This was unexpected because the predictive validities for the carefully selected models were high. Also, large differences between Swiss clinics are documented in literature [24] and by a heterogeneity in risk potential between the clinics of up to 40%. Nevertheless, neither of the risk adjustment models had a discernible effect on the observed to expected ratios of the seven outcome parameters, neither in their absolute orientation (above or below 1) or in their distance to 1 (1 meaning that observed and expected are equal). The differences between units that remains after risk adjustment can therefore not be attributed to the quality of care alone. In neonatology, for instance, there are factors that contribute to the differences between

Table 4 Odds ratios (OR) with standard errors (SE) of the risk adjustment parameters for each outcome and each risk adjustment (RA) approach

Outcome	RA approach	GA[a]		GA^2		BW[b] z-score		Male sex		Multiples		Apgar1		Major malformation		outborn		SES[c]	
		OR	SE	OR	SE	OR	SE	OR	SE	OR	SE	OR	SE	OR	SE	OR	SE	OR	SE
Mortality	Indirect standardization	0.52	0.02	-	-	-	-	-	-	-	-	-	-	-	-	-	-	-	-
	Logistic regression	0.20	0.12	1.10	0.01	0.88	0.06	1.07	0.11	1.03	0.12	0.74	0.02	7.88	0.19	0.76	0.27	-	-
	Multilevel	0.19	0.12	1.10	0.01	0.84	0.06	1.09	0.11	1.03	0.12	0.74	0.02	8.62	0.20	0.74	0.28	-	-
In hosp. Mortality	Indirect standardization	0.57	0.03	-	-	-	-	-	-	-	-	-	-	-	-	-	-	-	-
	Logistic regression	0.31	0.15	1.06	0.01	0.81	0.06	1.13	0.11	1.08	0.13	0.79	0.02	4.65	0.24	0.94	0.27	-	-
	Multilevel	0.28	0.15	1.07	0.01	0.79	0.06	1.16	0.12	1.06	0.13	0.80	0.02	5.34	0.24	0.89	0.28	-	-
Late onset sepsis	Indirect standardization	0.68	0.02	-	-	-	-	-	-	-	-	-	-	-	-	-	-	-	-
	Logistic regression	1.11	0.14	0.96	0.01	0.71	0.06	0.95	0.10	0.83	0.12	1.03	0.02	1.32	0.28	1.08	0.24	-	-
	Multilevel	1.02	0.15	0.96	0.01	0.68	0.06	0.96	0.10	0.79	0.12	1.03	0.02	1.48	0.29	0.98	0.24	-	-
NEC[d]	Indirect standardization	0.81	1.04	-	-	-	-	-	-	-	-	-	-	-	-	-	-	-	-
	Logistic regression	1.12	1.30	0.98	1.02	0.78	1.11	1.12	1.21	1.13	1.23	0.91	1.04	1.00	1.69	1.30	1.46	1.11	1.04
	Multilevel	1.09	1.30	0.98	1.02	0.78	1.11	1.13	1.21	1.11	1.23	0.91	1.04	1.01	1.69	1.32	1.46	1.11	1.04
sIVH[e]	Indirect standardization	0.65	0.03	-	-	-	-	-	-	-	-	-	-	-	-	-	-	-	-
	Logistic regression	0.64	0.16	1.01	0.01	1.30	0.07	1.28	0.12	1.18	0.13	0.85	0.03	0.69	0.41	1.37	0.25	-	-
	Multilevel	0.63	0.16	1.01	0.01	1.31	0.07	1.27	0.12	1.19	0.13	0.85	0.03	0.69	0.41	1.33	0.25	-	-
BPD[f]	Indirect standardization	0.62	0.03	-	-	-	-	-	-	-	-	-	-	-	-	-	-	-	-
	Logistic regression	0.79	0.17	0.98	0.01	0.53	0.07	1.60	0.12	1.03	0.13	0.94	0.02	3.91	0.27	1.18	0.27	-	-
	Multilevel	0.73	0.17	0.99	0.01	0.52	0.07	1.60	0.12	1.01	0.13	0.94	0.02	4.40	0.27	1.11	0.27	-	-
sROP[g]	Indirect standardization	0.47	1.07	-	-	-	-	-	-	-	-	-	-	-	-	-	-	-	-
	Logistic regression	0.45	1.42	1.01	1.03	0.75	1.16	1.23	1.28	1.26	1.31	0.93	1.05	1.06	2.17	1.51	1.73	0.98	1.05
	Multilevel	0.35	1.44	1.03	1.03	0.75	1.16	1.31	1.28	1.06	1.31	0.94	1.05	0.97	2.19	1.56	1.76	0.98	1.05

[a]*GA* gestational age
[b]*BW* birthweight
[c]*SES* socio-economic status
[d]*NEC* Necrotizing enterocolitis
[e]*sIVH* intra−/periventricular hemorrhage grade 3–4
[f]*BPD* bronchopulmonary dysplasia
[g]*sROP* retinopathy of prematurity grade 3 and above

clinics other than risk or quality of care. Even though there are national guidelines toward treatment at the limit of viability, [31] the Swiss clinics are known to adopt different approaches towards the care of infants born below 25 weeks GA. Clinics with a more active approach towards resuscitation in the delivery room will have a lower mortality but a higher risk for morbidities as the decision about whether to provide active treatment at birth is a critical predictor of subsequent outcomes in itself [32]. This can partially be adjusted for by stratified analysis of outcome of infants receiving active treatment, in our case "admitted to ward". But a more active approach which yields a higher risk may still lead to higher survival without impairment as recently shown by Rysavy et al. [33].

In 1997, Iezzoni reported on a series of studies comparing the effect of different severity of illness scores on risk adjustment and concluded that although hospitals vary in their unadjusted death rates, severity failed to explain these differences fully leaving the central question unresolved: "does severity adjustment isolate that residual quantity, namely quality of care differences across hospitals?" [34] Also using a severity score, Thomas et al. found that hospital mortality performance was significantly related to quality of care for only 3 of 10 conditions evaluated [35]. The primary finding of a recent Monte Carlo simulation on the relationship between the predictive validity of the risk-adjustment model and the accuracy of hospital quality reports found that the relationship was, at best, modest [36]. The same researchers maintain that even if perfect risk-adjustment was possible, random error will result in some hospitals being misclassified [37]. The main rationale behind their claims is that the often used AUC is a measure of discrimination: the degree to which the model can discriminate between those patients with the outcome of interest and those without the outcome of interest. As a consequence it will be higher in a setting in which there is greater heterogeneity in risk [36]. Thus, models with low risk heterogeneity will be read as having low predictive validity regardless of their ability to adjust for risk.

Nevertheless, most published approaches to risk adjustment still rely exclusively on factors known for their high predictive validity such as severity of illness scores like SNAP or CRIB in neonatology [11]. These examples reflect NICU practices that were common at the time of their development (1993), require up to 28 physiological data characteristics from up to the first 24 h of the new-born's lives, a period during which they are in the care of the clinics under observation for quality of performance, and require blood whereas differences in the timing of blood taking may affect risk adjustment [8]. Another hindering issue is the difficulty to achieve data completeness for all infants.

The SwissNeoNet selection of risk adjusters is therefore geared towards predictive validity, availability, and measurability and is the result of a consensus process among network members, by agreeing which factors the clinics should not be held responsible for in quality improvement and which factors should not be corrected for as they are under the control of the clinics. For the latter reason, we did not include caesarean section or antenatal steroids because we did not want to attribute a higher risk to clinics with lower rates in either of them. Particularly in the case of antenatal steroids, the units would have lost an opportunity to isolate a potential for improvement. Because the effect of risk adjustment is limited, members of the SwissNeoNet compare their outcomes in standardized mortality / morbidity ratio charts for stratified collectives and over pooled years. Stratifying can involve limiting the evaluation to a specific patient group such as from overall mortality to in-hospital-mortality, or separate analysis for infants born in different GA or birthweight groups. The crude observed-expected ratio (together with its 95% confidence interval) is displayed alongside its risk adjusted correspondent (Fig. 1). We also add the AUC value and link to documentation for the interpretation of the diagrams.

The strengths of our study lie in the quality and completeness of our population based data, in the data being covered for all live-born infants until death or primary discharge home, and in separating the data into training and validation sets. Switzerland provides wide regional diversity expressed by 26 cantons with 26 health care authorities, 4 languages, and 40% inhabitants with migration background. This diversity is also reflected in the up to 40% risk heterogeneity documented for mortality. The high proportion of missing SES data required imputation in a setting where data was not missing at random. Thus, we cannot be certain that excluding SES from mortality risk adjustment is correct. For the other outcome models, SES was missing at random.

Almost 20 years ago, Iezzoni maintained that answering the question on how to isolate quality-of-care differences requires expensive, time-consuming, logistically difficult, and methodologically complicated research and that only a handful of studies had addressed this question, most with equivocal results [34]. Risk adjustment for quality improvement spans all medical disciplines from alternative medicine to surgery and is performed by researchers, administrators, government agencies and health insurances. Yet we have not found a published solution on how to effectively isolate quality-of-care differences since Iezzoni's comment other than approaches that entailed visiting the participating clinics and assessing the attributional validity of their risk adjustment model on site, such as the DAVROS group [13]. But besides having its own bias issues, this approach, requiring independent experts, is personnel and time intensive. We could not afford copying it for one outcome let alone seven. It is therefore not so surprising that most of the literature on risk adjustment relies on predictive validity alone and measures neither change in attributional validity nor attributional validity itself. It would no less be important to know if quality improvement collaboratives with larger populations and/or differences in case-mix risk show a larger effect of risk adjustment and more effectively isolate quality differences.

Conclusions

To summarize, all three approaches to risk adjustment revealed comparable results with high predictive validity for mortality and several major morbidities. The indirect standardization approach was surprisingly similar to the other approaches.

In general, however, we conclude that risk adjustment has a limited effect when comparing the outcome of clinics with the same degree of specialization. We therefore propose that clinic outcomes be compared both in risk-adjusted and un-adjusted form. The predictive validity of the risk-adjustment should be quantified and reported. To correct for confounding, stratification into risk groups (such as gestational age or sex) could be used as an alternative to risk-adjustment. Rather than relying on the purely methodological approach of risk-adjustment alone,

as done ubiquitously by organizations delivering risk-adjusted annual reports, our experience shows that building small groups of clinic representatives and combining their expertise with methodologically transparent presentation of epidemiological data is very helpful in isolating relevant quality improvement potential.

Abbreviations

AUC: Area under receiver operating characteristics curve; BPD: Bronchopulmonary dysplasia; BW z-score: Birthweight z-score; GA: Gestational age; GA2: GA squared; N: Sample size for analysis; NEC: Necrotizing enterocolitis; SES: Socio economic status; sIVH: Intra–/periventricular haemorrhage grade 3–4; SMR: Standardized mortality/morbidity ratio; sROP: Retinopathy of prematurity grade 3 and above

Acknowledgements

We thank the following units for collaborating in the SwissNeoNet: Aarau: Cantonal Hospital Aarau, Children's Clinic, Department of Neonatology (Philip Meyer, Claudia Anderegg); Basel: University Children's Hospital Basel, Department of Neonatology (Sven Schulzke); Berne: University Hospital Berne, Department of Neonatology (Mathias Nelle), Department of Paediatrics (Bernhard Wagner); Chur: Children's Hospital Chur, Department of Neonatology (Thomas Riedel); Fribourg: Cantonal Hospital Fribourg, Department of Neonatology (Gregor Kaczala); Geneva: Department of child and adolescent, University Hospital (HUG), Neonatology Units (Riccardo E. Pfister); Lausanne: University Hospital (CHUV), Department of Neonatology (Jean-Francois Tolsa, Matthias Roth-Kleiner); Lucerne: Children's Hospital of Lucerne, Neonatal and Paediatric Intensive Care Unit (Martin Stocker); Neuchatel: Cantonal Hospital Neuchatel, Department of Paediatrics (Bernhard Laubscher); St. Gallen: Cantonal Hospital St. Gallen, Department of Neonatology (Andreas Malzacher), Children's Hospital St. Gallen, Neonatal and Paediatric Intensive Care Unit (John P. Micallef); Winterthur: Cantonal Hospital Winterthur, Department of Neonatology (Lukas Hegi); Zurich: University Hospital Zurich (USZ), Department of Neonatology (Dirk Bassler, Romaine Arlettaz), University Children's Hospital Zurich, Department of Neonatology (Vera Bernet).

Funding

The authors received no specific funding for this work.

Authors' contributions

MA was involved in study design, data collection, analysis and interpretation of the results and wrote the manuscript. DB and HUB were involved in data collection and study design and reviewed the manuscript together with JB, VvW and MAP who additionally assisted with biostatistics methodology and interpretation of the results. The Swiss Neonatal Network collected and contributed the data and, together will all co-authors, approved the final manuscript.

Competing interests

The authors declare that they have no competing interests.

Ethics approval and consent to participate

Data collection and evaluation for this study were approved by the Swiss Federal Commission for Privacy Protection in Medical Research and the ethical review board of the Canton of Zurich on behalf of all Swiss ethical review boards (KEK-ZH-Nr2014–0552) according to federal regulation. Up until 2014, the patients' parents/guardians were informed about the use of data for research and data of patients whose parents/guardians vetoed collection were not collected or removed if objection was raised at a later time point. A signed informed consent was not required.

References

1. Vohr BR, Wright LL, Dusick AM, Perritt R, Poole WK, Tyson JE, et al. Center differences and outcomes of extremely low birth weight infants. Pediatrics. 2004;113:781–9.
2. Draper ES, Zeitlin J, Fenton AC, Weber T, Gerrits J, Martens G, et al. Investigating the variations in survival rates for very preterm infants in 10 European regions: the MOSAIC birth cohort. Arch Dis Child Fetal Neonatal Ed. 2009;94:F158–63.
3. Isayama T, Lee SK, Mori R, Kusuda S, Fujimura M, Ye XY, et al. Comparison of mortality and morbidity of very low birth weight infants between Canada and Japan. Pediatrics. 2012;130:e957–65.
4. Payne NR, LaCorte M, Karna P, Chen S, Finkelstein M, Goldsmith JP, et al. Reduction of Bronchopulmonary dysplasia after participation in the Breathsavers Group of the Vermont Oxford network neonatal intensive care quality improvement collaborative. Pediatrics. 2006;118:S73–7.
5. Horbar JD, Soll RF, Edwards WH. The Vermont Oxford network: a community of practice. Clin Perinatol. 2010;37:29–47.
6. Gould JB. The role of regional collaboratives: the California perinatal quality care collaborative model. Clin Perinatol. 2010;37:71–86.
7. Grover TR, Pallotto EK, Brozanski B, Piazza AJ, Chuo J, Moran S, et al. Interdisciplinary teamwork and the power of a quality improvement collaborative in tertiary neonatal intensive care units. J Perinat Neonatal Nurs. 2015;29:179–86.
8. Kuhlthau K, Ferris TGG, Iezzoni LI. Risk adjustment for pediatric quality indicators. Pediatrics. 2004;113:210–6.
9. Richardson D, Tarnow-Mordi WO, Lee SK. Risk adjustment for quality improvement. Pediatrics. 1999;103:255–65.
10. Zupancic JAF, Richardson DK, Horbar JD, Carpenter JH, Lee SK, Escobar GJ. Revalidation of the score for neonatal acute physiology in the Vermont Oxford network. Pediatrics. 2007;119:e156–63.
11. Patrick SW, Schumacher RE, Davis MM. Methods of mortality risk adjustment in the NICU: a 20-year review. Pediatrics. 2013;131:S68–74.
12. Silva LK. Validity of the risk adjustment approach to compare outcomes. Cad Saúde Pública. 2003;19:287–95.
13. Wilson R, Goodacre SW, Klingbajl M, Kelly A-M, Rainer T, Coats T, et al. Evaluation of the DAVROS (development and validation of risk-adjusted outcomes for systems of emergency care) risk-adjustment model as a quality indicator for healthcare. Emerg Med J. 2014;31:471–5.
14. SwissNeoNet. Data definitions [Internet]. Available from: http://www.neonet.ch/en/neonatal-network/data-collection/. Accessed 10 Apr 2017.
15. Profit J, Soll RF. Neonatal networks: clinical research and quality improvement. Semin Fetal Neonatal Med. 2015;20:410–5.
16. Bell MJ, Ternberg JL, Feigin RD, Keating JP, Marshall R, Barton L, et al. Neonatal necrotizing enterocolitis. Therapeutic decisions based upon clinical staging. Ann Surg. 1978;187:1–7.
17. Papile L-A, Burstein J, Burstein R, Koffler H. Incidence and evolution of subependymal and intraventricular hemorrhage: a study of infants with birth weights less than 1,500 gm. J Pediatr. 1978;92:529–34.
18. JAMA Network | JAMA Ophthalmology | The International Classification of Retinopathy of Prematurity Revisited [Internet]. [cited 2015 Dec 8]. Available from: http://archopht.jamanetwork.com/article.aspx?articleid=417157.
19. Jobe AH, Bancalari E. Bronchopulmonary dysplasia. Am J Respir Crit Care Med. 2001;163:1723–9.
20. Tyson JE, Parikh NA, Langer J, Green C, Higgins RD. Intensive Care for Extreme Prematurity — moving beyond gestational age. N Engl J Med. 2008;358:1672–81.
21. Largo RH, Pfister D, Molinari L, Kundu S, Lipp A, Due G. Significance of prenatal, perinatal and postnatal factors in the development of Aga preterm infants at five to seven years. Dev Med Child Neurol. 1989;31:440–56.
22. Schokkaert E, Van de Voorde C. Direct versus indirect standardization in risk adjustment. J Health Econ. 2009;28:361–74.
23. Dickinson LM, Basu A. Multilevel modeling and practice-based research. Ann Fam Med. 2005;3:s52 60.
24. Steurer MA, Adams M, Bacchetti P, Schulzke SM, Roth-Kleiner M, Berger TM, et al. Swiss medical centres vary significantly when it comes to outcomes of neonates with a very low gestational age. Acta Paediatr. 2015;104:872–9.
25. Voigt M, Fusch C, Olbertz D, Hartmann K, Rochow N, Renken C, et al. Analyse des Neugeborenenkollektivs der Bundesrepublik Deutschland. Geburtshilfe Frauenheilkd. 2006;66:956 70.

26. Rüegger C, Hegglin M, Adams M, Bucher HU, for the SNN. Population based trends in mortality, morbidity and treatment for very preterm- and very low birth weight infants over 12 years. BMC Pediatrics. 2012;12:17.
27. Buuren S van, Groothuis-Oudshoorn K. mice: Multivariate Imputation by Chained Equations in R. Journal of Statistical Software [Internet]. 2011 [cited 2015 Dec 18];45. Available from: http://www.jstatsoft.org/v45/i03
28. R: a language and environment for statistical computing [Internet]. GBIF.ORG. [cited 2015 Dec 18.] Available from: http://www.gbif.org/resource/81287
29. Harrison DA, Brady AR, Parry GJ, Carpenter JR, Rowan K. Recalibration of risk prediction models in a large multicenter cohort of admissions to adult, general critical care units in the United Kingdom*: Crit Care Med. 2006;34:1378–88.
30. Profit J, Kowalkowski MA, Zupancic JAF, Pietz K, Richardson P, Draper D, et al. Baby-MONITOR: a composite indicator of NICU quality. Pediatrics. 2014; 134:74–82.
31. Berger T, Bernet V, El Alama S, Fauchère J, Hösli I, Irion O, et al. Perinatal care at the limit of viability between 22 and 26 completed weeks of gestation in Switzerland. Swiss Medical Weekly [Internet]. 2011 [cited 2015 Dec 18]; Available from: http://doi.emh.ch/smw.2011.13280.
32. Marlow N. The elephant in the delivery room. N Engl J Med. 2015;372:1856–7.
33. Rysavy MA, Li L, Bell EF, Das A, Hintz SR, Stoll BJ, et al. Between-hospital variation in treatment and outcomes in extremely preterm infants. N Engl J Med. 2015;372:1801–11.
34. Iezzoni LI. The risks of risk adjustment. JAMA. 1997;278:1600–7.
35. Thomas JW, Holloway JJ, Guire KE. Validating risk-adjusted mortality as an indicator for quality of care. Inquiry. 1993;30:6–22.
36. Austin PC, Reeves MJ. The relationship between the c-statistic of a risk-adjustment model and the accuracy of hospital report cards: a Monte Carlo study. Med Care. 2013;51:275–84.
37. Austin PC, Brunner LJ. Optimal Bayesian probability levels for hospital report cards. Health Serv Outcomes Res Method. 2007;8:80–97.

5

Prevalence, severity and early outcomes of hypoxic ischemic encephalopathy among newborns at a tertiary hospital, in northern Tanzania

Irene N. Simiyu[1], Deborah N. Mchaile[1,2,7*], Kahindo Katsongeri[1,3], Rune N. Philemon[2,4] and Sia E. Msuya[4,5,6]

Abstract

Background: Hypoxic Ischemic Encephalopathy (HIE) remains a problem of great concern worldwide especially in developing countries. The occurrence of a neurological syndrome can be an indicator of insult to the brain. We aimed to determine the prevalence, HIE proportions, neurological signs and early outcomes of newborns that developed birth asphyxia at KCMC Tanzania.

Methods: A prospective study was conducted at KCMC from November 2014 to April 2015 among newborns with birth asphyxia. Sarnat and Sarnat score was used to assess newborns immediately after birth to classify HIE and were later followed daily for 7 days or until discharge.

Results: Of the 1752 deliveries during the study period, 11.5% (*n* = 201) had birth asphyxia. Of the 201 newborns, 187 had HIE. Of these 187 with HIE; 39.0% had moderate HIE and 10.2% had severe HIE according to the Sarnat and Sarnat classification.

Neurological signs that were observed during the study period were; weak/absent reflexes (46.0%), hypotonia (43.3%) and lethargy (42.2%).

Mortality was 9.1% among the 187 newborns with HIE. Mortality was higher among newborns with severe HIE 84.2% (16/19) compared to those with moderate HIE 1.4% (1/73). On the 7th day after delivery, 17.1% (32/187) of the newborns did not show any change from the initial score at delivery.

Conclusion: Prevalence of birth asphyxia is high in our setting and most of the newborns (49%) end up with moderate/severe HIE. Good obstetric care and immediate resuscitation of newborns are vital in reducing the occurrence of HIE and improving the general outcome of newborns.

Keywords: Hypoxic ischemic encephalopathy, HIE, Birth asphyxia, Neuro-muscular signs, Neonates, Early outcomes, Tanzania

Background

Birth anoxia remains a vital cause of morbidity and mortality in neonates. Hypoxic ischemic encephalopathy affects the tissues of the body and can lead to permanent brain damage. Hypoxic ischemic encephalopathy results from lack of oxygen before, during or after birth [1].

The countdown report of 2015 estimated that neonatal deaths account for 45% of the 5.9 million child deaths that occurred in 2015 globally. Birth asphyxia is responsible for a large number of neonatal deaths after preterm births [2]. Perinatal asphyxia is thus a serious problem for child survival globally, more in developing countries. Apart from increased mortality, perinatal asphyxia results in serious neurological consequences ranging from cerebral palsy and mental retardation to epilepsy [3]. Reaching the sustainable development goal of 2030 of reducing preventable neonatal mortality to less than 12

* Correspondence: deborahsia@hotmail.com
[1]Kilimanjaro Christian Medical University College (KCMUCo), Moshi, Tanzania
[2]Department of Paediatrics, Kilimanjaro Christian Medical Centre (KCMC), Moshi, Tanzania

deaths per 1000 live births requires research and evidence interventions that target neonatal period [4].

Deaths due to perinatal asphyxia causes shock and pain to the mother and family at large. However, it can sometimes be avoided by close monitoring during the birth process with several assessments which include umbilical pH, 1 h post delivery blood gas, Apgar scores and neurological changes ranging from twitching, hypotonia, and seizures [3]. An Apgar scores at 5 min provides useful prognostic data before other evaluations are available. Low Apgar scores at 1, 5 and 10 min have been found to be markers with possible increased risk of death or chronic motor disability [3].

Neonatal encephalopathy preceded by perinatal hypoxic ischemic insult is a main contributor to global child mortality and morbidity. Brain injury in infants is a process that evolves over hours to days providing an opportunity for neuro-protective interventions. Advances in neuroimaging, techniques in monitoring of the brain and tissue biomarkers have improved the ability to diagnose, monitor and care for newborn infants. However, challenges remain in the availability of these imaging modalities in low income settings like Tanzania [5].

The gap between developed and developing countries with regards to neonatal mortality still remains wide. A child born in a developing country is 14 times more likely to die during the first 28 days of life than a baby born in a developed country; with sub-Saharan Africa and South East Asia being most affected [6]. These could be attributed to the lack of investigating and monitoring modalities. The aim of this study was to determine the prevalence, describe the severity and early neonatal outcomes of hypoxic ischemic encephalopathy among newborns with birth asphyxia (Apgar score < 7 at 5 min) at KCMC referral hospital born between November 2014 and April 2015.

Methods

Study design and area

This was a prospective study which enrolled newborns immediately after delivery and followed them daily for a period of 7 days after delivery. The study was conducted at the labor ward and newborns followed up at the neonatal ward (P3) at KCMC referral hospital situated in northern Tanzania. KCMC is a teaching and referral hospital in Moshi urban district. As a zonal referral center, KCMC receives normal and complicated cases from the local community in Kilimanjaro region and nearby regions in the Northern Tanzania and from nearby districts in Kenya.

The neonatal ward at KCMC hospital is a modest 6 room ward. Of these, 3 rooms are for acute cases with approximately 60 cots whilst the other 3 rooms have 15beds mainly for recovering newborns awaiting discharge. The neonatal ward admits a considerable number of neonates per year with most of those delivered being from within the facility. The unit does not have high tech advanced diagnostic facilities like most of SSA countries. Babies with asphyxia as assessed by the Sarnat and Sarnat staging are usually kept in the cool area of the ward where heaters are not switched on. Management offered is usually observation, oxygen therapy depending on the severity of hypoxia and prevention of sepsis. Blood PH, mechanical ventilation, Electroencephalogram (EEG), brain imaging or therapeutic cooling/hypothermia is not available at this set up.

Study population, sampling and enrollment procedure

The study population was all newborns seen at KCMC between November 2014 and April 2015 who had an Apgar score < 7 at the 5th minute. Newborns with birth asphyxia but with obvious congenital malformations were excluded from the study.

The formula for precision by Leslie Kish was used to calculate the sample size [7]. The minimum sample size required was 327 based on prevalence of HIE of 30.9% observed in Dar es Salaam [8], confidence interval of 95% and error set at 5%.

At the labor ward a standardized data extraction sheet was used to collect information from the patients' files and records of birth registry. Information collected was on maternal demographic information, gestation age at delivery based on last menstrual period, duration of labor, mode of delivery, birth complications, birth weight, Apgar score and occurrence of signs of HIE. Sarnat and Sarnat classification (Table 1), was used to record neurological signs and classify the severity of HIE of the newborns with birth asphyxia immediately after birth, and daily up to 7th day after birth or discharge from the neonatal ward.

Data processing and analysis

Data collected was entered and analyzed using the statistical package for the social science (SPSS) version 20. Categorical data was summarized using proportions, while mean and median with their measures of dispersion were used to summarize continuous data.

Categorization of severity of HIE

Newborns who were born with birth asphyxia were classified according to the Sarnat and Sarnat scoring criteria for HIE. The tool has 8 items which are assessed. Neonates scoring 1-10 were classified as having mild HIE, 11-14 as moderate HIE while those scoring 15-22 were classified as having severe HIE. The highest score obtained on any of the 7 days of follow up was used to assess the severity of birth asphyxia.

Table 1 Sarnat and Sarnat Scoring System

	1 2 3 4 5 6 7	1 2 3 4 5 6 7	1 2 3 4 5 6 7
	1	2	3
Consciousness	Hyper alert	Lethargic	Stuporous
Neuromuscular	Normal	Mild hypotonia	Flaccid
Reflexes	Weak > Normal	Weak	Absent
Pupils	Dilated	Constricted	Variable
Heart rate	Tachycardia	Bradycardia	Variable
Secretions	Sparge	Profuse	Variable
GIT motility	Normal	Increased	Variable
Convulsions	None	Common	Common early less common later
Duration	24 h	2-14 days	Weeks

Ethical approval

Approval to conduct the study was obtained from KCMUCo Research and Ethics Committee. Permission to conduct the study was also obtained from the Executive Director of KCMC Hospital and the heads of department of Pediatrics and Obstetrics and Gynecology. Consent was obtained from mothers. All newborns were managed in the neonatal ward following the standardized protocol for the unit.

Results

Prevalence of birth asphyxia

A total of 1752 newborns were delivered at the labor ward during the study period (November 2014 – April 2015). Of these newborns, 201 (11.5%) had birth asphyxia which was defined by an APGAR score less than 7 at 5 min after birth. Of the 201 newborns with asphyxia, 187 had hypoxic ischemic encephalopathy (HIE) giving a prevalence of 10.7% (187/1752). These 187 neonates with HIE were followed up daily for 7 days or until discharge if it happened before 7 days.

Characteristics of the participants

The median gestation age at delivery of the 187 newborns was 38 weeks (range 27 - 43). Their median birth weight was 2900 g (range 1100 - 5000). More than half 52.9% of the participants were females and delivered by cesarean section (70.1%), see Table 2. Of 131 cesarean sections, 96% were emergencies.

Severity of HIE

According to the Sarnat and Sarnat classification, majority of the 187 newborns with HIE had mild HIE 50.8% (n = 95) and 10.2% (19) had severe HIE, Table 3.

Higher proportion of severe HIE was noted among females 11.1% (n = 11) compared to males 9.1% (n = 8), but this difference was not a significant difference OR 1.25 (95% CI: 0.48 – 3.26). Severe HIE was also observed among LBW (< 2500 g) 14.3% than normal weight (≥ 2500 g), OR 1.90 (95% CI: 0.73 – 4.95).

Common neurological signs observed

Figure 1 shows common clinical signs that were observed in the newborns with HIE. Weak/absent reflexes (46.0%), hypotonia (43.3%) and lethargy (42.2%) were the most common observed signs. Among the least

Table 2 Characteristics of newborns with hypoxic ischemic encephalopathy at KCMC between Nov 2014 and April 2015 (N = 187)

Variable	Frequency	%
Sex		
Male	88	47.1
Female	99	52.9
Birth Weight		
Low Birth weight (<2500 g)	63	33.7
Normal (2500-4500 g)	123	65.8
Over weight (>4500 g)	1	0.5
Gestational age at delivery		
Pre term (<37 weeks)	61	32.6
Term (37-42 weeks)	121	64.7
Post Term (>42 weeks)	5	2.7
Apgar score at 5 min		
4-6	176	94.1
1-3	11	5.9
Referral		
Yes	123	65.8
No	64	34.2
Mode of delivery		
Spontaneous vaginal delivery	52	27.8
Cesarean section	131	70.1
Instrumental delivery	4	2.1

Table 3 Proportions of newborns with asphyxia who had mild, moderate or severe HIE per Sarnat and Sarnat classification ($N = 187$)

Variable	Frequency	%
Mild (1-10)	95	50.8
Moderate (11-14)	73	39.0
Severe (15-22)	19	10.2

occurring signs observed were; dilated pupils (0.5%), profuse secretions (1.6%), and constricted pupils (2.1%).

Early outcomes of newborns with HIE

Majority 73.7% ($N = 138$), of the 187 neonates with HIE were discharged within the 7 days of observation and 17.1% ($N = 32$) showed no clinical response. A total of 17 newborns died during the time of study which accounted for a general mortality of 9.1% among the neonates with HIE. Majority of the newborns who died were those with severe HIE 84.2%, than those with moderate HIE 1.4%, with no deaths among neonates with mild HIE, Table 4. Newborns with low birth weight had significantly higher mortality (15.9%) compared to those born with a normal weight (5.7%) [OR 3.15, (95% CI: 1.1 -8.7)].

Marked improvement and discharge was observed in newborns that had mild and moderate HIE (98.8 and 60.2%) respectively.

Neonates with moderate HIE and premature newborns were still hospitalized by the 7th day with no response or change in HIE status compared to others, Table 4.

Discussion

In this study 11.5% of the neonates had birth asphyxia and 10.7% were found to have HIE. The prevalence of HIE observed is lower compared with the findings of a study done in Tanzania at Muhimbili National Hospital in 2007 where the prevalence was found to be 30.9% [8]. It's however higher than among the studies done in high income countries. In Spain the prevalence of HIE was found to be 2.42 per 1000 infants between 2000 and 2008 [9]. Birth asphyxia is among the leading causes of death in the neonatal period and in Tanzania it contributes to 23% of the neonatal deaths. Apart from mortality, neonates who develops HIE have a risk of serious long term neuro-motor sequelae like cerebral palsy and epilepsy among the survivors. Hence improvement in monitoring of mothers in labor and of the newborns with HIE should be strengthened in our setting.

Most newborns who had HIE in this study had the mild form (50.8%). This is similar to findings done in South India where the proportion of newborns with mild HIE was 56% [10] and from another study conducted in Rotunda hospital in Ireland where of the 237 newborn assessed, 65.4% had the mild form of HIE [11]. Of note to practitioners' majority (98%) of newborns with mild HIE in this study improved and were discharged similar to observations at Muhimbili National Hospital in Tanzania, in Pakistan and India respectively where a total of 92.3% of the newborns were discharged to their mothers [5, 10, 12]. This indicates that with the appropriate care newborns with HIE can improve sufficiently to be discharged early.

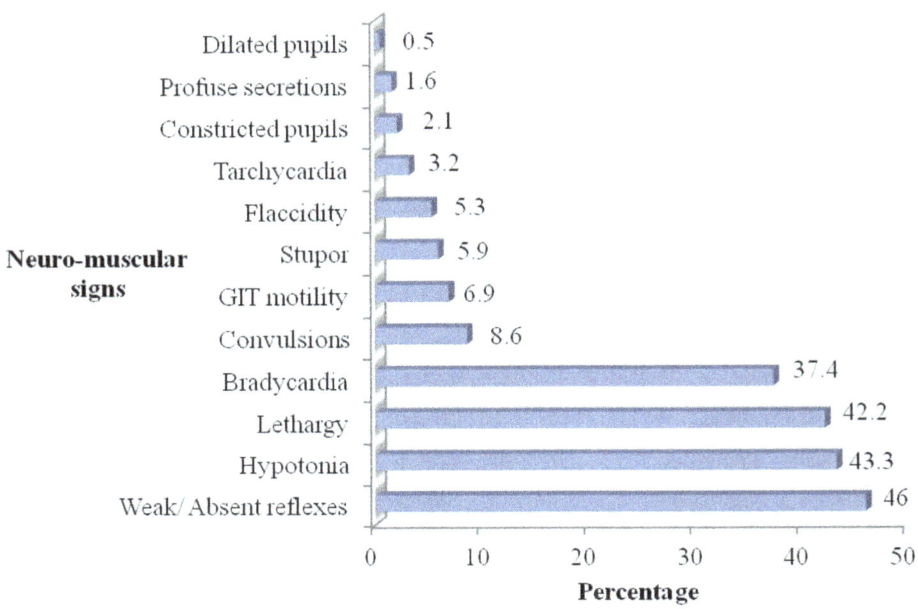

Fig. 1 Neurological signs seen among the newborns who had HIE

Table 4 Immediate outcomes by HIE classification, level of maturity and birth weight among newborns with birth asphyxia at KCMC hospital

	N	Discharge(*n* = 138)	Death (*n* = 17)	No Response in 7 days (*n* = 32)
Mild HIE	95	94 (98.9%)	0 (0.0%)	1 (1.1%)
Moderate HIE	73	44 (60.2%)	1 (1.4%)	28 (38.4%)
Severe HIE	19	0 (0.0%)	16 (84.2%)	3 (15.8%)
Premature (<37 weeks)	61	26 (42.6%)	7 (11.5%)	28 (45.9%)
Full term (37+)	126	112 (88.8%)	10 (7.9%)	4 (3.2%)
Low birth weight (<2500 g)	63	27 (42.9%)	10 (15.9%)	26 (41.3%)
Normal (2500-4500 g)	124	110 (89.4%)	7 (5.7%)	6 (4.9%)

During the study period, the most commonly occurring neurological signs were; weak/absent reflexes, hypotonia and lethargy. This compares closely with the findings from Liaquat University Hospital in Pakistan where among the most observed signs were depressed neonatal reflexes, lethargy and papillary abnormalities [12]. However, in Besat hospital in Iran, seizures (9.1%) were a common presenting sign, unlike in this study where only 8.6% of the participants had seizures being among the least occurring sign [13]. Presence of these signs should alert the health care providers at all levels to monitor newborns closely or timely referral from lower level health facilities.

Overall mortality observed among newborns with HIE was 9.1%. This finding is within observations of previous studies at Mulago Hospital in Uganda 12.9% [14], in Cameroon 10% [6], at tertiary hospital in Johannesburg South Africa 14.3% [3], at Liaquat teaching hospital in Pakistan 15% [12] and at Ayub Teaching hospital in Pakistan 16% [1]. Mortality was high among LBW newborns and those with severe HIE. This means strategies to reduce low birth weight should be reinforced. Further improving quality of monitoring labor cannot be overemphasized to prevent intrapartum related asphyxia.

Nearly 4 in 10 newborns with mild HIE had not responded by 7th day in the ward, so as 41% of LBW and 46% of preterm newborns. At seventh day of follow up, overall 17.1% (32) of the newborns had shown no response compared to initial assessment. The risk of long term sequelae is high in these 3 groups and this shows the need for long term follow up of children with HIE.

Limitations

Inclusion of preterm babies could have influenced some of the findings especially the neurological signs and mortality. Clinical assessment alone was used to categorize the severity of HIE which does not give a complete picture of the effect of hypoxia on the brain. Future studies should complement clinical assessment with EEG or CT scan for complete monitoring and evaluation of newborns with HIE.

Conclusions

The overall prevalence of hypoxic ischemic encephalopathy at KCMC tertiary hospital was found to be 10.7%. Most newborns presented with the mild form of HIE (50.8%) and were discharged to their mothers during the study period. Mortality during the first week of life was 9.1%, highest among neonates with the severe form of HIE and with low birth weight. At 7th day approximately 4 out of 10 neonates with moderate HIE, who were preterm or LBW did not show any improvement in response to treatment offered.

We recommend widespread usage and monitoring of newborns with asphyxia using the Sarnat and Sarnat classification chart in low income settings where sophisticated monitoring is not possible. Essential practices to improve monitoring of labor (before and during) are needed. As well as much emphasis on appropriate care of newborns with HIE.

Limitations

Usage of the Sarnat and Sarnat score as compared to other scored that have been clinically validated may have lead to either overestimation or under-estimation of the prevalence.

Abbreviations

EEG: Electroencephalogram; HIE: Hypoxic Ischaemic Encephalopathy; KCMC: Kilimanjaro Christian Medical College; KCMUCo: Kilimanjaro Christian Medical University College; LBW: Low birth weight

Acknowledgements

The authors express their heartfelt gratitude to the women who agreed to let their newborns participate in the study. Special thanks to all the staff at labor ward and neonatal ward at KCMC hospital for their help.

Funding

No funding was obtained for this study.

Authors' contributions

INS, RNP and SEM designed the study; INS, KK, RNP and DNM, inputs in the study design and conduct; INS, KK data collection; INS, SEM input in the analysis; INS, DNM, KK, RNP, SEM, read the final manuscript for scientific content of the paper. All authors read and approved the final manuscript.

Competing interests
The authors declare that they have no competing interests. All authors of the manuscript have read and agreed to its contents.

Author details
[1]Kilimanjaro Christian Medical University College (KCMUCo), Moshi, Tanzania. [2]Department of Paediatrics, Kilimanjaro Christian Medical Centre (KCMC), Moshi, Tanzania. [3]Department of Obstetrics and Gynaecology, Kilimanjaro Christian Medical Centre, Moshi, Tanzania. [4]Department of Community Health, KCMUCo, Institute of Public Health, Moshi, Tanzania. [5]Community Health Department, Kilimanjaro Christian Medical Centre, Moshi, Tanzania. [6]Department of Epidemiology & Biostatistics, KCMUCo, Institute of Public Health, Moshi, Tanzania. [7]KCMC Hospital, Moshi, Tanzania.

References
1. Qureshi AM, Rehman A, Siddiqi TS. Hypoxic ischemic encephalopathy in neonates. Ayub Med Coll. 2010;22(4):541–5.
2. WHO & UNICEF (2015). Countdown to 2015: a decade of.
3. Padayachee N, Ballot DE. Outcomes of neonates with perinatal asphyxia at a tertiary academic hospital in Johannesburg, South Africa. S Afr J Child Health. 2013;7(3):89-94.
4. WHO. Health in 2015: from millennium development goals (MDGs) to sustainable development goals (SDGs). In: WHO press. Geneva; 2015. *Switzerland* Newborn a.
5. Mwakyusa SD, Manji KP, Massawe A. The hypoxic ischemic encephalopathy score in predicting Neurodevelopmental outcomes among infants with birth asphyxia at the Muhimbili National Hospital, Dar-es Salaam. Am J. 2008;43(7):432–47.
6. Mah E, Mungyeh N, Chiabi A, Tchokoteu P, Ngeufack S, Bogne JB, Mbonda E. Neonatal mortality in a referral hospital in Cameroon over a seven year period; trends, associated factors and causes. Afr Health Sci. 2014;14(3):517–25.
7. Kish L. Survey sampling. New York: John Wiley and Sons, Inc.; 1965.
8. Juma A. Prevalence and immediate outcomes of hypoxic ischemic encephalopathy among infants admitted at the neonatal Ward of Muhimbili National Hospital in Dar es Salaam Tanzania. In: Official publication of the Tanzania Medical students' association; 2007.
9. Gracia-Alex VT, Madero R. Neonatal hypoxic encephalopathy; incidence and prevalence in the first decade of the 21st century. Anales de Pediatra. 2009; 7(14):319–26.
10. Lally PJ, Price DL, Pauliah SS, Bainbridge A, Kurien J. Neonatal Encephalopathic cerebral injury in South India assessed by Perinatal magnetic resonance biomarker and early childhood Neurodevelopmental outcome. PLoS One. 2014;9(2):e87874.
11. Hayes BC, Palsdottir N, Futrakul U. Hypoxic ischemic encephalopathy in newborn infants at >36 weeks' gestation. BMC Pediatr. 2013;14:207.
12. Shazia M, Seema B. To compare the outcome (early) of neonates with birth asphyxia in relation to place of delivery and age at time of admission. J Pak Med Assoc. 2012;62(12):1277–81.
13. Sabzehei KM, Behnaz B, Hassan B. The etiology, clinical type, and short outcome of seizure in newborns hospitalized in Besat hospital/Hamadan/ Iran. Iran J Pediatr. 2013;23(6):675–80.
14. Ondoa-Onama C, Tumwine JK. Immediate outcomes of babies with low Apgar score in Mulago hospital, Uganda. East Afr Med J. 2003;80:22–9.

6

Neonatal respiratory morbidity following exposure to chorioamnionitis

Amy Metcalfe[1*], Sarka Lisonkova[2], Yasser Sabr[2,3], Amelie Stritzke[4] and KS Joseph[2,5]

Abstract

Background: There are conflicting results in the literature on the impact of chorioamnionitis on neonatal respiratory morbidities. However, most studies are based on small clinical samples and fail to account for the competing risk of perinatal death. This study aimed to determine whether chorioamnionitis affects the incidence of respiratory distress syndrome (RDS) and bronchopulmonary dysplasia (BPD) after accounting for the increased risk of death.

Methods: Retrospective cohort study using linked birth and infant death registration and hospitalization records from Washington State between 2002 and 2011 (n = 763,671 singleton infants and n = 56,537 singleton preterm infants). Logistic regression models based on the traditional and fetuses-at-risk approaches were used to model two composite outcomes namely RDS and perinatal death and BPD and perinatal death. Confounders adjusted for in the models included maternal age, race, diabetes, hypertension, antenatal corticosteroids, mode of delivery and infant sex.

Results: While models using the traditional approach found a significant association only between chorioamnionitis and composite BPD and perinatal death (OR = 1.23, 95% CI: 1.01–1.50); using the fetuses-at-risk approach, there was a significant association between chorioamnionitis and both composite outcomes (RDS and perinatal death OR = 2.74, 2.50–3.01; BPD and perinatal death OR = 5.18, 95% CI: 4.39–6.11).

Conclusion: The fetuses-at-risk approach models the causal impact of chorioamnionitis on the development of the fetal lung and shows an increased risk of RDS, BPD and perinatal death associated with such maternal infection.

Keywords: Chorioamnionitis, Bronchopulmonary dysplasia, Respiratory distress syndrome, Fetuses at risk

Background

The impact of chorioamnionitis on fetal lung development and subsequent neonatal respiratory outcomes is controversial. A 2009 narrative review of the impact of histological chorioamnionitis on respiratory outcomes in premature infants found heterogeneous results [1]. Four (of 10) studies showed a decreased incidence of respiratory distress syndrome (RDS) following fetal exposure to histological chorioamnionitis, while 6 (of 10) studies found no difference [1]. Six (of 18) studies found an increased risk of bronchopulmonary dysplasia (BPD) following fetal exposure to histological chorioamnionitis, 1 (of 18) study found a decreased risk, and 11 (of 18) studies found no effect [1]. However, a 2012 systematic review and meta-analysis of 59 studies concluded that chorioamnionitis was a significant risk factor for BPD [2]. Despite differing conclusions about the role of chorioamnionitis on neonatal respiratory outcomes, the authors of both studies commented on substantial between-study heterogeneity related to the definitions of chorioamnionitis (clinical vs. histological) and BPD [1, 2]. There were also important differences in management of RDS, inclusion criteria and failure to adjust for confounding variables such as gestational age and exposure to antenatal steroids, as well as evidence of publication bias [1–3].

Some authors have proposed an 'early protection, late-damage' mechanism of action whereby antenatal inflammation promotes lung maturation in the premature infant, thus reducing the risk of RDS, and simultaneously causing an acute injury and leaving the lung vulnerable to additional post-natal injuries (such as those caused by mechanical ventilation and infection), and thereby

* Correspondence: amy.metcalfe@albertahealthservices.ca
[1]Department of Obstetrics and Gynecology, University of Calgary, Foothills Medical Centre, 4th Floor North Tower, 1403 29th St NW, Calgary, AB T2N 2T9, Canada

increasing the risk of BPD [4–7]. The apparently protective effect of chorioamnionitis on RDS was first documented by Watterberg and colleagues based on a study of 53 mechanically ventilated infants admitted to NICU in the late 1980s [8]. However, the relevance of this study given changing practices in neonatology has been questioned [1]. None of the infants in the Watterberg study received antenatal corticosteroids or surfactant – two practices that are commonplace today. Furthermore, changes to gentler means of ventilation (such as continuous positive airway pressure (CPAP)) may also help reduce further insults to the developing lung [1]. Additionally, the synthesis of epidemiological findings in both the 2009 and 2012 reviews did not unanimously support this hypothesis, and postmortem examinations of stillbirths affected by chorioamnionitis and infants who died from RDS are similar, suggesting that chorioamnionitis does not protect the fetal lung [9]. Understanding of the role of chorioamnionitis in neonatal respiratory morbidities is also complicated because stillborn fetuses and live born infants who die during the neonatal period are typically excluded from studies examining the impact of chorioamnionitis on respiratory outcomes. This is problematic as chorioamnionitis has been shown to increase the risk of neonatal death [10]. While clinical chorioamnionitis affects between 16 and 66% of premature babies born at <34 weeks of gestation, its causative role in stillbirth is estimated to play a role in only about a quarter of cases in developed countries [11, 12]; thus the systematic exclusion of these infants induces selection bias. To our knowledge, only one study has examined the impact of chorioamnionitis on the composite outcome of BPD or death and found a significant association (OR = 2.73, 95% CI: 1.00–7.42) [4], and no studies have used the composite outcome of RDS or death. This study aimed to determine whether chorioamnionitis affects the incidence of neonatal respiratory outcomes such as respiratory distress syndrome and bronchopulmonary dysplasia (after accounting for effects on perinatal death).

Methods

This study used individual-level de-identified routinely collected data on births (Birth Events Records Database (BERD)), hospitalizations (Comprehensive Hospital Abstract Records Database (CHARS)) and infant deaths in Washington State, USA. Singleton births (livebirths and stillbirths) without congenital anomalies (International Classification of Disease, 9th version clinical modification (ICD-9-CM) codes 740–759) that occurred between January 1, 2002 and December 31, 2011 were identified in BERD and CHARS data. The study focus was restricted to singleton preterm births with a recorded gestational age between 22 and 36 weeks since RDS and BPD are diseases of prematurity (n = 56,537 singleton preterm infants). This restricted population of interest was analyzed within the context of the full cohort of births that occurred between 22 and 42 weeks of gestation (n = 763,671 singleton infants) in order to estimate outcome rates under the fetuses-at-risk formulation (see below). An exemption for ethical review was granted by the Washington State Institutional Review Board as this study was considered research involving routine, publicly available, anonymized data.

Women with chorioamnionitis were identified by reviewing their hospitalization records for the ICD-9-CM code 658.4 (infection of amniotic cavity), their infant's hospitalization records for the ICD-9-CM code 762.7 (fetus or newborn affected by complications of placenta, cord and membranes: chorioamnionitis), or documentation of chorioamnionitis on the birth certificate. This case definition refers to clinical chorioamnionitis in the assessment of the clinician treating the mother and/or infant, as rates and results of pathological placental investigations could not be determined from these data sources [13]. The definition of clinical chorioamnionitis is subject of ongoing debate and is variably diagnosed by presence of the following criteria: maternal intrapartum fever, maternal and/or fetal tachycardia, purulent amniotic or vaginal fluids, uterine tenderness and maternal leukocytosis [14]. BPD was identified using ICD-9-CM code 770.7 (chronic respiratory disease arising in the perinatal period) in the infant's hospitalization records, while RDS was identified using ICD-9-CM code 769 (respiratory distress syndrome). While the database does not give further diagnostic detail, the definition of BPD followed the Eunice Kennedy Shriver National Institute of Child Health and Human Development consensus definition [15]. The clinical definition of RDS was presumably based on the requirement for surfactant.

Two methodological issues were addressed in this analysis in order to provide insight into the conflicting findings in the literature. First, potential confounding of the chorioamnionitis-respiratory outcome relation by gestational age was addressed using two alternative formulations, namely, the traditional perinatal formulation (with the denominator for gestational age-specific rates being total births) and the fetuses-at-risk formulation (denominator for gestational age-specific rates being fetuses in-utero). For instance, the gestational-age-specific outcome rates at 22 weeks were calculated using total births at 22 weeks at the denominator, whereas all live births and stillbirths at 22 weeks and beyond were used as the denominator for the calculation of gestational-age-specific outcome rates under the fetuses-at-risk formulation. Secondly, associations between chorioamnionitis and RDS, and chorioamnionitis and BPD were re-evaluated with the outcomes revised to encompass the composite outcomes of RDS and perinatal death (stillbirth or neonatal death), and BPD and perinatal death.

Using both the traditional and fetuses-at-risk formulations, descriptive statistics were used to characterize the population and logistic regression was used to evaluate the association between chorioamnionitis and the composite outcomes of RDS/perinatal death and BPD/perinatal death following adjustment for potential confounders. Potential confounders included race, maternal age, diabetes, hypertension, fetal sex, antenatal steroids and mode of delivery. Under the traditional approach, logistic regression analysis included gestational age as a covariate, while under the fetuses-at-risk approach, gestational age at birth was considered a factor on the causal pathway between chorioamnionitis and the outcomes, and therefore not included in the regression model. All analyses were conducted using Stata SE version 14 (College Station, Texas).

Results

Overall, 2631 out of 56,537 (4.65%, 95% CI: 4.48–4.83) pregnancies resulting in a preterm birth were complicated by chorioamnionitis. Under the fetuses-at-risk approach, the incidence rate of chorioamnionitis was stable until 30 weeks of gestation, at which point it increased in a linear fashion; whereas, under the traditional approach, the incidence rate of chorioamnionitis peaked at 23–24 weeks and declined steadily until 36 weeks of gestation (Fig. 1). Significant differences were also observed in the socio-demographic and clinical characteristics of pregnancies affected by chorioamnionitis (Table 1). Women with chorioamnionitis were significantly more likely to also have preterm premature rupture of membranes ($p < 0.001$), receive antenatal corticosteroids ($p < 0.001$), and have their infant admitted to a neonatal intensive care unit ($p < 0.001$), while their infants had lower gestational ages ($p < 0.001$) and were more likely ventilated ($p < 0.001$) (Table 1).

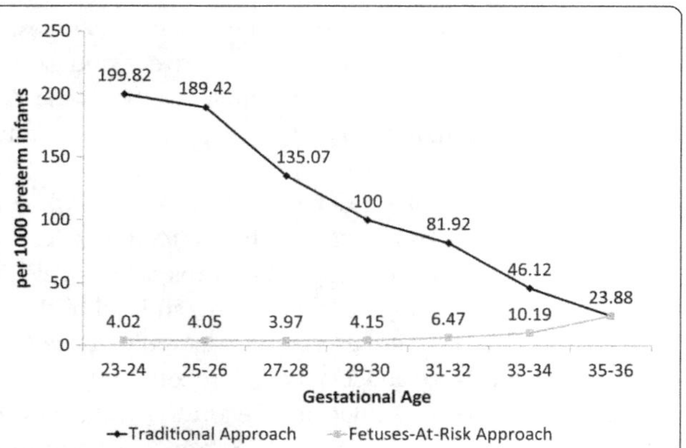

Fig. 1 Incidence rate of chorioamnionitis by gestational age. Washington State Preterm Births 2002–2011 n = 56,537

Under both the traditional and fetuses-at-risk approaches the pattern in the incidence of BPD was very similar for fetuses affected by chorioamnionitis, namely highest in the lowest gestational age ranges (Fig. 2a and b). However, under the traditional model, the incidence of composite BPD and perinatal mortality peaked at early preterm gestations (Fig. 2c), while under the fetuses-at-risk approach, this pattern was only observed for pregnancies affected by chorioamnionitis (Fig. 2d). This differed from the pattern seen for RDS (Fig. 3), whereby the traditional models for both RDS (Fig. 3a) and composite RDS and perinatal death (Fig. 3c) demonstrated a peak in the early preterm period irrespective of the presence of chorioamnionitis and then a steady decline until term gestation. On the other hand, the fetuses-at-risk models (Figs. 3b and d) show a similar pattern with a steady increase throughout the preterm gestation for RDS alone and composite RDS and perinatal death for pregnancies not affected by chorioamnionitis and an early peak with slight decrease for pregnancies complicated by chorioamnionitis.

Using the traditional approach, the crude model showed a statistically significant association between chorioamnionitis and BPD (OR = 5.61, 95% CI: 4.79–6.58) and the composite outcome of BPD and perinatal death (OR = 2.73, 95% CI: 2.42–3.09) (Table 2). Following adjustment for confounders, this relationship was attenuated, but remained statistically significant (BPD aOR = 1.34, 95% CI: 1.09–1.66; BPD or perinatal death aOR = 1.23, 95% CI: 1.01–1.50). Results from the fetuses-at-risk model were similar, albeit much stronger – a significant association was observed between chorioamnionitis and BPD (aOR = 6.25, 95% CI: 5.25–7.44), and between chorioamnionitis and the composite outcome of BPD and perinatal death (aOR = 5.18, 95% CI: 4.39–6.11) following adjustment for relevant confounders (Table 2).

The adjusted traditional and fetuses-at-risk models yielded divergent results for RDS (Table 2). Under the traditional approach, adjustment for confounders resulted in non-significant associations between chorioamnionitis and RDS (aOR = 0.99, 95% CI: 0.87–1.13) and between chorioamnionitis and composite RDS and perinatal death (aOR = 0.98, 95% CI: 0.86–1.12). However, under the fetuses-at-risk model the associations between chorioamnionitis and the two respiratory outcomes were significant (RDS OR = 2.78, 95% CI: 2.54–3.06, composite RDS and perinatal death OR = 2.74, 95% CI: 2.50–3.01) (Table 2).

Discussion

This is the first study examining the association of chorioamnionitis with common neonatal respiratory outcomes using a large administrative population-based database and taking perinatal mortality into account. Using the fetuses-at-risk approach takes all fetuses in

Table 1 Population characteristics – Washington State preterm births 2002–2011 n = 56,537

Variable	Mother did not have chorioamnionitis % (95% CI)	Mother had chorioamnionitis % (95% CI)	*p*-value
Maternal Race			<0.001
Non-hispanic white	56.8 (53.4–57.2)	54.4 (52.5–56.3)	
Non-hispanic black	4.3 (4.2–4.5)	6.5 (5.6–7.5)	
Hispanic	17.5 (17.2–17.8)	15.8 (14.5–17.3)	
Other/unknown	21.4 (21.0–21.7)	23.2 (21.6–24.8)	
Infant Sex			
Male	54.2 (53.7–54.6)	52.7 (50.7–54.7)	
Female	45.8 (45.4–46.2)	47.3 (45.3–49.3)	0.16
Preterm premature rupture of membranes	19.7 (19.4–20.0)	45.8 (43.9–47.7)	<0.001
Small for gestational age (<10th percentile)	13.4 (13.1–13.7)	7.1 (6.2–8.2)	<0.001
Antenatal steroids	1.0 (0.9–1.0)	19.2 (17.6–20.9)	<0.001
Admission to neonatal intensive care unit	36.9 (36.4–37.3)	59.8 (57.7–61.8)	<0.001
Mechanical ventilation of the neonate	7.6 (7.3–7.8)	14.6 (13.3–16.0)	<0.001
Respiratory distress syndrome	11.3 (11.1–11.6)	25.1 (23.5–26.8)	<0.001
Bronchopulmonary dysplasia	1.5 (1.4–1.6)	7.7 (6.8–8.8)	<0.001
Stillbirth	3.2 (3.1–3.4)	4.7 (4.0–5.6)	<0.001
Infant Death	0.4 (0.3–0.4)	0.3 (0.2–0.7)	0.80
	Mean (Standard Deviation)	Mean (Standard Deviation)	
Maternal age (years)	28.0 (6.3)	27.4 (6.4)	<0.001
Gestational age at delivery (weeks)	34.1 (2.9)	31.1 (4.5)	<0.001
Birth weight (grams)	2587.2 (1185.3)	2086.9 (1447.9)	<0.001

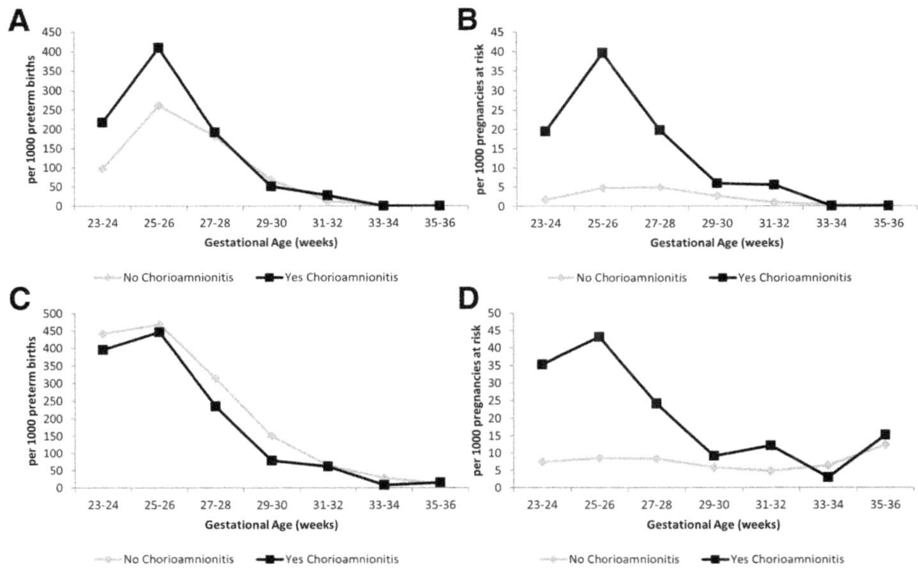

Fig. 2 Incidence of bronchopulmonary dysplasia (Panels **a** & **b**) and composite bronchopulmonary dysplasia and perinatal mortality (Panels **c** & **d**) using the traditional (Panels **a** & **c**) and fetuses-at-risk (Panels **b** & **d**) approach. Washington State Preterm Births 2002–2011 n = 56,537

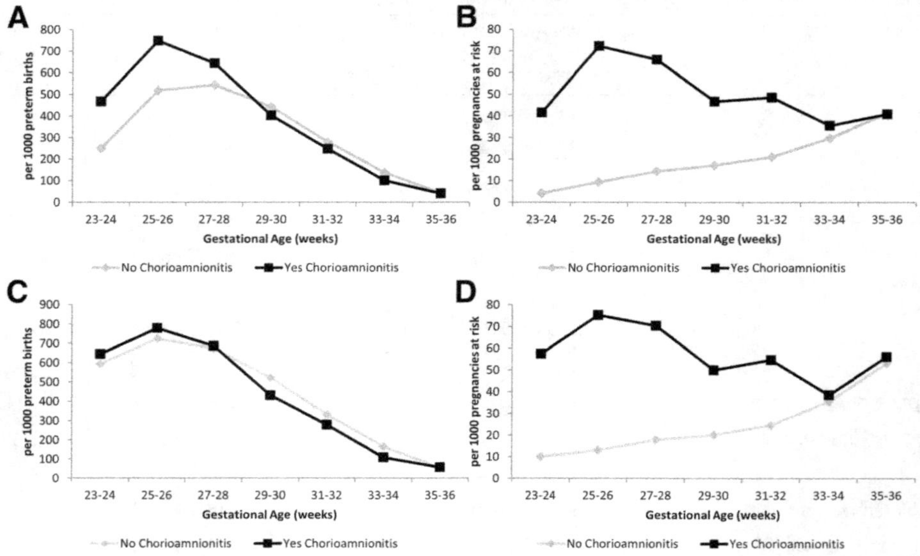

Fig. 3 Incidence of respiratory distress syndrome (Panels **a** & **b**) and composite respiratory distress syndrome and perinatal mortality (Panels **c** & **d**) using the traditional (Panels **a** & **c**) and fetuses-at-risk (Panels **b** & **d**)approach. Washington State Preterm Births 2002–2011 n = 56,537

utero at a particular gestational age into account, thereby explaining our finding of a slow rise in chorioamnionitis after 30 weeks of gestation, as only a few fetuses are affected at each gestational age. Taking only delivered neonates into account in the denominator, the traditional approach shows a much higher incidence and earlier peak since almost all extremely premature infants are universally affected to some degree by chorioamnionitis [11].

Similarly, in the traditional approach, for both RDS and BPD, both their isolated and composite outcomes combined with perinatal death, are highest in the early gestational ages, irrespective of the presence of chorioamnionitis. However, in the fetuses-at-risk approach the peak in the early gestational ages is largely maintained in the subgroup with chorioamnionitis, suggesting it may itself be associated with preterm delivery. Infants without chorioamnionitis in this model seem to be affected by RDS at later gestational ages which may be accounted for by a higher proportion of infant now born without concerns about chorioamnionitis.

The traditional perinatal model showed that chorioamnionitis appears to be associated with BPD, but not RDS after adjustment for relevant confounders and after accounting for the competing risk of perinatal death. On the other hand, the fetuses-at-risk approach shows a significantly increased risk of BPD and RDS following exposure to chorioamnionitis. Different results using the traditional and fetuses-at-risk approach are not unexpected. The traditional approach models the *prognostic* impact of chorioamnionitis on the development of the fetal lung, while the fetuses-at-risk approach models the *causal* effect of chorioamnionitis on respiratory outcomes. Part of the causality may be the inclination to proceed to delivery earlier with the presence of clinical symptoms of

Table 2 Logistic regression models examining the association between maternal chorioamnionitis and neonatal respiratory outcomes and perinatal death in preterm infants

	Traditional approach		Fetuses-at-risk approach[b]	
	OR (95% CI)	OR (95% CI)	OR (95% CI)	OR (95% CI)
	BPD	BPD or Perinatal mortality	BPD	BPD or Perinatal mortality
Crude Model	5.61 (4.79–6.58)	2.73 (2.42–3.09)	8.79 (7.53–10.26)	4.22 (3.76–4.73)
Adjusted Model[a]	1.34 (1.09–1.66)	1.23 (1.01–1.50)	6.25 (5.25–7.44)	5.18 (4.39–6.11)
	RDS	RDS or Perinatal Mortality	RDS	RDS or Perinatal Mortality
Crude Model	2.62 (2.39–2.87)	2.45 (2.25–2.68)	3.75 (3.46–4.07)	3.43 (3.19–3.70)
Adjusted Model[a]	0.99 (0.87–1.13)	0.98 (0.86–1.12)	2.78 (2.54–3.06)>	2.74 (2.50–3.01)

[a]Other potential confounders include: diabetes, hypertension, infant sex, maternal age, maternal race, mode of delivery, antenatal steroids. Traditional models are also adjusted for gestational age at delivery

[b]The fetuses-at-risk model included all fetuses-at-risk of respiratory outcomes and perinatal death (n = 763,671)

BPD bronchopulmonary dysplasia, *RDS* respiratory distress syndrome

chorioamnionitis. Delivery at lower gestational ages remains the strongest risk factor for development of BPD. The results from this study contradict the early protection, late damage hypothesis, and instead show an increased risk of RDS following chorioamnionitis.

Our results for BPD are congruent with the meta-analysis involving 59 studies and 15,295 infants which showed a significant association between chorioamnionitis and BPD (OR = 1.58, 95% CI: 1.11–2.24) [2]. To our knowledge, only one other study has examined the impact of chorioamnionitis on the composite outcome of BPD or death. This study of 301 infants, which did not adjust for confounders, found a significant crude association between chorioamnionitis and BPD (OR = 3.40, 95% CI: 1.02–11.3) and composite BPD or neonatal death (OR = 2.72, 95% CI: 1.00–7.42) [4]. Comparison of our findings related to RDS with other studies is more difficult as, to our knowledge, no studies have examined the composite outcome of RDS or death. Although one narrative review concluded that chorioamnionitis decreased the incidence of RDS [1], the review did not provide summary statistics. More studies included in the review found a null crude relationship between chorioamnionitis and RDS (6 studies involving 2310 infants) than those that found a significant risk reduction (4 studies involving 1310 infants) [1]. Although adjustment for a variety of confounders showed a negative relationship in some studies, most studies included in the review did not adjust for confounders [1].

Our study has both strengths and limitations. The large population-based sample allowed us to control for multiple potential confounders. Additionally, the use of a recent time period optimizes the applicability of our findings to contemporary neonatal populations. Definitions are based on the most recent consensus document [15], which is particularly relevant for BPD as multiple definitions exist clinically and in the scientific literature [2]. The primary limitations of this study are related to the use of administrative data. Administrative data has not been frequently used to study chorioamnionitis or neonatal respiratory outcomes. A validation study of BPD concluded that ICD-9 codes had sufficient specificity to recommend their routine use to identify this condition [16]. Cases of BPD that were missed tended to be milder in nature [16], which would bias our results towards the null. Similarly, another validation study reported a positive predictive value for 97.0% for the identification of neonatal RDS in administrative data [17], indicating the acceptability of administrative data to identify this condition. To our knowledge, no studies have validated ICD codes for chorioamnionitis. Only one study could be located that used ICD-based codes to identify chorioamnionitis (ICD-9-CM 762.7×, 658.4×) [18]. This population-based study found that chorioamnionitis affected 1.5% of first pregnancies resulting in a live birth and 3.7% of first pregnancies resulting in a stillbirth [18], which is comparable to the overall incidence of 4.65% observed in our study, given that our sample was restricted to preterm births. Our data source did not include information on clinical definitions or the severity of condition and we were unable to differentiate histological and clinical chorioamnionitis. It is estimated that only 8–52% of women with histological chorioamnionitis will display symptoms of clinical chorioamnionitis [10, 19, 20]. However, these results should be interpreted with caution as they come from a selected subsample of placentas that were sent for histological examination and may not reflect the true correlation between clinical and histological chorioamnionitis. Understanding the role of clinical chorioamnionitis which is diagnosed prospectively in the antenatal period (as compared to histological chorioamnionitis which is diagnosed retrospectively after delivery) on infant outcomes is important as it provides clinicians with an opportunity to possibly intervene during pregnancy (using antenatal corticosteroids to promote lung development, or maternal antibiotics). To our knowledge, this is the largest study of the effect of chorioamnionitis on neonatal respiratory outcomes to date. It is also one of very few that accounts for the competing risk of death associated with early chorioamnionitis.

Conclusions

The fetuses-at-risk analysis used in this study indicates that antenatal inflammation associated with chorioamnionitis leaves the lung vulnerable to RDS and additional post-natal injuries, thus increasing the risk of BPD. Our findings dispute the hypothesis that antenatal inflammation may protect the fetal lung, thus reducing the incidence of RDS. Our study provides evidence confirming that chorioamnionitis increases the risk of RDS, BPD and perinatal death, and pregnancies with chorioamnionitis should be monitored closely and delivered in a facility with appropriate respiratory support and therapy available for infants.

Abbreviations

BERD: Birth events records database; BPD: Bronchopulmonary dysplasia; CHARS: Comprehensive Hospital Abstract Records Database; CI: Confidence interval; CPAP: Continuous positive airway pressure; ICD-9-CM: International classification of disease version 9 – clinical modification; OR: Odds ratio; RDS: Respiratory distress syndrome

Authors' contributions

AM: acquired the data, conducted the analysis, interpreted the data, drafted the manuscript, approved the final version of the manuscript, agrees to be accountable for all aspects of this work. SL: interpreted the data, critically revised the manuscript, approved the final version of the manuscript, agrees to be accountable for all aspects of this work. YS: interpreted the data, critically revised the manuscript, approved the final version of the manuscript, agrees to be accountable for all aspects of this work. AS: interpreted the data, critically revised the manuscript, approved the final version of the manuscript, agrees to be accountable for all aspects of this work. KSJ: conceived the study, interpreted the data, critically revised the manuscript, approved the final version of the manuscript, agrees to be accountable for all aspects of this work.

Competing interests

The authors declare that they have no competing interests.

Ethics and consent to participate

An exemption for ethical review and a waiver of consent for participant consent was granted by the Washington State Institutional Review Board as this study was considered research that does not involve human subjects in accordance with 45 CFR 46 section 102(f)(2). This exemption was granted as this research did not involve any direct contact with individuals or the receipt of identifiable private information from confidential records. This exemption was granted in accordance with The Belmont Report: Ethical Principles and Guidelines for the Protection of Human Subjects of Research (1979) and Washington State Agency administrative procedures.

Author details

[1]Department of Obstetrics and Gynecology, University of Calgary, Foothills Medical Centre, 4th Floor North Tower, 1403 29th St NW, Calgary, AB T2N 2T9, Canada. [2]Department of Obstetrics and Gynecology, University of British Columbia, Vancouver, BC, Canada. [3]Department of Obstetrics and Gynecology, King Saud University and King Khalid University Hospital, Riyadh, Saudi Arabia. [4]Department of Pediatrics, Section of Neonatology, University of Calgary, Calgary, AB, Canada. [5]School of Population and Public Health, University of British Columbia, Vancouver, BC, Canada.

References

1. Been JV, Zimmermann LJ. Histological chorioamnionitis and respiratory outcome in preterm infants. Arch Dis Child Fetal Neonatal Ed. 2009; 94(3):F218–25.
2. Hartling L, Liang Y, Lacaze-Masmonteil T. Chorioamnionitis as a risk factor for bronchopulmonary dysplasia: a systematic review and meta-analysis. Arch Dis Child Fetal Neonatal Ed. 2012;97(1):F8–f17.
3. Lacaze-Masmonteil T. That chorioamnionitis is a risk factor for bronchopulmonary dysplasia–the case against. Paediatr Respir Rev. 2014;15(1):53–5.
4. Been JV, Rours IG, Kornelisse RF, Jonkers F, de Krijger RR, Zimmermann LJ. Chorioamnionitis alters the response to surfactant in preterm infants. J Pediatr. 2010;156(1):10–15.e11.
5. Kramer BW, Kallapur S, Newnham J, Jobe AH. Prenatal inflammation and lung development. Seminars in fetal & neonatal medicine. 2009;14(1):2–7.
6. Prendergast M, May C, Broughton S, Pollina E, Milner AD, Rafferty GF, Greenough A. Chorioamnionitis, lung function and bronchopulmonary dysplasia in prematurely born infants. Arch Dis Child Fetal Neonatal Ed. 2011;96(4):F270–4.
7. Lee J, Oh KJ, Park CW, Park JS, Jun JK, Yoon BH. The presence of funisitis is associated with a decreased risk for the development of neonatal respiratory distress syndrome. Placenta. 2011;32(3):235–40.
8. Watterberg KL, Demers LM, Scott SM, Murphy S. Chorioamnionitis and early lung inflammation in infants in whom bronchopulmonary dysplasia develops. Pediatrics. 1996;97(2):210–5.
9. Zanardo V, Vedovato S, Cosmi E, Litta P, Cavallin F, Trevisanuto D, Chiarelli S. Preterm premature rupture of membranes, chorioamnion inflammatory scores and neonatal respiratory outcome. BJOG. 2010;117(1):94–8.
10. Ogunyemi D, Murillo M, Jackson U, Hunter N, Alperson B. The relationship between placental histopathology findings and perinatal outcome in preterm infants. J Matern Fetal Neonatal Med. 2003;13(2):102–9.
11. Lahra MM, Jeffery HE. A fetal response to chorioamnionitis is associated with early survival after preterm birth. Am J Obstet Gynecol. 2004; 190(1):147–51.
12. Goldenberg RL, McClure EM, Saleem S, Reddy UM. Infection-related stillbirths. Lancet. 2010;375(9724):1482–90.
13. Bommarito KM, Gross GA, Willers DM, Fraser VJ, Olsen MA. The Effect of Clinical Chorioamnionitis on Cesarean Delivery in the United States. Health Serv Res. 2016;51(5):1879–95.
14. Higgins RD, Saade G, Polin RA, Grobman WA, Buhimschi IA, Watterberg K, Silver RM, Raju TN, Chorioamnionitis Workshop P. Evaluation and Management of Women and Newborns With a Maternal Diagnosis of Chorioamnionitis: Summary of a Workshop. Obstet Gynecol. 2016;127(3):426–36.
15. Ehrenkranz RA, Walsh MC, Vohr BR, Jobe AH, Wright LL, Fanaroff AA, Wrage LA, Poole K, National Institutes of Child H, Human Development Neonatal Research N. Validation of the National Institutes of Health consensus definition of bronchopulmonary dysplasia. Pediatrics. 2005;116(6):1353–60.
16. Landry JS, Croitoru D, Menzies D. Validation of ICD-9 diagnostic codes for bronchopulmonary dysplasia in Quebec's provincial health care databases. Chronic Dis Inj Can. 2012;33(1):47–52.
17. Ford JB, Roberts CL, Algert CS, Bowen JR, Bajuk B, Henderson-Smart DJ, group N. Using hospital discharge data for determining neonatal morbidity and mortality: a validation study. BMC Health Serv Res. 2007;7:188.
18. Getahun D, Lawrence JM, Fassett MJ, Strickland D, Koebnick C, Chen W, Jacobsen SJ. The association between stillbirth in the first pregnancy and subsequent adverse perinatal outcomes. Am J Obstet Gynecol. 2009;201(u):378 e371–6.
19. Paul DA, Zook K, Mackley A, Locke RG. Reduced mortality and increased BPD with histological chorioamnionitis and leukocytosis in very-low-birth-weight infants. J Perinatol. 2010;30(1):58–62.
20. Sebire NJ, Goldin RD, Regan L. Histological chorioamnionitis in relation to clinical presentation at 14-40 weeks of gestation. J Obstet Gynaecol. 2001;21(3):242–5.

7

Early characteristics of infants with pulmonary hypertension in a referral neonatal intensive care unit

Shilpa Vyas-Read[1,5*], Usama Kanaan[1,2], Prabhu Shankar[1], Jane Stremming[3], Curtis Travers[4], David P. Carlton[1] and Anne Fitzpatrick[1]

Abstract

Background: Approximately 8–23% of premature infants develop pulmonary hypertension (PH), and this diagnosis confers a higher possibility of mortality. As a result, professional societies recommend PH screening in premature infants. However, the risk factors for and the outcomes of PH may differ depending on the timing of its diagnosis, and little evidence is available to determine at-risk infants in the referral neonatal population. The objective of this study was to define clinical and echocardiographic characteristics of infants with pulmonary hypertension during the neonatal hospital course and at or near-term.

Methods: Infants who had the following billing codes: < 32 weeks, birth weight < 1500 g, neonatal unit, and echocardiograph had records abstracted from a data warehouse at Children's Healthcare of Atlanta. The outcome was defined as late PH on the final echocardiogram for all patients, and, separately, for patients with multiple studies. Descriptive statistics, univariable, and multivariable models were evaluated, and odds ratios and 95% confidence intervals are expressed below as (OR, CI).

Results: 556 infants were included in the overall study, 59 had PH on their final echocardiogram (11%). In multivariable analyses, atrial septal defect (2.9, 1.4–6.1), and intrauterine growth restriction (2.7, 1.2–6.3) increased the odds of late PH, whereas caffeine therapy decreased PH (0.4, 0.2–0.8). When the analyses were restricted to 32 infants who had multiple echocardiograms during their hospitalization, the association between atrial septal defect (5.9, 2.0–16.5) and growth restriction (3.7, 1.3–10.7) and late PH was strengthened, but the effect of caffeine therapy was no longer significant. In this smaller subgroup, infants with late PH had their final echocardiogram at a median of 116 days of life, and 42–74% of them had right ventricular pathology.

Conclusions: Early clinical variables are associated with PH persistence in a referral neonatal population. Identification of early clinical factors may help guide the ascertainment of infant risk for late PH, and may aid in targeting sub-groups that are most likely to benefit from PH screening.

Keywords: Very low birth weight, Growth restriction, Caffeine, Pulmonary hypertension, Atrial septal defect

* Correspondence: svyasre@emory.edu
[1]Pediatrics, Emory University School of Medicine, Atlanta, GA, USA
[5]Division of Neonatology, Emory University School of Medicine, 2015 Uppergate Dr. NE, 3rd floor, 30322 Atlanta, GA, USA

Background

For infants who are born early in the third trimester of pregnancy or before, fetal factors coupled with prematurity and postnatal injury may combine to result in pulmonary vascular disease, a process which manifests clinically as pulmonary hypertension (PH) [1–4]. The incidence of PH in very low birth weight infants is estimated to range between 16 and 43% [5–8], and infants with bronchopulmonary dysplasia and PH have been suggested to have up to a 4.6-fold higher odds of mortality than those infants with bronchopulmonary dysplasia without PH [5–7, 9]. Further, infants who were born prematurely continue to have an increased risk for PH that persists into childhood and adolescence [10].

Given the potential for neonatal and post-neonatal mortality, professional societies' such as the American Heart Association and the American Thoracic Society recommend screening premature infants for the development of PH [11]. Unfortunately, few predictors for the development of PH are known. The most widely studied predictor for PH is bronchopulmonary dysplasia (BPD). Among infants with the most severe form of BPD, 29 to 53% also had a diagnosis of PH, and infants with severe BPD have over a 6-fold increased odds of PH when compared to infants with less severe lung disease [1, 12–15]. Intrauterine growth restriction has also been associated with PH, suggesting that fetal vascular programming may play a role in the development of hypertension [5, 16–18]. Few other potential predictors have been identified other than these, postnatal infection, and possibly illicit drugs [14, 19, 20].

In this study, we utilized observational data from very low birth weight, premature infants within our referral population to determine if early clinical factors are associated with pulmonary hypertension. To our knowledge, this cohort is the largest sample of neonates who received echocardiograms to be studied for PH. Because factors that contribute to the development of PH, such as infant growth and mortality, may differ in Identification of early clinical factors that are associated with neonatal PH may aid in identifying an "at risk" population that may require more echocardiographic surveillance during the hospital stay or more formal follow-up after hospital discharge.

Methods

Study design

This study was approved by the Institutional Review Board at Emory University and at Children's Healthcare of Atlanta. The study population was a retrospective, observational cohort of patients at two hospitals in Atlanta (Children's Healthcare of Atlanta, Egleston or Scottish Rite campus) from January 2010 to September 2014. Infants who were less than 32 weeks gestational age at birth, had a birth weight of less than 1500 g, were in the neonatal intensive care unit, and had an echocardiogram were identified using ICD-9 codes and were included. Patients were excluded if medical records were missing or if they had multiple anomalies/aneuploidy, congenital heart disease (other than atrial septal defect, ventricular septal defect, or patent ductus arteriosus), or congenital lung disease.

Definitions of exposures and outcomes

Outcomes

The primary outcome was late pulmonary hypertension (late PH) on the final echocardiograph prior to death or discharge from the neonatal intensive care unit. Pulmonary hypertension (PH) was defined as an echocardiogram that showed: 1) a moderate-to-large patent ductus arteriosus (PDA) with bidirectional or right-to-left shunting; 2) a tricuspid regurgitation jet gradient of ≥32 mmHg with septal flattening, right ventricular hypertrophy, or right ventricular dilation; or 3) a tricuspid regurgitation jet velocity of ≥45 mmHg [16, 19, 21]. Echocardiographs were ordered at the discretion of the attending neonatologist and interpreted by pediatric cardiologists.

Clinical variables

The following variables were abstracted from the infant medical record: 1) maternal drug use, the use of tobacco and/or alcohol; 2) illicit drug use, including the use of illegal drugs such as cannabis, amphetamines, or other substances; 3) infant race and gender; and 4) prenatal and intrapartum complications. The following discrete variables were abstracted from the clinical data warehouse using ICD-9 codes: 1) intraventricular hemorrhage; 2) necrotizing enterocolitis; 3) retinopathy of prematurity; 4) medication use; 5) respiratory support; and 6) positive blood culture. Death was defined as mortality from any cause during the hospital course.

Echocardiographic variables

The echocardiographic characteristics of infants with late PH were determined by the final echocardiogram of the hospital stay. For infants with only one study, the final echocardiogram was the infant's first study in our neonatal hospital system. For infants with more than one study, the final echocardiogram was the infant's last study in our neonatal hospital system. Directionality of the shunt through an ASD, ventricular septal defect, or patent ductus arteriosus (PDA) was determined by the pediatric cardiologist at the time of the echocardiogram as 1) left-to-right or none 2) bidirectional or 3) right-to-left. The tricuspid regurgitation jet velocity (TRJV) was graded as 1) normal, < 32 mmHg 2) mild, 32–44 mmHg 3) moderate 45–60 mmHg and 4) severe ≥60 mmHg at that time. Septal flattening was defined subjectively as none, any, or severe by the pediatric cardiologist performing the echocardiogram. Right ventricular dilatation, hypertrophy, and dysfunction were defined as either present or absent. Atrial septal defects were categorized as 1) none or patent foramen ovale (PFO), 2) patent foramen ovale versus atrial septal defect (PFO vs. ASD), or 3) atrial septal defect (ASD). PDA was defined as 1) none or small or ligated versus 2) moderate-to-large on the first study echocardiogram. Ventricular septal defects were defined as 1) intact, tiny, and small or 2) moderate-to-large or multiple.

Descriptive statistics

Two-sample t-tests for normally distributed variables, and Wilcoxon rank sum tests for skewed distributions were utilized. For categorical variables, chi-square tests of proportion were used to compare outcome groups unless the cell frequency was ≤ 5, in which case the Fisher's exact test was used.

Univariable and multivariable analyses

To determine the effect of echocardiographic and early hospital characteristics on the outcome of late PH, univariable logistic regression was used to arrive at odds ratios, and 95% confidence intervals.

A multivariable model was constructed by the manual addition of each significant variable to the intercept and gestational age variable. The -2Log likelihood values were determined, and the value of each additional variable was determined using a likelihood ratio test with $p \geq 0.05$ as a stopping rule. A final model that included gestational age, atrial septal defect (ASD vs. None or PFO), intrauterine growth restriction (yes or no), caffeine (yes or no), and positive-pressure ventilation at 28 days (yes vs. no) was derived. Although gestational age and positive-pressure ventilation were not statistically significantly different between groups, they were forced into the model as important risk factors for the development of late PH. Additionally, the defined multivariable model was evaluated again in infants who had more than one echocardiogram performed, and who had evidence of late PH on this final study. Odds ratios and 95% confidence intervals were constructed. All statistical procedures were performed using SAS 9.4 statistical software and the level of significance for comparisons was a p-value <0.05.

Results

Patient selection

An initial search of the electronic health record (Clarity) database from January 2010 to January 2015 yielded 586 infants that met the inclusion criteria of having a gestational age of less than 32 weeks at birth, having a birthweight less than 1500 g at birth, being admitted to the neonatal intensive care unit, and having an echocardiographic procedure (Fig. 1). Of these, 25 infants were excluded from the study population due to multiple anomalies or aneuploidy (8 infants), congenital heart disease other than PDA, ASD or VSD (11 infants), congenital lung disease (2 infants), or missing medical information (4 infants). Five patients were excluded due to missing outcome data, and 556 infants were included in the study cohort. Ninety-two infants (16%) in the overall cohort had at least one echocardiogram that met criteria for pulmonary hypertension (PH) during the hospital course. Infants who had echocardiographic evidence of pulmonary hypertension on their last neonatal study were defined as having late pulmonary hypertension (late PH). If an infant had only one study, then the first study determined the infant's classification into outcome groups. If an infant had more than one study, then the final echocardiogram result determined whether he/she was classified as having late PH. The majority of infants with and without late PH had an echocardiogram after 30 days of life, and 29–31% of infants had early echocardiograms before 30 days of life (Fig. 2). The median day of life for infants with over one study was 116 days for infants with late PH, and 101 for infants without late PH, indicating that PH on the final echocardiogram was detected beyond 3 months of life for this group (Fig. 2, panel B). All infants in both groups received at least one echocardiogram. Twenty-five percent of infants with late PH, and 27% of infants without late PH also had a second echocardiogram. A higher proportion of infants in the late PH group had over 2 echocardiograms when compared with infants without late PH (29% vs. 19%). Forty-six percent of infants in the late PH group had evidence of PH on their first and only echocardiogram, and 54% of infants had over one study and the final echocardiogram showed PH.

Echocardiographic characteristics of infants with late PH

Of the 556 infants evaluated, 59 patients had late PH on their final echocardiogram (10.6% of the total cohort, 64% of the infants with an initial diagnosis of PH), and 497 infants did not (Table 1). The median timing of the echocardiogram was 77 days of life for infants in the late PH group, and 41 days of life for infants without late PH. Infants who had an atrial septal defect (ASD) had 4.6-fold higher odds of late PH, when compared with infants without an ASD. The association between patent ductus arteriosus size and late PH was not significant. Forty-three percent of infants with late PH had an ASD with bidirectional or right-to-left shunting, indicating that patients in our PH group had poor right ventricular compliance likely due to the effect of chronically

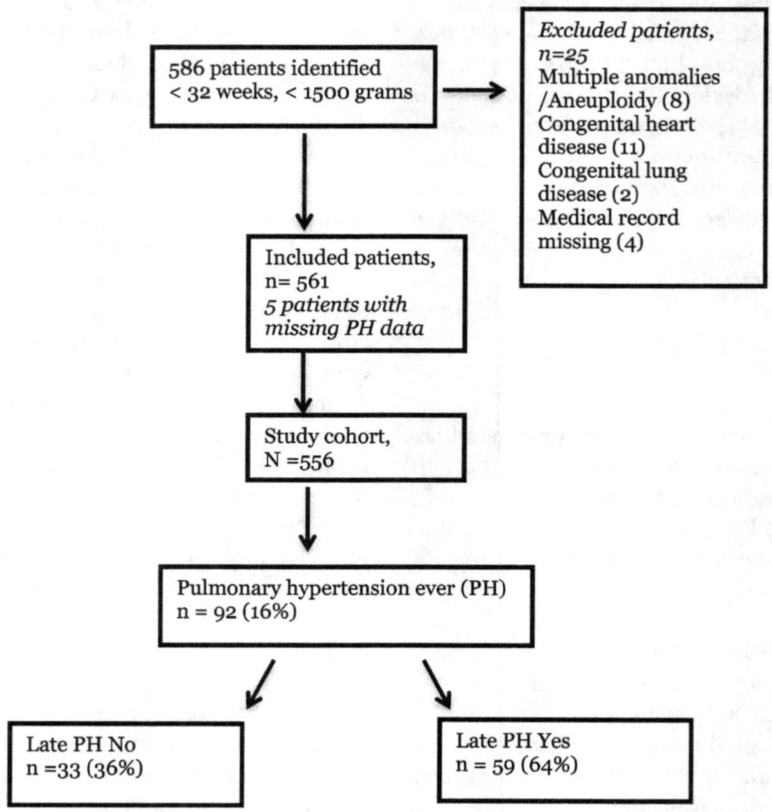

Fig. 1 Flowchart of study patient selection. An electronic health record database query was performed for <32 weeks gestation at birth, < 1500 g birthweight, neonatal intensive care unit, and echocardiographic procedure. 586 infants were identified, and 25 of these met exclusion criteria. 556 patients were included in the study, and 92 (16%) had PH on any one echocardiogram while in the neonatal intensive care unit. Of the 92 infants with PH, 59 (64%) also had PH on their final echocardiogram of the hospital stay. Of these 59 infants, 32 had more than one echocardiogram and the last study during the neonatal stay showed PH

elevated pulmonary pressure. Eighty-one percent of infants with late PH had tricuspid jet velocities of ≥32 mmHg, compared with 2% of patients without late PH. The 11 infants with "normal" tricuspid regurgitation in the late PH group also had a patent ductus arteriosus, making interpretation of the jet gradient difficult. The majority of infants with late PH had some evidence of either right ventricular dilation (55% vs. 8%) or right ventricular hypertrophy (56% vs. 10%), and one-third had right-ventricular dysfunction (33% vs 3%), respectively, when compared with those without late PH. Ventricular septal defects and left ventricular dysfunction did not differ between the late PH groups.

Associations between neonatal characteristics and late PH

In univariable analysis, infants with late PH overall had lower birthweight than infants who did not have PH persistence (0.75 ± 0.24 kg vs. 0.83 ± 0.25 kg, $p = 0.02$) (Table 2). For each kilogram increase in an infant's birthweight, the odds of PH dropped significantly (OR 0.2, 95% CI 0.1–0.7), and infants with intrauterine growth restriction had higher odds of developing late PH than normally grown infants (OR 2.9; 95% CI 1.3–6.2). Interestingly, an association between caffeine and late PH was also seen. Fifty-one percent of infants with late PH received caffeine, compared with 69% of infants without late PH (OR 0.5; 95% CI 0.3–0.8). Despite this discrepancy in caffeine use, we did not detect a difference in the level of respiratory support at 28 days of life or at 36 weeks corrected gestational age between groups. Nineteen percent of infants with late PH were treated with sildenafil, and 3% also were treated with bosentan. Other birth variables and early hospital characteristics did not differ between the comparison groups.

Because outcomes and predictors may differ based on the timing of PH diagnosis, we then evaluated early clinical and echocardiographic factors in infants who had multiple studies and had an echocardiogram showing PH on their final study [21]. This subgroup of 32 infants had their final echocardiogram between 101 days

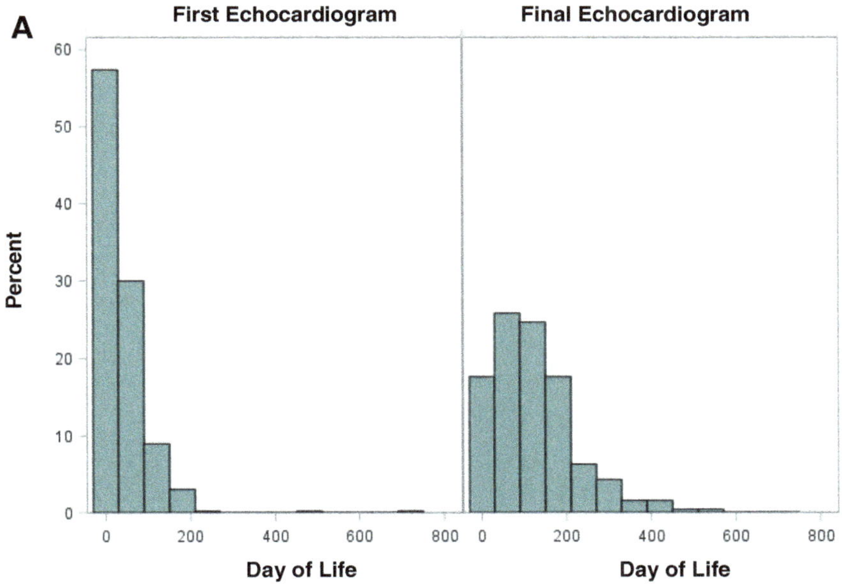

B

Study Cohort Characteristics	Infants with Late PH, n=59	Infants without Late PH, n = 497
Timing of echocardiogram n, %		
< 30 days of life*	17, 29%	154, 31%
> 30 days of life*	34, 58%	290, 58%
Study Number for echocardiogram n, %		
1#	57, 97%	495, 100%
2	15, 25%	134, 27%
> 2	17, 29%	95, 19%
Day of life of echocardiogram (Median, IQR)		
First	15 (7 - 77)	27 (15 - 48)
Final (for infants with > 1 study)	116 (61 - 170)	101 (38 - 174)
Echocardiogram sequence		
First	27, 46%	273, 55%
Final (for infants with > 1 study)	32, 54%	224, 45%

Fig. 2 Description of the timing and number of echocardiograms in infants with and without late PH. Infants were categorized as having late pulmonary hypertension (late PH) if their final echocardiogram in the hospital showed PH. For infants with only one echocardiogram, the final study was their first echocardiogram. For infants with more than one study, the final echocardiogram of the neonatal course was captured. Echocardiograms were performed by clinical pediatric cardiologists and quantitative variables (tricuspid regurgitation jet velocity) and qualitative variables (shunt directions, septal flattening, degree of right ventricular dysfunction/dilation/hypertrophy) were measured. Panel **a** shows the distribution of the day of life for the first and final echocardiogram of the infants in the entire cohort. Panel **b** shows the day of life that the echocardiograms were obtained, the number of studies by group, and the day of life and sequence of the first and final echocardiogram. * missing day of life information in the late PH group (n = 8), and in the without late PH group (n = 53). #2 infants had missing study number information in both groups

(infants without late PH) and 116 days (infants with late PH) (Table 3). The gestational age of infants with multiple studies ranged from 25.7 to 25.9 weeks in both groups, placing the final echocardiogram between 39 and 41 weeks corrected gestational age. Infants in this subgroup with late PH had an Apgar score that was significantly lower than their counterparts who did not have late PH (3.0 vs. 4.3, p = 0.01). More than double the infants with multiple studies and late PH had a history of intrauterine growth restriction, when compared with infants without late PH (23% vs. 9%, p = 0.03). In this subgroup that was evaluated later in the neonatal course, caffeine therapy was not associated with the outcome of late PH (63% vs. 68%, p = 0.55). Interestingly, the use of respiratory support at 28 days or 36 weeks again did not differ between groups.

Table 1 Echocardiographic characteristics of infants with late pulmonary hypertension

Echocardiographic parameters	Infants with Late PH, *n* = 59	Infants without Late PH, *n* = 497	Odd ratio (95% CI)	*p* - value
Timing of final echo Median (IQR)	77 (13–136)	41 (21–105)	1.0 (1.0–1.0)	0.39
Atrial septal defects				
None/PFO	43, 73%	434, 87%	ref	
PFO vs. ASD	4, 7%	24, 5%	1.7 (0.6–5.1)	0.68
ASD	10, 17%	22, 4%	4.6 (2.0–10.3)	<0.01*
Atrial shunt direction (n, %)				
None or left-to-right	29, 57%	312, 87%	ref	
Bidirectional/Right-to-Left	22, 43%	47, 13%	5.0 (2.7–9.5)	<0.01*
Patent Ductus Arteriosus				
None	16, 36%	217, 54%	ref	
Small	11, 24%	69, 17%	2.2 (1.0–4.9)	0.28
Moderate/Large	18, 40%	116, 29%	2.1 (1.0–4.3)	0.27
Patent ductus arteriosus shunt direction (n, %)				
None or left-to-right	12, 43%	177, 99%	ref	
Bidirectional/Right-to-Left	16, 57%	1, < 1%	236.0 (29–1933)	<0.01*
Tricuspid regurgitation jet velocity (n, %)				
Normal, < 32 mmHg	11, 19%	474, 98%	ref	
Mild, 32–44 mmHg	23, 39%	12, 2%	83.0 (33–207)	< 0.01*
Mod, 45–60 mmHg	15, 25%	0, 0%	________	____
Severe, > 60 mmHg	10, 17%	0, 0%	________	____
Septal flattening (n, %)				
None	1, 2%	96, 43%	ref	
Any	48, 98%	126, 57%	36.6 (5.0–269.7)	< 0.01*
Right ventricular dilation (n, %)				
None	25, 45%	436, 92%	ref	
Any	31, 55%	36, 8%	15.0 (8.0–28.1)	< 0.01*
Right ventricular hypertrophy (n, %)				
None	22, 44%	427, 90%	ref	
Any	28, 56%	50, 10%	10.9 (5.8–20.4)	< 0.01*
Right ventricular dysfunction (n, %)				
None	38, 67%	472, 97%	ref	
Any	19, 33%	14, 3%	16.9 (7.8–36.2)	< 0.01*
Ventricular Septal Defect				
None/Small	51, 96%	421, 97%	ref	
Mod/Large	2, 4%	11, 3%	1.5 (0.3–6.9)	0.60
Left ventricular dysfunction (n, %)	7, 12%	31, 6%	2 (0.8–4.8)	0.11

Infants were categorized as having late pulmonary hypertension (late PH) if their final echocardiogram in the hospital showed PH. Echocardiograms were performed by clinical pediatric cardiologists and quantitative variables (tricuspid regurgitation jet velocity) and qualitative variables (shunt directions, septal flattening, degree of right ventricular dysfunction/dilation/hypertrophy) were measured. Odds ratios were defined using univariable logistic regression, *$p < 0.05$ is significant

Four times the proportion of infants with multiple studies and late PH had atrial septal defects, when compared with those without late PH (28% vs. 7%, $p < 0.001$). Although death rates during the neonatal hospitalization were similar in late PH groups, the proportion of infants with bidirectional or right-to-left

Table 2 Evaluation of birth and early hospital characteristics of infants with late PH

Birth/early hospital characteristics	Infants with Late PH, *n* = 59	Infants without Late PH, *n* = 497	Odds ratio (95% CI)	*p* - value
Apgar 1 min. Mean ± SD	3.5 ± 2.8	4.1 ± 2.6	0.9 (0.8–1.0)	0.10
Apgar 5 min. Mean ± SD	6.3 ± 2.4	6.5 ± 2.2	1.0 (0.8–1.1)	0.44
Birthweight (kg) Mean ± SD	0.75 ± 0.24	0.83 ± 0.25	0.2 (0.1–0.7)	0.02*
Gestational age (wks) Mean ± SD	26.1 ± 2.4	26.1 ± 2.2	1.0 (0.9–1.1)	0.99
Mode of Delivery (n, %)				
C/S	44, 77%	327, 66%	1.7 (0.9–3.3)	0.10
Vaginal	13, 23%	166, 34%	ref	
Gender (n, %)				
Male	33, 56%	289, 42%	0.9 (0.5–1.6)	0.71
Female	26, 44%	205, 42%	ref	
Intrauterine growth restriction (n, %)	10, 18%	35, 7%	2.9 (1.3–6.2)	< 0.01*
Placental abruption (n, %)	9, 16%	49, 10%	1.7 (0.8–3.7)	0.17
Chorioamnionitis (n, %)	3, 5%	50, 10%	0.5 (0.2–1.7)	0.27
Maternal betamethasone (n, %)				
2 or more doses	27, 57%	267, 62%	0.8 (0.4–1.5)	0.52
0–1 doses	20, 43%	162, 38%	ref	
Race (n, %)				
Black	36, 61%	290, 60%	1.1 (0.6–1.8)	0.84
White/Asian/Hispanic	23, 39%	196, 40%	ref	
Illicit drug use (n, %)	3, 6%	41, 9%	0.6 (0.2–2.2)	0.47
Multiples (n, %)	12, 21%	91, 18%	1.2 (0.6–2.3)	0.68
Maternal drug use	5, 10%	39, 9%	1.2 (0.4–3.1)	0.76
Caffeine (n, %)	29, 51%	341, 69%	0.5 (0.3–0.8)	< 0.01*
Any respiratory support, 28 days (n, %)	26, 44%	212, 43%	1.0 (0.6–1.8)	0.87
Positive pressure ventilation, 28 days (n,%)	26, 44%	203, 41%	1.1 (0.7–2.0)	0.63
Any respiratory support, 36 weeks (n, %)	26, 44%	199, 40%	1.2 (0.7–2.2)	0.45
Sildenafil (n, %)	11, 19%	19, 4%	5.8 (2.6–12.8)	< 0.01*
Bosentan	2, 3%	0, 0%	______	______

The birth and early hospital characteristics of infants who had late PH were compared to those infants who did not have late PH using univariable logistic regression. Odds ratios were defined using univariable logistic regression, *$p < 0.05$ is significant

shunts through an ASD or PDA was much higher in infants who had late PH on their final echocardiogram (46% vs. 12% and 57% vs. 0%, respectively). Further, a large proportion of infants with multiple studies and late PH had some degree of septal flattening (97% vs. 53%, $p < 0.001$), right ventricular dilation (69% vs. 11%, $p < 0.001$), right ventricular hypertrophy (74% vs. 17%, $p < 0.001$), or right ventricular dysfunction (42% vs. 5%, $p < 0.001$) on their final echocardiogram, indicating this that this subgroup was a very high-risk and high-acuity group within a sick, referral neonatal population.

Multivariable model for the outcome of late PH

To assess how each co-variate found to be significant in our univariable model affected the outcome of late PH when other early characteristics were adjusted for, we generated a multivariable model that evaluated gestational age, atrial septal defect, intrauterine growth restriction, caffeine therapy, and positive-pressure ventilation at 28 days on late PH (Table 4, A). Gestational age, instead of birth weight, was utilized as a co-variate because of potential collinearity between birth weight and intrauterine growth restriction. When other factors were controlled, infants with ASD had a 2.9-fold higher

Table 3 Comparison of characteristics between infants who had multiple studies by late PH status

Birth/early hospital characteristics	Infants with multiple studies and late PH n = 32	Infants with multiple studies without late PH n = 224	p - value
Apgar 1 min. Mean ± SD	3.0 ± 2.4	4.3 ± 2.5	0.01*
Apgar 5 min. Mean ± SD	6.0 ± 2.3	6.5 ± 2.2	0.27
Birthweight (kg) Mean ± SD	0.68 ± 0.19	0.80 ± 0.24	<0.01*
Gestational age (wks) Mean ± SD	25.7 ± 2.3	25.9 ± 2.2	0.73
Mode of Delivery – C/S (n, %)	23, 72%	145, 65%	0.44
Gender – Male (n, %)	16, 50%	129, 58%	0.42
Intrauterine growth restriction (n, %)#	7, 23%	20, 9%	0.03*
Placental abruption (n, %)#	4, 13%	24, 11%	0.76
Chorioamnionitis (n, %)#	2, 6%	22, 10%	0.75
Maternal betamethasone (n, %)	16, 59%	122, 63%	0.72
Multiples (n, %)#	3, 9%	46, 21%	0.16
Caffeine (n, %)	20, 63%	152, 68%	0.55
Any respiratory support, 28 days (n, %)	17, 53%	113, 51%	0.81
Any respiratory support, 36 weeks (n, %)	21, 66%	117, 52%	0.35
Death (n, %)	12, 20%	86, 17%	0.56
Day of life, death or discharge Mean ± SD	113 ± 81	126 ± 74	0.61
Race (n, %)			0.52
Black	21, 66%	132, 60%	
Other	11, 34%	89, 40%	
Atrial septal defects (n, %)	9, 28%	16, 7%	<0.001*
Bidirectional/right-to-left atrial shunt (n, %)	12, 46%	18, 12%	<0.001*
Patent Ductus Arteriosus (n, %)			
Moderate/Large#	4, 19%	22, 14%	0.51
Bidirectional/R-to-L#	4, 57%	0, 0%	< 0.001*
Septal flattening (n, %)	29, 97%	79, 53%	<0.001*
Right ventricular dilation (n, %)	20, 69%	23, 11%	<0.001*
Right ventricular hypertrophy (n, %)	20, 74%	36, 17%	<0.001*
Right ventricular dysfunction (n, %)	13, 42%	11, 5%	<0.001*
Ventricular Septal Defect – Mod/Lgt# (n, %)	1, 4%	2, 1%	0.35
Left ventricular dysfunction (n, %)#	3, 9%	16, 7%	0.67

For infants who had more than one study in the neonatal intensive care unit, clinical characteristics were compared between late PH groups. Two-sample t-tests or Wilcoxon rank sum test for continuous variables, or Chi-square/Fisher's exact test for categorical variables were used. *$p < 0.05$ for comparison groups. #Fisher's Exact Test used

odds of late PH, compared to infants with no significant atrial shunts (95% CI 1.4–6.1). In this cohort, gestational age did not significantly increase the odds of late PH. However, infants with intrauterine growth restriction continued to have a 2.7-fold higher odds for late PH, even when other significant variables were controlled (95% CI 1.2–6.3). Infants receiving caffeine therapy had a lower probability of late PH than those who did not receive caffeine (OR 0.4; 95% CI 0.2–0.8). Positive-pressure ventilation was not significantly associated with late PH, when other factors were controlled (OR 1.5, 95% CI 0.8–2.9).

When the model was evaluated in the sicker subgroup of infants who had multiple studies, infants with an ASD had even higher odds of late PH than those who did not have significant ASD, with other variables being held constant (OR 5.9, 95% CI 2.0–16.5). Similarly, infants with multiple studies who had growth restriction had a

Table 4 Multivariable model for the outcome of late PH in all infants and in infants with multiple studies

Variable	Odds ratio	95% CI	*p*-value
Overall multivariable model for the outcome of late PH			
Gestational age	0.9	0.8–1.1	0.22
Atrial septal defect (ASD vs. None)	2.9	1.4–6.1	<0.01*
Growth restriction	2.7	1.2–6.3	0.02*
Caffeine	0.4	0.2–0.8	0.01*
Positive-pressure ventilation	1.5	0.8–2.9	0.16
Multivariable model for the outcome of late PH, among infants with multiple studies			
Gestational age	0.9	0.7–1.1	0.18
Atrial septal defect (ASD vs. None)	5.9	2.0–16.5	<0.001*
Growth restriction	3.7	1.3–10.7	0.01*
Caffeine	0.8	0.3–1.8	0.53
Positive-pressure ventilation	1.4	0.6–3.3	0.38

A) The association between significant co-variates and the outcome of late pulmonary hypertension was evaluated. B) The association between significant co-variates and the outcome of late pulmonary hypertension in infants with multiple studies was evaluated. Gestational age and positive-pressure ventilation were forced into the model. Multivariable logistic regression was used to derive odds ratios and 95% confidence intervals. $^*p \leq 0.05$ was significant

3.7-fold increase in the odds of late PH, when compared with normally grown infants (95% CI 1.3–10.7). Interestingly, the effect of caffeine on late PH was no longer significant in this small subgroup of infants, when gestational age, ASD, growth restriction and positive-pressure ventilation were controlled (OR 0.8, 0.3–1.8).

Discussion

In this study, we identify important risk factors for PH in a referral neonatal population including birthweight, the presence of an atrial septal defect, intrauterine growth restriction, and caffeine therapy. Further, we have shown that atrial septal defect and intrauterine growth restriction are significantly associated with late PH in infants who are at or near-term gestation.

In our multivariable model, the presence of an atrial septal defect increased the odds of late PH significantly, even when gestational age, growth restriction, caffeine use, and positive-pressure ventilation were controlled. Further, this association was strengthened in a subgroup of infants who had their final echocardiogram showing PH at or near term. Supporting these findings, other investigators have also found an association between the presence of an ASD and the development of PH in infants with BPD, a diagnosis that conferred an increased risk of mortality [22, 23]. Animal models of chronic left-to-right shunting have increased pulmonary vascular resistance and arteriolar medial thickness, implying biologic plausibility to the association between ASD and PH [24, 25]. Epidemiologically, ASDs account for 8–10% of congenital heart defects, though the majority of these close spontaneously in the first year of life [26]. For those with persistent defects, small studies have suggested that infants with BPD may have improved respiratory outcome following transcatheter closure of left-to-right shunts at approximately 6 months of age [27, 28]. Unfortunately, our finding that ASDs were associated with PH development is difficult to interpret causally. ASDs may cause right heart enlargement and diastolic septal flattening due to volume load, which may be confused with systolic septal flattening due to PH. In a similar manner, the presence of a large PDA may complicate the diagnosis of PH by echocardiography by elevating the right ventricular pressure due to transmission of aortic pressure to the pulmonary artery in the absence of elevated pulmonary resistance. However, 43–57% of infants in our analyses had bidirectional or right-to-left shunts, offering some reassurance that our findings are the result of elevated pulmonary resistance and not echocardiographic detection bias due to left-to-right shunting. Further, over half of the infants with late PH also had either right ventricular dilation or hypertrophy, supporting our hypotheses that these infants suffered from chronically elevated pulmonary resistance.

Intrauterine growth restriction was associated with pulmonary hypertension in descriptive analyses in our investigation, and it continued to be associated with PH when other clinical factors were controlled. Infants who had intrauterine growth restriction had a 2.9-fold higher odds of late PH when compared to normally grown infants, and this association was enhanced in our subgroup of infants who had late PH near term (OR 5.9 for late PH). In a single center study by Check et al., infants with BPD, who had a birth weight for gestational-age ratio percentile of less than 25%, had a 3.9-fold increase in the odds of PH at 36 weeks' gestation. When this model was further controlled for gestational age, multiple gestation, gender and race, the odds of PH for growth-restricted infants were increased to 5.9, similar to our findings [16]. Our population differed slightly from that in the prior study, in that we did not restrict our cohort only to infants with BPD, and the overall proportion of infants with intrauterine growth restriction was only 8% (compared with 30%). Because evidence suggests that fetal factors potentially influence the propensity for disease in childhood and adulthood, the association between intrauterine growth restriction and PH should likely be interrogated further [29–31].

Interestingly, caffeine therapy strongly decreased the odds of late PH in our study overall. When gestational age, ASD status, growth restriction, and positive-pressure ventilation were controlled, the potentially protective effect of caffeine therapy on late PH was significant (OR 0.4, 95% CI 0.2–0.8). However, when the cohort was restricted to infants who had late PH later in life (the multiple studies group), the effect of caffeine on the outcome was no longer significant (OR 0.8, 95% CI 0.3–1.8). This differential effect in the association between caffeine therapy and the outcome of late PH may be secondary to the smaller numbers and potentially inadequate power in our subgroup analysis. Alternatively, it is possible that the effect of caffeine therapy on PH during the neonatal hospitalization is mediated through bronchopulmonary dysplasia. In support of this possibility, others have shown that caffeine therapy, particularly when initiated early in life, is associated with a reduction in bronchopulmonary dysplasia and ventilation time for premature neonates [32–34]. Additionally, it is possible that infants who are corrected to near-term and continue to have late PH are a different population than their younger counterparts, and the neonatal predictors of pulmonary hypertension at differing points during the postnatal hospital stay should continue to be carefully characterized.

We acknowledge that pulmonary hypertension based on echocardiographic parameters is challenging to define due to difficulty in obtaining a measurable tricuspid regurgitation jet velocity, and poor sensitivity and specificity for the detection of PH [35]. However, echocardiography is widely used in neonatal intensive care units because safety considerations prohibit the use of cardiac catheterization as a screening tool and clinical decisions are often made based on echocardiographic findings [36]. Further, the definitions of PH applied in our study are comparable to those used in other investigations, and studies have shown strong agreement between clinical and research echocardiograms for the detection of PH [7, 8, 12, 37]. In our cohort, infants were defined as having PH if they had a bidirectional or right-to-left patent ductus arteriosus shunt (indicating systemic or supra-systemic pulmonary vascular resistance), or a mildly elevated tricuspid regurgitation jet velocity with septal flattening, right ventricular hypertrophy or dilation, or a tricuspid regurgitation jet velocity of over 45 mmHg. Although a discrete number for the tricuspid regurgitation jet velocity may be difficult to obtain, we were able to group infants into having a tricuspid regurgitation jet that was "normal" (< 32 mmHg) or "abnormal" (> 32 mmHg). In other investigations, a measurable tricuspid jet velocity in combination with septal flattening, right ventricular hypertrophy, or right ventricular dilation had a positive predictive value of 89–100% [35]. Given these values, our patients who were classified as having PH echocardiographically would also be likely to have PH if they underwent catheterization. Longer-term follow-up and serial echocardiography may be useful to increase the positive prediction of echocardiogram for the development of PH. Additionally, although the optimal echocardiographic parameters for infants at risk of PH is not known, algorithms to detect the disease in a systematic manner are now being developed based on available literature [36].

The strengths of our study include its evaluation of a referral population of high-acuity neonates at particular risk for PH. To our knowledge, this is the largest sample of premature neonates who have received echocardiograms to be studied for pulmonary hypertension. Additionally, we included objective clinical variables in our models that would be readily available early in the neonatal hospital course, and steered away from variables that have traditionally been associated with PH but are present later in the neonatal course. We focused on utilizing these variables to begin to assess if early clinical factors can be utilized to determine infant risk for PH. Further, we have found strong associations between ASD and late PH and growth restriction and late PH, raising the question of whether premature infants with these particular risk factors should be evaluated earlier or more frequently for pulmonary hypertension, than those without these risks.

In summary, in this study, we have confirmed clinical variables that were known to be associated with the development of PH in premature infants, such as intrauterine growth restriction, and we have identified new factors that are associated with PH persistence, such as caffeine use and atrial septal defect. Our multivariable model for persistence of PH utilizes only readily available clinical variables, rather than solely relying on echocardiographic or respiratory characteristics, to establish risk for PH. Echocardiographic and respiratory variables may vary by clinician judgement, and utilizing these variables for prediction of PH may prove to be challenging and difficult to generalize. Our study utilized only fixed and demographic variables that can be validated in larger, prospective studies to define infant risk for PH during the neonatal course. In this way, clinicians could target serial echocardiography to higher-risk infants, and potentially impact postnatal PH surveillance and management in a timely manner.

Conclusions

The presence of an atrial septal defect and intrauterine growth restriction strongly increased the odds of pulmonary hypertension that persists at or near-term in very low birthweight premature infants. Premature infants in referral neonatal intensive care units with these risk factors should potentially have PH evaluations performed earlier or more frequently in their hospital course.

Abbreviations

BPD: Bronchopulmonary dysplasia; late PH: Late pulmonary hypertension

Acknowledgments

The authors would like to acknowledge Karen Parker for her aid in the submission of this manuscript.

Funding

Supported by the National Center for Advancing Translational Sciences of the National Institutes of Health under Award Number UL1 TROOO454. The content is solely the responsibility of the authors and does not necessarily represent the official views o/the National Institutes of Health.

Authors' contributions

SVR: conception and design, acquisition of data, interpretation of data, drafting of the manuscript, final approval of the manuscript, and accountability ensuring accuracy and integrity of the work; UK: echocardiographic parameter selection and interpretation, critical revision of the manuscript, final approval of the manuscript, and accountability ensuring accuracy and integrity of the work; PS: abstraction of data from clinical data warehouse, final approval of the manuscript, and accountability ensuring accuracy and integrity of the work; JS: acquisition of data, final approval of the manuscript, and accountability ensuring accuracy and integrity of the work; CT: database creation, interpretation of the data, final approval of the manuscript, and accountability ensuring accuracy and integrity of the work; DPC: interpretation of data, critical revision of the manuscript, final approval of the manuscript, and accountability ensuring accuracy and integrity of the work; AF: conception and design, interpretation of data, critical revision of the manuscript, final approval of the manuscript, and accountability ensuring accuracy and integrity of the work.

Competing interests

The authors have no competing interests in the design, implementation, analysis or preparation of this manuscript. The NIH was not involved in the 1) study design; 2) the collection, analysis, and interpretation of data; 3) the writing of the report; and 4) the decision to submit the manuscript for publication. Shilpa Vyas-Read wrote the first draft of the manuscript and no form of payment was given to anyone to produce the manuscript.

Author details

[1]Pediatrics, Emory University School of Medicine, Atlanta, GA, USA. [2]Sibley Heart Center, Pulmonary Hypertension Program, Atlanta, GA, USA. [3]Department of Pediatrics, University of Colorado, Denver, CO, USA. [4]Biostatistics, Pediatric Research Alliance, Atlanta, GA, USA. [5]Division of Neonatology, Emory University School of Medicine, 2015 Uppergate Dr. NE, 3rd floor, 30322 Atlanta, GA, USA.

References

1. Mourani PM, Abman SH. Pulmonary hypertension and vascular abnormalities in bronchopulmonary dysplasia. Clin Perinatol. 2015;42:839–55.
2. Berkelhamer SK, Mestan KK, Steinhorn RH. Pulmonary hypertension in bronchopulmonary dysplasia. Semin Perinatol. 2013;37:124–31.
3. Baker CD, Abman SH. Impaired pulmonary vascular development in bronchopulmonary dysplasia. Neonatology. 2015;107:344–51.
4. Abman SH. Bronchopulmonary dysplasia: "a vascular hypothesis". Am J Respir Crit Care Med. 2001;164:1755–6.
5. An HS, Bae EJ, Kim GB, Kwon BS, Beak JS, Kim EK, et al. Pulmonary hypertension in preterm infants with bronchopulmonary dysplasia. Korean Circ J. 2010;40:131–6.
6. Khemani E, McElhinney DB, Rhein L, Andrade O, Lacro RV, Thomas KC, et al. Pulmonary artery hypertension in formerly premature infants with bronchopulmonary dysplasia: clinical features and outcomes in the surfactant era. Pediatrics American Academy of Pediatrics. 2007;120:1260–9.
7. Slaughter JL, Pakrashi T, Jones DE, South AP, Shah TA. Echocardiographic detection of pulmonary hypertension in extremely low birth weight infants with bronchopulmonary dysplasia requiring prolonged positive pressure ventilation. J Perinatol. 2011:31:635–40.
8. Bhat R, Salas AA, Foster C, Carlo WA, Ambalavanan N. Prospective analysis of pulmonary hypertension in extremely low birth weight infants. Pediatrics. 2012;129:e682–9.
9. Murthy K, Savani RC, Lagatta JM, Zaniletti I, Wadhawan R, Truog W, et al. Predicting death or tracheostomy placement in infants with severe bronchopulmonary dysplasia. J Perinatol. 2014;34:543–8.
10. Naumburg E, Soderstrom L, Huber D, Axelsson I. Risk factors for pulmonary arterial hypertension in children and young adults. Pediatr Pulmonol. 2017;52:636–41.
11. Abman SH, Hansmann G, Archer SL, Ivy DD, Adatia I, Chung WK, et al. Pediatric pulmonary hypertension: guidelines from the American Heart Association and American Thoracic Society. Circulation. 2015;132:2037–99.
12. Kim D-H, Kim HS, Choi CW, Kim EK, Kim BI, Choi J-H. Risk factors for pulmonary artery hypertension in preterm infants with moderate or severe bronchopulmonary dysplasia. Neonatology. 2012;101:40–6.
13. Mirza H, Ziegler J, Ford S, Padbury J, Tucker R, Laptook A. Pulmonary hypertension in preterm infants: prevalence and association with bronchopulmonary dysplasia. J Pediatr. 2014;165:909–14.e1.
14. Ali Z, Schmidt P, Dodd J, Jeppesen DL. Predictors of bronchopulmonary dysplasia and pulmonary hypertension in newborn children. Dan Med J. 2013;60:A4688.
15. Al-Ghanem G, Shah P, Thomas S, Banfield L, Helou El S, Fusch C, et al. Bronchopulmonary dysplasia and pulmonary hypertension: a meta-analysis. J Perinatol. 2017;37:414–9.
16. Check J, Gotteiner N, Liu X, Su E, Porta N, Steinhorn R, et al. Fetal growth restriction and pulmonary hypertension in premature infants with bronchopulmonary dysplasia. J Perinatol. 2013;33:553–7.
17. Mestan KK, Check J, Minturn L, Yallapragada S, Farrow KN, Liu X, et al. Placental pathologic changes of maternal vascular underperfusion in bronchopulmonary dysplasia and pulmonary hypertension. Placenta. 2014;35:570–4.
18. Farrow KN, Steinhorn RH. Pulmonary hypertension in premature infants. Sharpening the tools of detection. Am J Respir Crit Care Med. 2015;191:12–4.
19. Waruingi W, Mhanna MJ. Pulmonary hypertension in extremely low birth weight infants: characteristics and outcomes. World J Pediatr. 2014;10:46–52.
20. Nagiub M, Kanaan U, Simon D, Guglani L. Risk factors for development of pulmonary hypertension in infants with bronchopulmonary dysplasia: systematic review and meta-analysis. Paediatr Respir Rev. 2017;23:27–32.
21. Mourani PM, Sontag MK, Younoszai A, Miller JI, Kinsella JP, Baker CD, et al. Early pulmonary vascular disease in preterm infants at risk for bronchopulmonary dysplasia. Am J Respir Crit Care Med. 2015;191:87–95.
22. Choi EK, Jung YH, Kim HS, Shin SH, Choi CW, Kim EK, et al. The impact of atrial left-to-right shunt on pulmonary hypertension in preterm infants with moderate or severe bronchopulmonary dysplasia. Pediatr Neonatol. 2015;56:317–23.
23. Weismann CG, Asnes JD, Bazzy-Asaad A, Tolomeo C, Ehrenkranz RA, Bizzarro MJ. Pulmonary hypertension in preterm infants: results of a prospective screening program. J Perinatol. 2017;37:572–7.
24. Rondelet B, Kerbaul F, Van Beneden R, Hubloue I, Huez S, Fesler P, et al. Prevention of pulmonary vascular remodeling and of decreased BMPR-2 expression by losartan therapy in shunt-induced pulmonary hypertension. Am J Physiol Heart Circ Physiol. 2005;289:H2319–24.
25. Lam C-F, Peterson TE, Croatt AJ, Nath KA, Katusic ZS. Functional adaptation and remodeling of pulmonary artery in flow-induced pulmonary hypertension. Am J Physiol Heart Circ Physiol. 2005;289:H2334–41.
26. Schwerzmann M, Pfammatter J-P. Approaching atrial septal defects in pulmonary hypertension. Expert Rev Cardiovasc Ther. 2015;13:693–701.
27. Wood AM, Holzer RJ, Texter KM, Hill SL, Gest AL, Welty SE, et al. Transcatheter elimination of left-to-right shunts in infants with bronchopulmonary dysplasia is feasible and safe. Congenit Heart Dis. 2011;6:330–7.
28. Thomas VC, Vincent R, Raviele A, Diehl H, Qian H, Kim D. Transcatheter closure of secundum atrial septal defect in infants less than 12 months of

age improves symptoms of chronic lung disease. Congenit Heart Dis. 2012;7:204–11.

29. Bassareo PP, Marras AR, Cugusi L, Zedda AM, Mercuro G. The reasons why cardiologists should consider prematurity at birth and intrauterine growth retardation among risk factors. J Cardiovasc Med (Hagerstown). 2016;17(5): 323–9.
30. Cruz-Lemini M, Crispi F, Valenzuela-Alcaraz B, Figueras F, Sitges M, Bijnens B, et al. Fetal cardiovascular remodelling persists at 6 months of life in infants with intrauterine growth restriction. Ultrasound Obstet Gynecol. 2016;48(3): 349–56.
31. Jayet P-Y, Rimoldi SF, Stuber T, Salmon CS, Hutter D, Rexhaj E, et al. Pulmonary and systemic vascular dysfunction in young offspring of mothers with preeclampsia. Circulation. 2010;122:488–94.
32. Taha D, Kirkby S, Nawab U, Dysart KC, Genen L, Greenspan JS, et al. Early caffeine therapy for prevention of bronchopulmonary dysplasia in preterm infants. J Matern Fetal Neonatal Med. 2014;27:1698–702.
33. Dobson NR, Patel RM, Smith PB, Kuehn DR, Clark J, Vyas-Read S, et al. Trends in caffeine use and association between clinical outcomes and timing of therapy in very low birth weight infants. J Pediatr. 2014;164:992–3.
34. Davis PG, Schmidt B, Roberts RS, Doyle LW, Asztalos E, Haslam R, et al. Caffeine for apnea of prematurity trial: benefits may vary in subgroups. J Pediatr. 2010;156:382–7.
35. Mourani PM, Sontag MK, Younoszai A, Ivy DD, Abman SH. Clinical utility of echocardiography for the diagnosis and management of pulmonary vascular disease in young children with chronic lung disease. Pediatrics. 2008;121:317–25.
36. Nagiub M, Lee S, Guglani L. Echocardiographic assessment of pulmonary hypertension in infants with bronchopulmonary dysplasia: systematic review of literature and a proposed algorithm for assessment. Echocardiography. 2015;32:819–33.
37. Carlton EF, Sontag MK, Younoszai A, DiMaria MV, Miller JI, Poindexter BB, et al. Reliability of Echocardiographic Indicators of Pulmonary Vascular Disease in Preterm Infants at Risk for Bronchopulmonary Dysplasia. J Pediatr. 2017;186:29–33.

8

Comparison of neonatal red cell transfusion reporting in neonatal intensive care units with blood product issue data

Jillian A. Patterson[1,2*], Jennifer R. Bowen[2,3], Sally Francis[4] and Jane B. Ford[1,2]

Abstract

Background: Infants in Neonatal Intensive Care Units represent a heavily transfused population, and are the focus of much research interest. Such research commonly relies on custom research databases or routinely collected data. Knowledge of the accuracy of transfusion recording in these databases is important. This study aims to assess the reporting of red blood cell transfusion neonatal intensive care unit data compared with routinely collected hospital blood bank ("Blood Watch") data.

Methods: Blood Watch data was linked with the NICUS Data Collection, and with routinely collected birth and hospital data for births between 2007 and 2010. The sensitivity, specificity, and positive and negative predictive values for transfusion were calculated, compared to the Blood Watch data. The agreement between the NICUS and Blood Watch datasets on quantity transfused was also assessed.

Results: Data was available on 3934 infants, of which 16.2% were transfused. Transfusion was reported in the NICUS Data Collection with high specificity (98.3%, 95% confidence interval (97.8%,98.7%)), but with some under-enumeration (sensitivity 89.2% (95% CI 86.5%,91.5%)). There was excellent agreement between the NICUS and Blood Watch datasets on quantity transfused (Kappa 0.90, 95% CI (0.88,0.92)). Transfusion reporting in the hospital data for these infants was also reliably reported (Sensitivity 83.7% (95% CI 80.6%,86.5%), specificity 99.1% (95% CI 98.7%,99.4%)).

Conclusions: Transfusion is reliably reported in the neonatal intensive care unit data, with some under-reporting, and quantity transfused is well recorded. The NICUS Data Collection provides useful information on blood transfusions, including quantity of blood transfused in a high risk population.

Keywords: Sensitivity, Neonatal intensive care, Transfusion, Validity

Background

Infants, particularly low birth weight and premature neonates represent a highly transfused population [1–3], with many of these transfusions occurring within neonatal intensive care units (NICU) [1]. Understanding the frequency of, and reasons and risk factors for transfusion in this population is important for service delivery, and to monitor the appropriateness of transfusion in these infants. The data needed to conduct such research are commonly sourced from medical record review [4, 5], routinely collected administrative databases [1], or custom research datasets [3, 6, 7]. It is important to know how accurately transfusion information is recorded in these databases when using any of these data sources for research. As these data sources are frequently collected for purposes other than clinical management, the reliability of the information they contain is unknown.

Where a high level of inaccuracies are present in the data it can affect research findings based on the data. In databases where transfusions are frequently recorded when they are not actually given (low sensitivity) or if a

* Correspondence: Jillian.patterson@sydney.edu.au
[1]Clinical and Population Perinatal Health Research, Kolling Institute, Northern Sydney Local Health District, St Leonards, NSW 2065, Australia
[2]Sydney Medical School Northern, University of Sydney, Sydney, Australia

large proportion of transfusions are not recorded for patients receiving them (low specificity) then risk estimates based on these data can be biased or diluted. This problem is exacerbated where the likelihood of a transfusion being recorded varies over time or according to the severity of the patient's condition. Comparison of transfusion reporting across databases allows the extent of over- and under-reporting to be estimated. In New South Wales (NSW), Australia, one custom research database on ill neonates is the Neonatal Intensive Care Units (NICUS) Data Collection. This data collection contains information abstracted from the medical record on selected infants admitted to NICU [8]. In 2007, information on red blood cell transfusion was included in this database for the first time, but the accuracy of the data collected has not been assessed. In this time period, hospital blood banks have been submitting information to a central database 'Blood Watch' on each red cell unit issued. Linkage of these databases, along with routinely collected hospital admission and birth data, provides the opportunity to assess the reporting of transfusion in the NICUS and hospital data.

Previous studies in general inpatient populations, and in obstetric populations have found that transfusion is reported with high specificity [9], but some under-enumeration [10, 11]. These studies have been based on routinely collected hospital data, which records only fact of transfusion, rather than quantity transfused. Quantity transfused is often an indicator of the severity of the condition of the infant. Both the NICUS and Blood Watch Data Collections contain additional information on the quantity of blood transfused, which could expand the scope of future studies on transfusion in this population. This study aims to identify the accuracy of using neonatal intensive care unit and hospital data to identify neonatal transfusions among babies admitted to neonatal intensive care.

Methods

The study population was all liveborn infants of at least 23 weeks gestation born in one of six NSW hospitals with Neonatal Intensive Care Unit (NICU) facilities and maternity services who submitted data to the Blood Watch database (two additional hospitals with NICU facilities do not have maternity services, and one did not have complete data available). Infants were eligible if they were admitted to NICU and had data available across the Perinatal, Admitted Patients and Neonatal Intensive Care Surveillance datasets. Only records pertaining to the hospital of birth were included; transfusions occurring following transfer to another hospital were not examined. Births were identified from the Perinatal Data Collection, a statutory collection of all births in NSW. Data on transfusion was available from three sources: the Clinical Excellence Commission 'Blood Watch' data, the Admitted Patient Data Collection ('hospital data'), and the Neonatal Intensive Care Units (NICUS) Data Collection. Data was available from 1 January 2007 to 31 December 2010.

The Blood Watch data incorporates information from the Australian Red Cross Blood Service on the type and number of products issued to a patient, and combines this with pathology test results available for the patient. This data is submitted electronically to a central database by laboratories in participating hospitals. Each unit of blood issued is an individual record in this data, allowing calculation of number of units transfused. Transfusion in this dataset was defined as the issue (without return) of one or more units of red cells to a patient. Standard issue red cell units and the smaller pedipacks (single unit split into 4) commonly used for infants and children are each counted as a single transfusion.

The Admitted Patient Data Collection is a census of admissions to NSW hospitals. Data on up to 50 diagnoses and procedures are collected and coded according to the International Classification of Diseases version 10, Australian Modification (ICD10-AM) and the Australian Classification of Health Interventions (ACHI) respectively. Transfusion was identified from a record of transfusion of red cells or exchange transfusion in the procedure codes. The number or volume of transfusions was not available from the hospital data. The Perinatal Data Collection was used to identify birth admissions (that is, the admission during which the delivery of the infant took place). The Perinatal Data Collection also provided information on the pregnancy and the birth of the infant.

Data on infants meeting one or more of the following criteria are recorded in the NICUS database: < 32 weeks gestation, birthweight ≤ 1500 g, requiring assisted ventilation, undergoing surgery requiring the opening of a body cavity, insertion of a central line or intentional hypothermia for infants with hypoxic ischaemic encephalopathy. From 1 January 2007, this database contains a record of each transfusion performed within the NICU in these infants. Not all infants admitted to NICU are eligible for inclusion in this database.

Probabilistic linkage was used to combine records from each database, belonging to the same infant, corresponding to their birth admission. Linkage was performed by the NSW Centre for Health Record Linkage using privacy preserving principles, with deidentified data provided to researchers.

Transfusion reported in the Blood Watch data was considered the "gold standard". Sensitivity, specificity and positive and negative predictive values were calculated comparing reporting of 'any red cell transfusion' in Blood Watch and the NICUS Data Collection, and are reported with exact binomial confidence limits. Agreement between quantity transfused was assessed using weighted Kappa statistics for Blood Watch and NICUS data, where kappa values less than 0.4 represent poor agreement, 0.4–0.75 good agreement and greater than 0.75 represent excellent agreement beyond chance [12]. Due to small numbers of infants and the narrow range of number of transfusions given, number of transfusions was grouped into 1–2, 3–4, 5–9 and 10+ to reflect clinical severity. Trends in rates were assessed using the Cochran-Armitage test for trend.

A secondary analysis was conducted comparing reporting of transfusion in the hospital data (compared with Blood Watch data) among this high risk population.

All references to transfusion in this manuscript refer to red cell transfusions. All analysis was performed in SAS 9.3. This study received ethical approval from the NSW Population and Health Services Research Ethics Committee.

Results

Between January 2007 and December 2010, there were 91,473 infants liveborn in tertiary hospitals. Of these 3934 (4.3%) had records across the birth, hospital and NICUS databases and were included for analysis (Fig. 1, also see Additional file 1: Table S1, which describes the characteristics of the population). Pre-transfusion haemoglobin measures were available for 505 (12.8%) infants, with the lowest recorded haemoglobin ranging from 39 g/L to 198 g/L (median 91 g/L). Almost half (1833, 46.6%) of NICU infants were ≥33 weeks gestation, 606 (15.4%) had a five minute Apgar score of <7 and 979 (24.9%) were from multifetal pregnancies.

The Blood Watch data reported information for 637 (16.2%) transfused infants in the NICUS Data Collection, and NICUS had transfusion data for 628 (15.9%) (Table 1). There was no significant change over time in transfusion rates reported in any dataset (Blood Watch $p = 0.08$, NICUS data $p = 0.14$, Hospital $p = 0.45$) Red cell transfusion was reliably reported in the NICUS Data Collection, but with some false positives (Sensitivity 89.2% (95% CI 86.5%,91.5%), Specificity 98.3% (97.8%,98.7%), PPV 90.9 (88.3%,93.0%)) (Table 2). The sensitivity of transfusion reporting was higher in the earlier years, and the decline in sensitivity was not associated with any particular hospital.

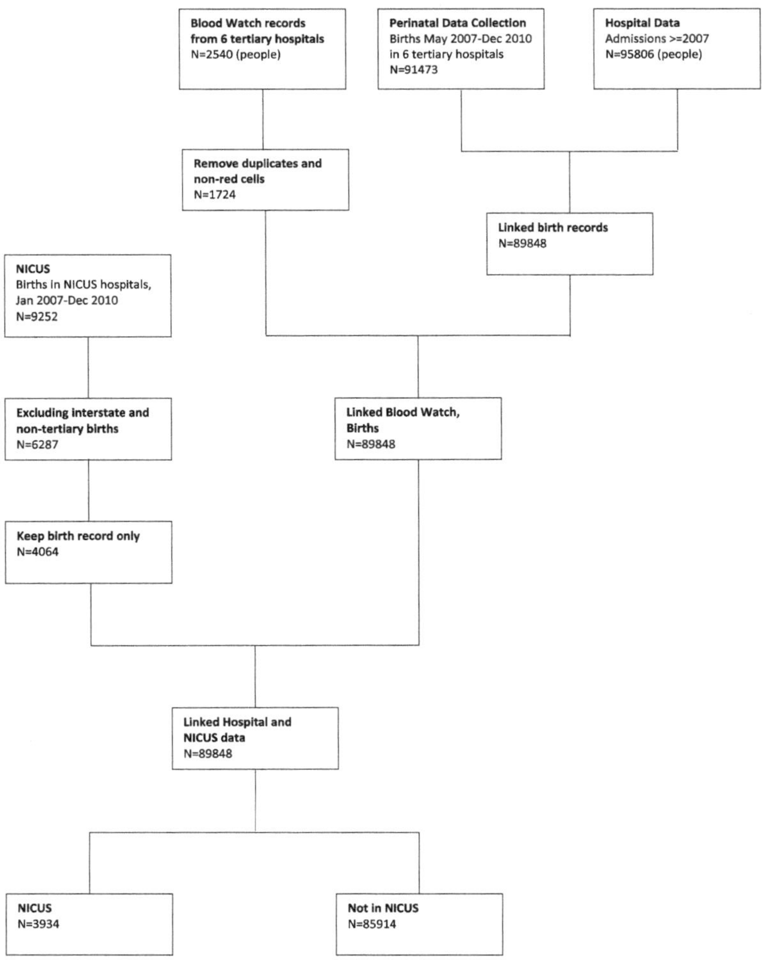

Fig. 1 Identification of related records for infants registered in the Neonatal Intensive Care Units' Data Collection

Table 1 Transfusion reporting in Blood Watch (hospital blood bank) vs Neonatal Intensive Care Units' (NICUS) Data Collection for infants registered in the NICUS Data Collection

		Blood Watch Data Collection	
		Transfusion	No Transfusion
NICUS Data Collection	Transfusion	568 (14.4)	57 (1.5)
	No Transfusion	69 (1.8)	3240 (82.4)

There was excellent agreement between the Blood Watch and NICUS databases in terms of quantity transfused (Weighted Kappa 0.90 (0.88,0.92)) (Table 3). The proportion of transfusions reported in the NICUS data increased as quantity transfused increased (Table 4), with all infants receiving transfusions of 10 or more units identified as transfused in the NICUS data. The proportion of 1 and 2 unit transfusions identified in the NICUS data was slightly better in earlier years, but the accuracy of the reporting of larger volume transfusions remained high across the study period.

Within this population of infants in NICU, the hospital data reported on 562 (14.3%) transfused infants. Compared with Blood Watch data, the reporting of transfusion in the hospital data for this subpopulation had sensitivity 83.7% (80.6%, 86.5%), specificity 99.1% (98.7%, 99.4%), and PPV 94.8% (92.7%, 96.5%) and showed a similar decline in accuracy of reporting over the study period to NICU data (PPV declined from 97.0% (92.5%, 99.2%) in 2007 to 90.5% (85.6%, 94.7%) in 2010) (See Appendix).

Of the 69 infants with transfusion reported in Blood Watch but not NICUS data (false negatives), 81% (N = 56) received 1–2 units of blood, 61% (N = 42) were ≤32 weeks gestation, and 20% (N = 14) were term infants. Of the 57 reported in NICUS but not in Blood watch (false positives), 70% received 1–2 units of blood, 54% (N = 31) were infants ≤32 weeks and 26% (N = 15) were term infants.

Discussion

Between 2007 and 2010 data was available on 3934 infants admitted to a NICU and included in the NICUS database. Of these infants, around one in six received a red cell transfusion. Overall, there was good reporting of transfusion in neonatal intensive care unit data, but with some under-enumeration (sensitivity 89.2%). Transfusion was reported with high specificity (98.3%), meaning that cases reported are likely to be true cases. Although the NICUS database is well established (with reporting commencing in 1992), blood transfusion information has only been collected from 2007. A one off linkage with the Blood Watch data submitted by hospital blood banks provided an important opportunity to understand previously un-validated data items in NICUS and hospital data. Validating transfusion reporting via medical record review would be labour intensive and costly, and thus potentially difficult to justify, however through linkage of datasets reporting transfusion using different sources, such validation becomes more feasible.

This relatively high transfusion rate of infants admitted to a NICU reflects the more serious condition of these infants compared with the general neonatal population which has a transfusion rate of 5.4 per 1000 births [1]. It is possible that reporting in this high risk population is not generalizable to all infants, however most infants are transfused in the NICU setting [1]. For the same group of infants, transfusion reporting in the hospital data was less complete, with sensitivity 83.7% and specificity of 99.1%. This degree of ascertainment is consistent with the reporting of transfusion in adults [9] and in the obstetric population [11]. The NICUS data, being a more specialized collection, was better able to identify transfused infants compared with hospital data. This may be due to differences between NICUS and hospital records in how the data is collected. Hospital transfusion is coded from the medical record, and relies on documentation of transfusion in the notes, whereas NICUS data is collected by clinical nurse specialists [13] who have ICU experience, and may be more familiar with finding this information in the medical record. Nevertheless, the hospital data has reasonable reporting of transfusion and, assuming overall consistency of reporting, provides a valuable data source

Table 2 Sensitivity and Specificity of transfusion reporting in Neonatal Intensive Care Units' (NICUS) Data Collection compared with Blood Watch (hospital blood bank) data collection for infants in the NICUS Data Collection

		Blood Watch data	NICUS rate	Sensitivity	Specificity	Positive Predictive Value	Negative Predictive Value
Total		637/ 3934 (16.2)	625/ 3934 (15.9)	89.2 (86.5, 91.5)	98.3 (97.8, 98.7)	90.9 (88.3, 93.0)	97.9 (97.4, 98.4)
Year	2007	154/ 905 (17.0)	149/ 905 (16.5)	92.9 (87.6, 96.4)	99.2 (98.3, 99.7)	96.0 (91.4, 98.5)	98.5 (97.4, 99.3)
	2008	172/ 980 (17.6)	172/ 980 (17.6)	89.5 (84.0, 93.7)	97.8 (96.5, 98.7)	89.5 (84.0, 93.7)	97.8 (96.5, 98.7)
	2009	157/ 992 (15.8)	147/ 992 (14.8)	87.3 (81.0, 92.0)	98.8 (97.8, 99.4)	93.2 (87.8, 96.7)	97.6 (96.4, 98.5)
	2010	154/ 1057 (14.6)	157/ 1057 (14.9)	87.0 (80.7, 91.9)	97.5 (96.2, 98.4)	85.4 (78.8, 90.5)	97.8 (96.6, 98.6)

Table 3 Agreement between Neonatal Intensive Care Units (NICUS) Data Collection and the Blood Watch (Hospital blood bank) Data Collection on quantity transfused for infants registered in the NICUS Data Collection

	Blood Watch				
NICUS Data Collection	0 units	1–2 units	3–4 units	5–9 units	10 plus units
None	3240	56	10	3	0
1–2 units	40	306	17	3	0
3–4 units	8	10	115	16	0
5–9 units	8	1	5	68	2
10 plus units	1	0	0	7	18
Weighted Kappa (95% CI)	0.90 (0.88, 0.92)	<.0001			

on transfusions outside of NICU (which represent at least 7% of transfusions) [1].

Excellent agreement was noted on quantity transfused between the Blood Watch and NICUS databases. Few databases collect quantity transfused, and so validation studies to date have examined only reporting of fact of transfusion [9–11]. Given the important additional detail provided by quantity transfused, it is reassuring to know that this information is reliably reported. Better reporting was observed in higher volume transfusions. This is consistent with the findings of other validation studies, where more serious conditions are more likely to be reported [11, 14–16].

Table 4 Proportion of Blood Watch (hospital blood bank) transfusions identified in the Neonatal Intensive Care Units' (NICUS) Data Collection, by volume transfused

		Quantity transfused (units)	NICUS Data Collection (N)	Blood Watch Data (N)	% of transfusions identified in the NICUS Data Collection Row %
Total		1 to 2	316	372	84.9
		3 to 4	137	147	93.2
		5 to 9	94	97	96.9
		10 or more	20	20	100.0
Year	2007	1 to 2	81	89	91.0
		3 to 4	32	34	94.1
		5 to 9	23	24	95.8
		10 or more	7	7	100.0
	2008	1 to 2	87	100	87.0
		3 to 4	29	33	87.9
		5 to 9	32	33	97.0
		10 or more	6	6	100.0
	2009	1 to 2	75	92	81.5
		3 to 4	35	37	94.6
		5 to 9	23	24	95.8
		10 or more	4	4	100.0
	2010	1 to 2	73	91	80.2
		3 to 4	41	43	95.3
		5 to 9	16	16	100.0
		10 or more	3	3	100.0

Over time, the sensitivity of transfusion reporting declined in the NICUS data. This decline seemed to be largely among the smaller volume transfusions. The reasons for this decline are unclear, however a similar decline was not seen when comparing hospital and Blood Watch data reporting, suggesting there has been little change to the reporting in the gold standard.

In some cases, false positives and negatives will be due to clerical error, however some differences were identified between infants who were identified as having transfusion compared with those who were not. False positives and negatives in the data were most frequently low volume transfusions. In some cases this may reflect situations where the blood was ordered but not transfused and not returned to the blood bank or the transfusion was not noted in the medical record. This is also consistent with the finding of better reporting in more severe cases, where transfusion is expected, and where multiple transfusion occasions make it more likely that a case will be identified. Transfusions among term infants were overrepresented in the false negatives, suggesting that where transfusion is unexpected, coders may not specifically look for evidence of transfusion.

This study has a number of strengths. By obtaining transfusion information from independent sources, the reliability of transfusion reporting between the sources was able to be assessed. In particular, as both Blood Watch and NICUS databases provide data on quantity of blood transfused, the agreement in quantity transfused was able to be assessed. A potential limitation of the study is the narrow definition of the study population, in that it does not include all infants admitted to NICU, and so the generalizability to other study populations may be limited, however most infants transfused would be expected to appear in the NICUS data. Another limitation is that there may be errors in reporting in the gold standard Blood Watch data, particularly where red cells were released from the blood bank, returned, but not recorded as such, although such instances would be rare. These cases would falsely lower the sensitivity of the NICUS data.

Conclusions

This study shows high consistency of reporting of transfusion, including quantity transfused, between the Blood Watch and NICUS databases. Although there is some under-enumeration, cases reported are likely to be true cases, as such, although the NICUS data may underestimate transfusion rates, it provides a valuable source of data for risk adjustment and analysis. The inclusion of quantity transfused in neonatal intensive care unit data provides reliable and useful additional information for research, compared with hospital data.

Appendix

Table 5 Sensitivity and Specificity of transfusion reporting in hospital data compared with Blood Watch (hospital blood bank) data for infants in the Neonatal Intensive Care Units (NICUS) database

		Blood Watch Data	Hospital data	Sensitivity	Specificity	Positive predictive value	Negative predictive value
Total		637/ 3934 (16.2)	562/ 3934 (14.3)	83.7 (80.6, 86.5)	99.1 (98.7, 99.4)	94.8 (92.7, 96.5)	96.9 (96.3, 97.5)
Year	2007	154/ 905 (17.0)	134/ 905 (14.8)	84.4 (77.7, 89.8)	99.5 (98.6, 99.9)	97.0 (92.5, 99.2)	96.9 (95.4, 98.0)
	2008	172/ 980 (17.6)	146/ 980 (14.9)	82.0 (75.4, 87.4)	99.4 (98.6, 99.8)	96.6 (92.2, 98.9)	96.3 (94.8, 97.5)
	2009	157/ 992 (15.8)	134/ 992 (13.5)	81.5 (74.6, 87.3)	99.3 (98.4, 99.7)	95.5 (90.5, 98.3)	96.6 (95.2, 97.7)
	2010	154/ 1057 (14.6)	148/ 1057 (14.0)	87.0 (80.7, 91.9)	98.4 (97.4, 99.1)	90.5 (84.6, 94.7)	97.8 (96.6, 98.7)

Abbreviations

NICU: Neonatal Intensive Care Unit; NICUS: Neonatal Intensive Care Units Data Collection; NSW: New South Wales; PPV: Positive predictive value

Acknowledgements

The authors would like to thank the Directors, NICUS members and Audit Officers of the Neonatal Intensive Care Units for providing data used in this study from the NICUS Data Collection. The authors would also like to thank the Clinical Excellence Commission for provision of the Blood Watch Data, the NSW Ministry of Health for access to the population health data and the NSW Centre for Health Record Linkage for linking the data sets.
This work was supported by a Partnership Grant from the Australian National Health and Medical Research Council NHMRC (#1027262), the Australian Red Cross and the NSW Clinical Excellence Commission. Jane Ford is supported by an Australian Research Council Future Fellowship (#120100069).
The funding bodies played no role in the design; the collection, analysis and interpretation of data; the writing of the manuscript; nor the decision to submit the manuscript for publication.

Authors' contributions

JP and JF designed the study, JP performed the analysis and drafted the manuscript and JB and SF provided clinical input. All authors were involved in the interpretation of results, revising the manuscript and approve this final 'to be published' version for submission.

Competing interests

The authors declare that they have no competing interests.

Author details

[1]Clinical and Population Perinatal Health Research, Kolling Institute, Northern Sydney Local Health District, St Leonards, NSW 2065, Australia. [2]Sydney Medical School Northern, University of Sydney, Sydney, Australia. [3]Royal North Shore Hospital, Northern Sydney Local Health District, St Leonards, NSW 2065, Australia. [4]BloodWatch Program, NSW Clinical Excellence Commission, Sydney, NSW 2000, Australia.

References

1. Bowen JR, Patterson JA, Roberts CL, Isbister JP, Irving DO, Ford JB. Red cell and platelet transfusions in neonates: a population-based study. Arch Dis Child Fetal Neonatal Ed. 2015 Sep;100(5):F411-5. https://doi.org/10.1136/archdischild-2014-307716. Epub 2015 May 14.
2. Murray NA, Roberts IA. Neonatal transfusion practice. Arch Dis Child Fetal Neonatal Ed. 2004;89(2):F101–7.
3. Keir AK, Yang J, Harrison A, Pelausa E, Shah PS, on behalf of the Canadian Neonatal Network. Temporal changes in blood product usage in preterm neonates born at less than 30 weeks' gestation in Canada. Transfusion (Paris). 2015;55(6):1340–6.
4. Widness JA, Seward VJ, Kromer IJ, Burmeister LF, Bell EF, Strauss RG. Changing patterns of red blood cell transfusion in very low birth weight infants. J Pediatr. 1996;129(5):680–7.
5. Berg A, Courtney R, Krishnamurti L, Triulzi DJ, Yazer MH. Is intensive monitoring during the first transfusion in pediatric patients necessary? Hematology. 2014;19(5):304–8.
6. Stritzke AI, Smyth J, Synnes A, Lee SK, Shah PS. Transfusion-associated necrotising enterocolitis in neonates. Arch Dis Child Fetal Neonatal Ed. 2013; 98(1):F10–4.

7. von Lindern JS, Khodabux CM, Hack KE, van Haastert IC, Koopman-Esseboom C, van Zwieten PH, Brand A, Walther FJ. Long-term outcome in relationship to neonatal transfusion volume in extremely premature infants: a comparative cohort study. BMC Pediatr. 2011;11:48.
8. Neonatal Intensive Care Units (NICUS). New South Wales Pregnancy and Newborn Services Network web site. http://www.psn.org.au/nicus. Accessed 15 June 2015.
9. Henderson T, Shepheard J, Sundararajan V. Quality of diagnosis and procedure coding in ICD-10 administrative data. Med Care. 2006;44(11):1011–9.
10. Joseph KS, Fahey J, Canadian Perinatal Surveillance System. Validation of perinatal data in the discharge abstract database of the Canadian Institute for Health Information. Chronic Dis Can. 2009;29(3):96–100.
11. Lain SJ, Roberts CL, Hadfield RM, Bell JC, Morris JM. How accurate is the reporting of obstetric haemorrhage in hospital discharge data? A validation study. Aust N Z J Obstet Gynaecol. 2008;48(5):481–4.
12. Woodward M: Measuring agreement. In: Epidemiology: study design and data analysis. 2nd edn. Edited by Chatfield C, Zidek JV. London: Chapman and Hall/CRC; 1999: 91.
13. Ford JB, Algert CS, Morris JM, Roberts CL. Decreasing length of maternal hospital stay is not associated with increased readmission rates. Aust N Z J Public Health. 2012;36(5):430–4.
14. Bell JC, Ford JB, Cameron CA, Roberts CL. The accuracy of population health data for monitoring trends and outcomes among women with diabetes in pregnancy. Diabetes Res Clin Pract. 2008;81(1):105–9.
15. Roberts CL, Bell JC, Ford JB, Hadfield RM, Algert CS, Morris JM. The accuracy of reporting of the hypertensive disorders of pregnancy in population health data. Hypertens Pregnancy. 2008;27(3):285–97.
16. Zwart JJ, Yazdani ST, Harvey MS, de Vries RR, van Roosmalen J. Underreporting of major obstetric haemorrhage in the Netherlands. Transfus Med. 2010;20(2):118–22.

9

Supporting play exploration and early developmental intervention versus usual care to enhance development outcomes during the transition from the neonatal intensive care unit to home

Stacey C. Dusing[1*], Tanya Tripathi[2], Emily C. Marcinowski[1], Leroy R. Thacker[3], Lisa F. Brown[4] and Karen D. Hendricks-Muñoz[5]

Abstract

Background: While therapy services may start in the Neonatal Intensive Care Unit (NICU) there is often a gap in therapy after discharge. Supporting Play Exploration and Early Development Intervention (SPEEDI) supports parents, helping them build capacity to provide developmentally supportive opportunities starting in the NICU and continuing at home. The purpose of this single blinded randomized pilot clinical trial was to evaluate the initial efficacy of SPEEDI to improve early reaching and exploratory problem solving behaviors.

Methods: Fourteen infants born very preterm or with neonatal brain injury were randomly assigned to SPEEDI or Usual Care. The SPEEDI group participated in 5 collaborative parent, therapist, and infant interventions sessions in the NICU (Phase 1) and 5 at home (Phase 2). Parents provided daily opportunities designed to support the infants emerging motor control and exploratory behaviors. Primary outcome measures were assessed at the end of the intervention, 1 and 3 months after the intervention ended. Reaching was assessed with the infant supported in an infant chair using four 30 s trials. The Early Problem Solving Indicator was used to evaluate the frequency of behaviors during standardized play based assessment. Effect sizes are including for secondary outcomes including the Test of Infant Motor Performance and Bayley Scales of Infant and Toddler Development.

Results: No group differences were found in the duration of toy contact. There was a significant group effect on ($F1,8 = 4.04$, $p = 0.08$) early exploratory problem-solving behaviors with infants in the SPEEDI group demonstrating greater exploration with effect sizes of 1.3, 0.6, and 0.9 at the end of the intervention, 1 and 3 months post-intervention.

Conclusions: While further research is needed, this initial efficacy study showed promising results for the ability of SPEEDI to impact early problem solving behaviors at the end of intervention and at least 3 months after the intervention is over. While reaching did not show group differences, a ceiling effect may have contributed to this finding. This single blinded pilot RCT was registered prior to subject enrollment on 5/27/14 at ClinicalTrials.Gov with number NCT02153736.

* Correspondence: scdusing@vcu.edu
[1]Department of Physical Therapy, Motor Development Lab, Virginia Commonwealth University, Office: 1200 E Broad St. B106, PO BOX 980224, Richmond, VA 23298, USA

Background

In the United States 1 in 8 infants are born prematurely (< 37 weeks gestation), placing the infants at increased risk for learning difficulties, lower quality of life, and motor disabilities with up to 50% of infant born very preterm requiring special education [1, 2]. Infants born preterm with neonatal white matter injury are also at higher risk of having cerebral palsy (CP), cognitive impairments, requiring more teacher attention, and having an increased need for special education support [3–6]. While survival of infants born preterm is more certain than ever, developmental services typically use a "wait and see" approach to start intervention and once enrolled provides low intensity intervention resulting in little to no lasting effects on motor and cognitive development [7, 8]. Basic science and clinical evidence suggest early and intense intervention is more effective than a long-term low intensity approach at promoting neural recovery in adults and children as well as in animal models of cerebral palsy [9–12]. Evidence-based, effective early intervention programs are needed to target early motor abilities that support motor and cognitive development in infants at high risk of having cerebral palsy or minor neurological dysfunctions.

Motor and cognitive development are tightly coupled, suggesting that delays in one domain could contribute to delays in other domains [13–17]. Motor experience provides infants an opportunity to learn about objects and interaction supports development in multiple domains [17–20]. The action perception model of development is governed by the theory that motor activity contributes to the infants attempts to attend to the environment, allowing the infant to receive and interpret important information, and solve problems by linking the mind and body in a cycle that supports development [21]. Children with motor impairments or delays have limited ability to interact with and interpret the environment, restricting their opportunities to learn through action [16]. Atypical postural control and impaired reaching abilities are common in infants born preterm and infants later diagnosed with development deficits such as CP, developmental coordination disorder, and minor neurological dysfunction [22–27]. Children born preterm with motor coordination disorders or CP score lower on problem-solving tasks than those without motor disabilities at school age [14, 15]. The relationship between motor and cognitive outcomes in infants born preterm supports the need for interventions that incorporate both the motor and cognitive domains and the interaction between these domains to maximize outcomes.

Developmental interventions for infants born preterm often focus on one approach; motor, cognitive, or parent-children interactions. A recent Cochrane review demonstrated that intervention to support motor development were slightly more effective when initiated in the NICU, and was more effective when intervention strived to impact both parent-child interaction and infant development [28].

The purpose of this study was to assess the initial efficacy of Supporting Play, Exploration, and Early Developmental Intervention (SPEEDI) an intervention that started in the NICU and continued for 12 weeks in the community. The goals of SPEEDI were to provide an enriched environment and increased opportunities for infant initiated movements through collaborative parent, therapist and infant interactions during the first months of life in order to enhance the infant's development during and after the intervention period (Additional file 1).

Therefore, the primary aims of this single blinded randomized controlled trial were to evaluate the short-term efficacy of SPEEDI at enhancing reaching and play based exploratory problem solving compared to infants receiving usual care. We hypothesized that compared to the usual care group, the SPEEDI intervention group would demonstrate increased reaching and early problem solving skills at the end of the intervention, 1 and 3 months after the intervention ended. The secondary aims were to explore the impact of SPEEDI on longer-term motor and cognitive development.

Methods

Design overview

This study is a single blinded randomized pilot clinical trial.

Setting and participants

Every infant admitted to a single level IV NICU during the enrollment period was screened for eligibility. Infants born extremely preterm (<29 weeks of gestation) and/or with neonatal diagnosis of a brain injury, who lived within 30 min of the hospital, and spoke English were eligible for this study. Brain injuries included intraventricular hemorrhage (grade 3 or 4), periventricular white matter injury, hypoxic ischemic encephalopathy or hydrocephalus requiring a shunt. Exclusion criteria included: a diagnosis of a genetic syndrome (e.g., Trisomy 21) or musculoskeletal deformity. (e.g., limb deficiency). Information was provided to parents of eligible infants between 35 and 40 weeks of gestation if the infant was off ventilator support by 40 weeks of gestation. Only one infant from eligible multiple births was enrolled in the study. The infant's medical records were used to document medical complications and score the Neonatal Medical Index [29]. All infants received a packet of age-appropriate infant toys and total of $100 to offset travel, parking, and time meeting with the study staff.

Randomization and interventions

Infants were randomized to the intervention or usual care group after a baseline assessment using a stratified (brain injury / no brain injury) randomization scheme. All infants, regardless of group assignment, participated in usual care as it was deemed unethical to withhold routine care. Usual care included referral to therapy services in the NICU at the medical team discretion and referral to their local Early Intervention (EI) program. EI was provided in accordance with state implementation guidelines under the United States Individuals with Disabilities Education Improvement Act (IDEIA) [30]. Parents were offered referral by NICU staff prior to discharge, during visits to the Neonatal Continuing Care Program, or by the study assessment team if requested by a parent. In order to document the usual care services provided outside of the study protocol, NICU medical records were reviewed and parents were asked to fill out a questionnaire at each assessment visit to document enrollment in and frequency of outpatient or EI therapy visits.

Infants enrolled in the usual care group received only usual care in the NICU and community. Infants enrolled in the SPEEDI group participated in a 2 phase intervention utilizing principles of the synactive theory of development and action perception theory to train parents to provide daily intervention to support the infant's development through environmental enrichment and active engagement (Additional file 1). The first phase, delivered face to face in the NICU, focused on helping parents identify ideal times to interact with their infant, provide developmentally appropriate interaction and start to consider how they will interact with their infant after NICU discharge [31, 32]. All sessions were designed to include some time with the infant, discussion of behavioral cues and development, and answering the parents' questions. Videos were provided for parents to review between sessions (Additional file 2). An activity booklet was reviewed with the parent during the last few visits in phase 1 in preparation for phase 2 (Additional file 3). Phase 2 focused on parents using the skill acquired during phase 1 to provide their infant with daily opportunities for motor and problem-solving based play with a goal of improving motor skills and early problem solving (Table 1). The Phase 2 intervention is based on action-perception theory which stresses the important role of early experience in shaping development [13]. SPEEDI applies this theory by engaging parents in providing early experiences that are the "just right challenge" for the infant that day, matching the demand with the infant's ability to support ongoing development. A focus was placed on allowing the infant to use self-directed movements, variability in movement pattern, and active infant engagement through parental support and environmental enrichment (Additional file 1 Key Principles). Parents were encouraged to progress the activities from easier (stage 1) to harder (stage 2) activities over the 12 weeks of phase 2 intervention. Study interventionists meet with parents in their home 5 times during phase 2 to

Table 1 SPEEDI Intervention Description

Phase 1 (21 days starting when medically stable)	Phase 2 (12 weeks starting at the end of phase 1)
In NICU	Primarily at home, but started in NICU if not ready for discharge on day 21 post baseline.
5 intervention sessions provided by the parent and therapist jointly and in response to the infant's behavioral cues based on the synactive theory of development [31, 32].	Parents were encouraged to provided activities daily, with a goal of at least 20 min per day of activities 5 days per week, provided by the parent
33 Videos of positive and negative interaction available to parents throughout the phase 1 intervention as examples (Additional file 2)	An activity booklet (Additional file 3), with pictures, simple text, and a log for parent to record daily activities and questions was used to encourage parents to provide motor and cognitive opportunities daily in a variety of play positions, environments, and with objects [13].
Coaching on behavioral states, self-calming, environmental modification, and choosing times for feeding and play based interactions using dolls or video clips if the infant was not alert or fatigued	Parent encourage to provide the "just right challenge" advancing from stage 1 to stage 2 activities as they observed their infant improving or discuss with therapist at each visit
Provide experience with variable and self-directed movements and social interaction without physiological or behavioral stress. Introduced phase 2 activities by end of phase1	Physical Therapist participated in 5 parent-infant activity session over 12 weeks and helped with advancing from stage 1 to stage 2 activities as the infant was ready.
Guided participation used in identifying cues to stop, alter, or delay interactions during caregiving, feeding, play activities	Parent was encouraged to develop a daily routine for encouraging developmental play.

Over arching theme: Encouraging parents to provide the "just right challenge" by pacing intervention and the experiences provided based on the infant's behavioral state, signs of stress including autonomic, motor, or attention changes and demonstrated readiness for increasing duration or difficulty of developmental play skills

Key principles: Encourage self-initiated movement, variability, object interaction, and social interaction. Do not impose movement on the infant. Observe and respond to the infant's behavioral cues. (Additional file 1)

Key Strategies to support motor development during interactions: provide graded postural support, observe spontaneous movement in response to your support, vary postural support to encourage different opportunities and sensory input, vary positioned with the minimal support to encourage variable movements

support the parents' abilities to progress the intervention. Parents were encouraged to contact their interventionist with any questions or concerns between visits. The visit schedule was flexible to meet the family's needs, but the same number of visits were provided for all infants.

The study interventionists were both board certified pediatric physical therapist with extensive experience providing intervention in the NICU and in the first months of life. They were trained using a detailed manual, having previously participated in a feasibility study of SPEEDI, and met at regular intervals to discuss intervention strategies. To ensure ongoing adherence to the key principles of the intervention, the interventionists: 1) completed a fidelity checklist self-reflecting on whether they had covered the key intervention principles and used key intervention strategies (Table 1) after each phase 1 visits, 2) reflected on the parents' use of the key principle and strategies during the collaborative sessions in phase 2, and 3) 30% of the intervention sessions were video recorded and fidelity scored by the other interventionist. In order to track adherence and approximate dose of intervention provided by parents the data from the daily activity log within the activity booklet was used to compare anticipated with actual days of intervention and progression from stage 1 to stage 2 activities (Additional file 3).

Outcomes and follow up

All infants enrolled in the study were assessed on the same schedule by a physical therapist blind to group assignment who completed extensive training and reached reliability on all outcome measures prior to the study. The assessment schedule was baseline, End phase 1 (21 days after baseline), End phase 2 (12 weeks after End Phase 1), Follow up 1 (1 month after End phase 1, and Follow up 2 (2 months after follow up 1 or 3 months after End phase 2) (Table 2). A priori power analysis using data from a feasibility study determined a sample size of 14 infants, 7 per group, was needed to detect group differenced on the primary outcomes with alpha 0.10 and 80% power [33]. The secondary outcomes were included in the protocol to allow for further analysis and the estimation of effect sizes for future research.

Primary outcomes

Reaching skill

Reaching was assessed at end phase 2 and both follow up visits. The infant was positioned in an infant seat that provided trunk support and was reclined to 20 degrees while two synchronized video cameras placed at 45 degrees on the left and right sides were used to record the anteriolateral views of the infant's behavior. Reaching skill was assessed using four 30 s trials. An infant rattle was presented to the midline of the infant's chest at 75% of the infant's arm length. An additional eleven trials were presented under 3 conditions to explore early arm use, however these results are not presented in this manuscript as they were not directly related to the primary or secondary aims. Behavioral coders marked each time the infants' hand was in contact with a toy and the duration of each behavior was calculated using behavioral coding software.[1] A toy contact was coded whenever any portion of the infant's hand, distal to the wrist, was in contact with a toy, regardless of hand position. The two coders were blind to group assignment. On 20% of visits, reliability was calculated using a percentage agreement at each visit: [agreed/ (agreed + disagreed)] * 100. Intra rater and inter rater agreement for toy contact 95.4 and 97.0, respectively.

Exploratory problem-solving behaviors

Problem-solving behaviors were assessed using the Early Problem Solving Indicator (EPSI) at end phase 2 and both follow up visits. The EPSI is the cognitive subtest of the Individual Growth and Development Indicators designed to measure infant and toddler play-based problem-solving from 6 to 36 months of age. While the

Table 2 Assessment schedule

Domain	Baseline	End Phase 1	End Phase 2	Follow up 1	Follow up 2	12 months Adjusted Age
	Day 0	Day 21	Day 111 (15 weeks)	Day 141 (20 weeks)	Day 201 (29 weeks)	Target Day 382 –clinical visit
Therapy or EI Services	EMR	EMR	Parent survey	Parent survey	Parent survey	Clinical records
Seated Exploration and Reaching			Hands midline and Reaching	Hands midline and Reaching	Hands midline and Reaching	
Problem Solving			EPSI	EPSI	EPSI	
Motor	TIMP	TIMP	TIMP	TIMP	Bayley	Bayley
Cognition					Bayley	Bayley
Language					Bayley	Bayley

infants in this study were initially less than 6 months of age, the final study visit was at about 6 months of age and two of the four behaviors coded as part of the EPSI are commonly observed in young infants. So this tool was deemed the best available to document early-problem solving behaviors during play. The EPSI defines problem-solving as consisting of visual exploration, object manipulation and memory [34]. Previous studies with the EPSI show adequate reliability and validity, and usefulness in documenting change over time [35, 36]. During the EPSI, the infant was video-recorded interacting with 3 standard toys: pop-up animals toy, 6 seriated plastic cups, and a pound a ball game with a hammer and 4 balls. Infants were given each toy for 2 min while the examiner supported the child in sitting (pop up and cups) and prone (pound a ball) in order to sample 2 common play positions. If needed the examiner used a standard set of prompts such as tapping on the toy at a consistent frequency to engage or re-engage the infant in the standardized toy without demonstrating the use of the toy. The lead author has been certified by the EPSI developer to train blinded examiners and coders.

The frequency of 4 behaviors (look, explore, function, solution) were coded using definitions from the EPSI protocol. These behaviors were mutually exclusive, so only one behavior is coded at any time. Look was coded when the infant was looking at the toy. Explore was coded when the infant touched, manipulated, mouthed, rubbed, shook, pushed, pulled, banged, threw, or dropped the toy. A function was coded if the infants used the toy in a manner in which it was intended but does not require that the child complete all of the functions of the toy (e.g., moved one lever to make an animal pop up or nesting any 2 cups). A solution was coded if the infant used the toy in a way that its full functionality was displayed (e.g., moved all levers and buttons, so that all animals popped up or nesting all the cups in order). Two coders who were blinded to the infant's group assignment, recoded 20% of visits, including some from each of the 4 study visits, with an inter rater agreement of 94.0% and intra rater agreement of 97.7%. The total number of problem solving behaviors was calculated as a sum of look, explore, function, and solution for each infant at each visit to represent that infant's problem solving abilities.

Secondary outcome measures

Neuromotor control and development

The Test of Infant Motor Performance (TIMP) and Bayley Scales of Infant and Toddler Development, third edition (Bayley) were included, because they are commonly used clinical assessments in the population and ages included in this study. The TIMP was administered at the baseline, end of each phase of intervention, and at the first follow-up visit. TIMP raw score can ranges from 0 to 142. The Bayley was administered at the final follow-up visit and 3 months after the intervention ended [37, 38]. Normative values on the Bayley include Composite Scores for Cognitive, Language, and Motor with a mean of 100 and a standard deviation of 15. In order to quantify the longer-term outcomes, Bayley scores from the Neonatal Continuing Care Program at 12 months of adjusted age were extracted from the infant's medical record if available. All infants in this study meet the criteria for referral to this clinic and appointments were scheduled at NICU discharge. In all but 1 case, the examiner in the clinic was blinded to group assignment at the clinic visit.

Statistical analysis

Descriptive statistics were used to describe the study sample. The planned sample size and statistical significance was a priori set with an α level of 0.10 level to reduce the risk of missing small, but important group differences in this first efficacy study of SPEEDI (i.e., Type II error). To assess the primary outcomes of Toy contact (reaching) and Frequency of total problem-solving behaviors a repeated measures ANOVA (RMANOVA) [39] was fit using a mixed linear model (MLM). The model fit included a between subjects factor (Group: Intervention, Control), one within subject factor (Time: Assessment time point of end phase 2, follow up 1, and follow up 2) and the interaction between Group and Time. Post-hoc analysis of the types of problem solving behaviors was completed to quantify changes in exploratory problem solving not reflected in the total problem-solving behavior score. Secondary outcome measures were assessed to estimate effect sizes. Effect sizes were calculated using change in TIMP raw score from baseline to end phase 2 and to evaluate group differences on the Bayley Motor, Language, and Cognitive Composites at 3 months post intervention and at 12 months adjusted age. Due to the preliminary nature of this study, no corrections for multiple comparisons were used.

Results

Fourteen infants meet the inclusion criteria and enrolled. Median birth weight, gestational age, gender, race, ethnicity, and number of infants with a brain injury were similar between groups (Table 3). In the SPEEDI intervention group mothers were significantly younger, infants were sicker (higher NMI scores) and started the study at an older age (Table 3). The majority of mother's in both the groups reported living in poverty and did not have a college education. The majority of the sample was African American (Table 3).

Table 3 Description of subjects

	Total *n* = 14	Control *n* = 7	SPEEDI *n* = 7	*p*-value[e]
Maternal Age[b]	29.50 (27.00, 31.00)	31.00 (29.00, 42.00)	27.00 (23.00, 31.00)	0.05[d]
Maternal Education[a]				0.14[c]
HS or Less	46% (6/13)	33% (2/6)	57% (4/7)	
Some College	23% (3/13)	50% (3/6)	0% (0/7)	
College or More	31% (4/13)	17% (1/6)	43% (3/7)	
Household Income[a]				
< $24,000 (poverty)	50% (7/14)	57% (4/7)	43% (3/7)	1.00[c]
$24,001 - $ 36,000	50% (7/14)	43% (3/7)	57% (4/7)	
> $36,001 (1.5 time poverty)	0% (0/14)	0% (0/7)	0% (0/7)	
Gender Male[a]	57% (8/14)	43% (3/7)	71% (5/7)	0.59[c]
Birth Weight (g)[b]	795.00 (615.00, 1190.00)	840.00 (700.00, 320.00)	680.00 (580.00, 1190.00)	0.48[d]
Gestational Age (wks)[b]	25.50 (25.00, 27.00)	26.00 (25.00, 28.00)	25.00 (24.00, 27.00)	0.44[d]
Race[a]				
Caucasian	14% (2/14)	14% (1/7)	14% (1/7)	
African American	72% (10/14)	72% (5/7)	72% (5/7)	
Biracial	7% (1/14)	0% (0/7)	14% (1/7)	
Other	7% (1/14)	14% (1/7)	0% (0/7)	
Ethnicity[a]				
Hispanic	7% (1/14)	14% (1/7)	0% (0/7)	
Non-Hispanic	93% (13/14)	86% (6/7)	100% (7/7)	
IVH (Any grade)[a]	36% (5/14)	14% (1/7)	57% (4/7)	0.27[b]
IVH Grade 3 or 4[a]	14% (2/14)	14% (1/7)	14% (1/7)	1.00[b]
HIE[a]	7% (1/14)	14% (1/7)	0% (0/7)	1.00[c]
PVL[a]	14% (2/14)	0% (0/7)	29% (2/7)	0.46[b]
Days in NICU[b]	116.50 (93.00, 125.00)	93.00 (65.00, 107.00)	125.00 (116.00, 126.00)	0.14[d]
NMI Rating[b]	5.00 (4.00, 5.00)	5.00 (4.00, 5.00)	5.00 (5.00, 5.00)	0.06[d]
Adjusted Age[b]				
Baseline (weeks of gestation)	38 (35, 39)	35 (35, 39)	39 (36, 40)	0.05[d]
End Phase 1 (weeks of gestation)	40 (38, 42)	38 (38, 41)	42 (40, 43)	0.05[d]
End phase 2 (weeks of adjusted age or beyond 40 weeks of gestational age)	13.5 (11.0, 15.0)	13.0 (11.0, 14.0)	15.0 (13.0, 15.0)	0.28[d]
Follow-up 1 (1 month after intervention)	18.0 (16.0, 19.0)	16.0 (15.0, 18.0)	19.0 (18.0, 20.0)	0.09[d]

Notes: [a]Percent (n/total)
[b]Median (IQR)
[c]Fisher's Exact Test
[d]Mann-Whitney U Test (Wilcoxon Rank-sum test)
[e]Between Group Differences Unadjusted for multiple comparisons

A total of 4 infants, 2 in each group and 2 with brain injury, did not complete the study. Three infants were lost while still in the NICU, 1 infant in each group was unable to continue for medical reasons and 1 infant in the intervention group withdrew after the baseline assessment. The data for these 3 infants were excluded from all outcome assessment. One additional infant, from the usual care group, could not be reached for follow up visits after NICU discharge thus only his baseline and end phase 1 data (TIMP only) were included (Fig. 1).

Description of usual care

Fifty percent of the infants enrolled in the study were receiving therapy services in the NICU at baseline. Infants received a mean of 6.0 visits (range 2–12) from PT and 3.8 visits (range 0–7) from OT during the 21 days of Phase 1

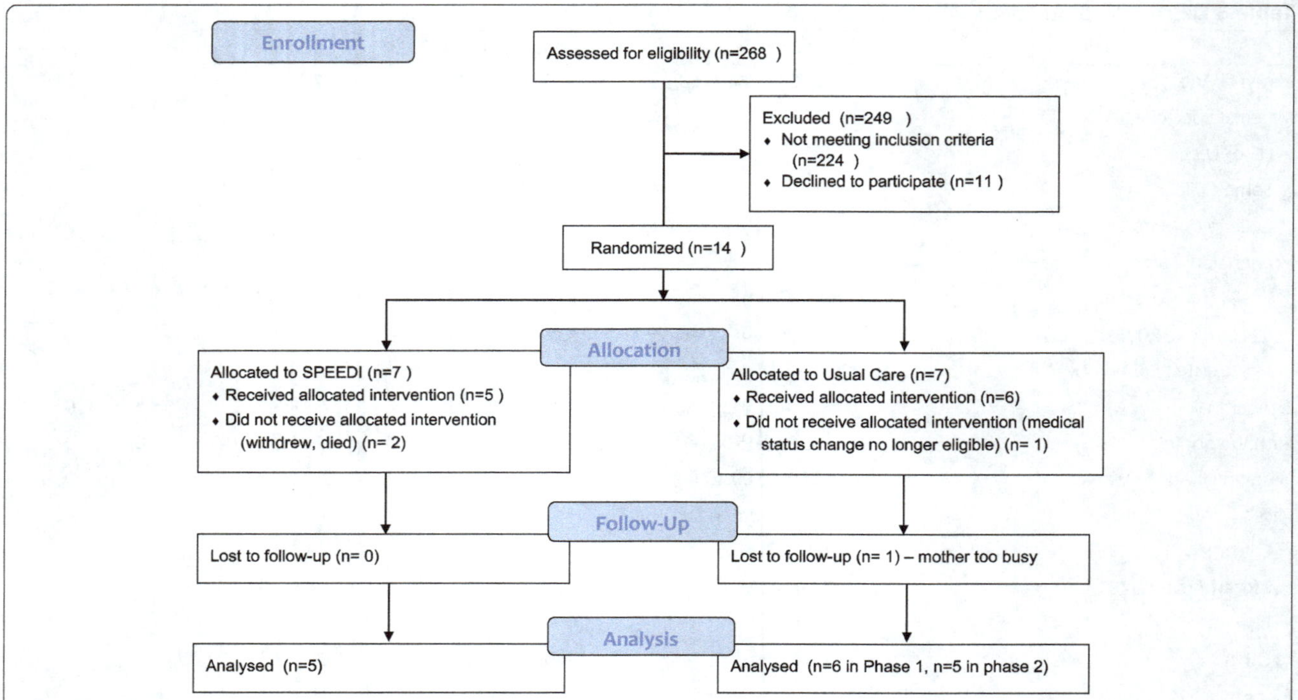

Fig. 1 CONSORT Flow chart. This flow chart showing the recruitment and retention of participants in each arm of the clinical trial

of this study. All infants, except 1 in the SPEEDI group, had been assessed for EI services by follow up 1. Only 4 of the infants were receiving direct therapy services, 3 in the control group, with an average of 1.4 therapy visits per month planned based on parent report.

Fidelity of SPEEDI intervention

The SPEEDI therapist's adherence to the key principles of SPEEDI was 87.9% on self report and 86.5% scored by a second rater. All phase 1 sessions were completed with a mean duration of 45 min. During 4 out of 25 sessions, limited infant alertness necessitated discussion and simulation rather than interaction with the infant. The 7 key principle of the intervention were reviewed an average of 3.6 times each during Phase 1. Each of the 4 intervention strategies were used an average of 3.7 times over the 5 sessions and an average of 3.0 strategies were used per sessions.

During Phase 2, infants received all 5 parent/therapist home based intervention sessions with a mean duration of 35 min. During 1 session with 3 different infants, the infant was too sleepy for the parent to demonstrate the SPEEDI intervention activities during the phase 2 sessions. The therapist and parent talked about the parents observations and simulated the activities as needed during these sessions. Parents addressed a mean of 5.6 key principles per session with principles being addressed a mean of 4.0 out of a possible 5 times during phase 2. Each of the 4 key intervention strategies were used an average of 3.9 times with an average of 3.1 key strategies used in each session.

Parent/infant dyads were expected to document 53 days of intervention between the end of phase 1 assessment visit and the last intervention visit. Parent documented a mean of 63.8 session (range 52–68) or 120% of the anticipated days of intervention. There was a gradual progression in the difficulty of the opportunities parents documented providing. Three of the 5 infants progressed through all activities while 2 infants continued to work on a stage 1 activity. Parents retained the activity booklet and were asked to continue the activities until the end of phase 2 outcome visit.

Primary outcomes

Reaching skill

Infants in both groups increased the duration they were in contact with the toy during the reaching trials with increasing age. ($F = 5.33$, $p = 0.02$) There was no significant Group-Time interaction ($F_{2,16} = 0.32$, $p = 0.73$) and no group differences in the duration of toy contact. However, infant in the SPEEDI group were in contact with the toy for a mean of 28.02 (16.3) out of 30 s in comparison to the usual care group 20.2 (21.45) seconds, 1 months after the intervention ended. Thus, the SPEEDI group approached a ceiling on this measure. The effect sizes for duration of toy contact were 0.11, 0.41, and 0.38 at endphase 2, followup 1 and followup 2 respectively suggesting a small but measureable effect of the intervention.

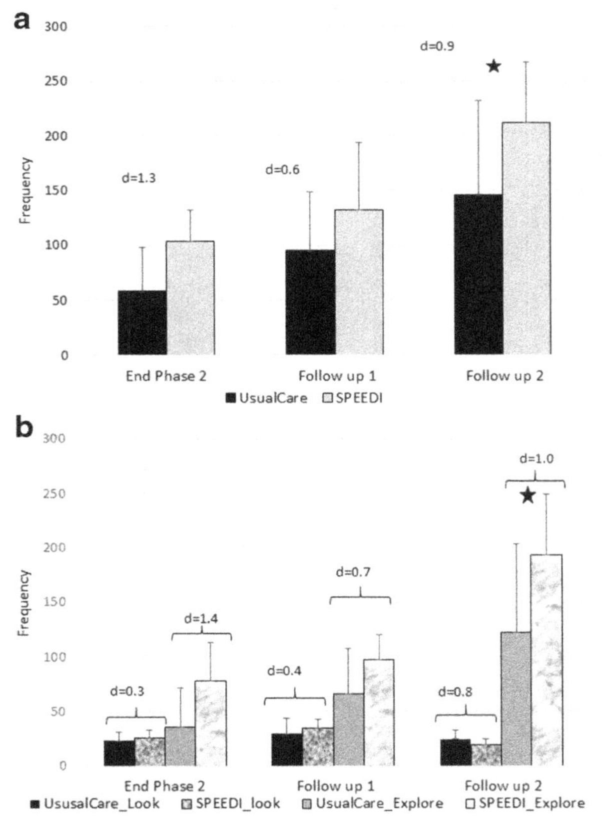

Fig. 2 Problem Solving Outcomes. The frequency of problem solving behaviors during a 6-min interaction with 3 standardized toys. A: total problem solving behaviors. B: frequency of looks and explores, 2 specific types of problem solving behaviors. Star represented statistically significant group differences. Error bar represent 1 standard deviation from the mean. The effect size (d) for each comparison is included

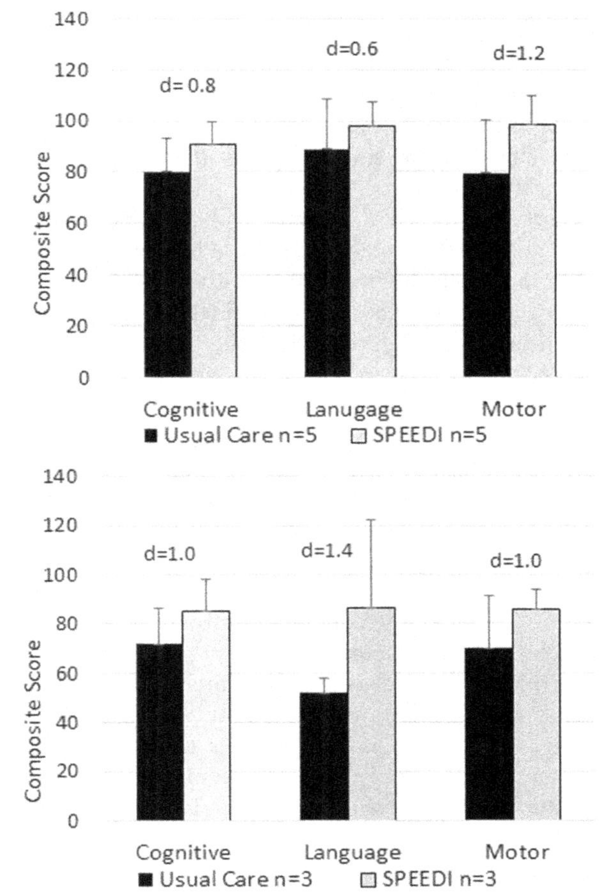

Fig. 3 Global Development Outcomes. The Bayley composite score 3 months post intervention and at 12 months of age, approximately 9 months post intervention are provided for the Cognitive, Language (expressive and receptive), and Motor (Gross and Fine) domains. The 9 month post intervention visits includes infants who attended the Neonatal Continuing Care Program clinic visit and had a completed Bayley. Two infant in the SPEEDI group and 1 in the usual care group did not attend the clinic visit. One infant in the usual care group attended the clinic but could not complete the Bayley due to significant motor impairments

Exploratory problem-solving behaviors

Early problem solving behaviors increased in frequency with age in both groups (Fig. 2a and b). There is no significant group-time interaction for the sum of all early problem solving behaviors. However there was a significant group ($F_{1,8} = 4.04$, $p = 0.08$) and time effect ($F_{2,17} = 9.76$, $p < 0.01$, Fig. 2a). The Cohen D effects size for total problem solving behaviors and explore at the end of the intervention and during follow up were moderate to large (range 0.6 to 1.4, Figure 2a and b).

Secondary outcomes

Neuromotor control and development

TIMP change in raw scores from baseline to the end of the intervention had a large effect size (d = 1.04). Longer-term global development outcomes on the Bayley had moderate to large effect sizes approximately 9 months post intervention at the 12 month adjusted age clinical assessment visit (Fig. 3a and b).

Discussion

This initial efficacy randomized clinical trial suggest that intervention, such as SPEEDI, empowering parents to implement a daily routine of parent supported movement opportunities and environmental enrichment, has the potential to enhance development, even after the intervention has ended. Recent rehabilitation research on the treatment of children with motor impairments has emphasized the need for task specific and self-initiated movements to enhance learning [12, 40–42]. Parents of infants in the SPEEDI group were encouraged to identify ideal times to interact, set up the environment to provide a "just right challenge," and support their infants self-initiated movements through a variety of activities. Based on parental adherence during collaborative parent, therapists, and infant sessions during phase 2 and the parent's activities logs, the parents were able to utilize this training and incorporate these principles into their daily routine.

Infants adapt their arm and hand movements weeks before the onset of reaching [43]. While infant in both group increased their contact with toys during the reaching trials, infants in the SPEEDI group appear to have hit a plateau limiting the ability to quantify group differences. However, moderate to large effect sizes for the TIMP and the motor composite of the Bayley suggest that infants in the SPEEDI group had motor outcome scores higher than the usual care group, which might be statistically different with a larger sample size or with additional assessment of reaching earlier in the study period.

The majority of cognitive or problem solving assessments in infants and children required and are influenced by a child's motor function [44, 45]. Likewise, a child's ability to learn through interaction with the world can be influenced by motor impairments. All infants in this study improved their exploratory problem solving, primarily their exploration of objects, over the 3 months following the end of the intervention. However, the large effect sizes at all assessments, and statistically significant difference at follow up 2, suggest that infants in the SPEEDI group were able to demonstrate a higher frequency of exploratory problem solving behavior than the infants in the usual care group. While there is a requirement for motor activity to "explore" on the EPSI that may have contributed to the improved scores, the infants in the SPEEDI group appear to have higher cognitive scores at 3 and 9 months after the intervention reflected by the large effect sizes on the Bayley, supporting these initial efficacy finding on the EPSI.

While the results of this study are not conclusive and further study is needed, the SPEEDI intervention is consistent with current motor learning and developmental theory increasing the likelihood these findings are not extraneous. SPEEDI focuses around a few central tasks including support for infant initiated midline head and arm control, reaching, and object exploration in supine, sidelying, and prone. When the intervention started, most infants were unable to perform any of these tasks independently. However, the infants in this study had been moving in the extra uterine world for up to 16 weeks before starting this study. While not assessed in this study, interventions like SPEEDI may provide opportunities for activity dependent neuroplasticity to enhance the retention of the corticospinal fibers in infants with brain injury or immaturity and limit negative plasticity associated with a lack of variable movements [11]. In combination with supporting parents ability to provide daily opportunities' to their infant, SPEEDI used a motor learning approach to increase repetitions of self-initiated movements that would not be possible in these infants without the environmental enrichment and support provided by the therapists or caregivers.

This initial evidence for the efficacy of SPEEDI challenges the current "wait and see" approach to early intervention and the medical community [9, 46]. SPEEDI is a feasible intervention if NICUs and state and federally supported early intervention program work together to ensure parents are given adequate information on the importance of providing an enriched environment, appropriately timed interactions, and support to enhance variable self-initiated movements. This cannot be done through a single session or generalized intervention strategies [47]. Parents appear to benefit from ongoing help to develop routines during the transition from the NICU to home that may lead to a decrease in the need for future services.

Limitations

As a pilot and first efficacy study of this intervention, we planned to use an $\alpha = 0.10$ for the primary outcome measures without correction of multiple comparisons in post-hoc testing. This limited our ability to conclude definitively on the efficacy of this intervention. The sample size was smaller than initially intended due to the loss of 4 enrolled infants. The inclusion of infant with significant brain injury and chronic lung disease resulted in 2 medical status changes that could not have been anticipated. These combined with the 2 voluntary drop outs reduced our sample to lower than the 7 infants per group needed to meet our planned power. We have included the effect sizes for the outcome assessments to enhance the readers' ability to interpret the results with this small sample size. In addition, the loss of 2 infants with brain injuries eliminated our ability to do any type of sub-analysis to look at the efficacy of SPEEDI for infants with and without brain injury. Thus further data is needed on the efficacy of SPEEDI for infants at the highest risk of having CP. The planned use of reaching as a primary outcome, when the infants in the SPEEDI group reached a plateau limited our ability to fully describe group differences on the primary outcome measures. Infants in the SPEEDI group were more medically fragile resulting in an older gestational age before initiating intervention. Thus, it is possible that the group differences are not the result of the intervention, but

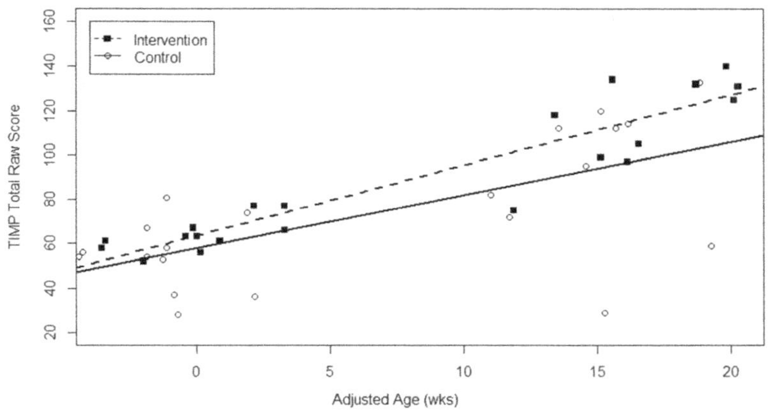

Fig. 4 Group Differences in Motor Development with Increasing Age. The individual scores on the TIMP and predicted regression lines from the post hoc MLM with a significant interaction term. Suggests the rate of development was impacted by changes in age and group assignment

are related to the older age of these infants at each data point. We addressed this where possible by evaluating change scores and plan to statistically control for age in future studies. In an attempt to evaluate the initial efficacy of SPEEDI controlling for age at assessment, we did a post-hoc analysis of the TIMP raw scores using a MLM including group, adjusted age at assessment, and an interaction term. The TIMP was our only measure that could be assessed from baseline to 1 month post intervention and thus was selected as the optimal measure for this post-hoc analysis. The interaction term was significant ($F_{1,29} = 3.24$, $p = 0.08$), Fig. 4. Using the predicted model from the MLM infants in the SPEEDI group gained 16.9 point more than the control group from baseline to 1 month post intervention ($p = 0.07$). This further supports the initial efficacy of SPEEDI, but requires additional research due to the preliminary and post-hoc nature of this analysis. While parent's impressions of this intervention were not systematically collected in this study, they were in the feasibility study. Parents in the feasibility study reports that completing the activities daily was hard immediately post discharge but helped it become part of their routine interaction within a few weeks [33]. Additional qualitative study of group differences in parental impressions of the interventions would be beneficial in future studies.

Future research is need on the efficacy of SPEEDI to impact long term developmental outcomes in infant born very preterm, the need for future rehabilitation services, and quantification of changes in parent child interactions. A larger study of SPEEDI, including a comparison of the efficacy of SPEEDI for infant at the highest risk of CP, is in development and is needed before the efficacy of SPEEDI can be fully described.

Conclusions

SPEEDI appears to have some benefit for infant born very preterm contributing to exploratory problem solving skills in the first months of life. Further research is needed, but preliminary evidence is promising, on the impact of SPEEDI on motor outcomes in infancy.

Additional files

Additional file 1: Guiding Principles for SPEEDI Intervention. Includes the theoretical model and list of key principles of the Supporting Play Exploration and Early Development Intervention (SPEEDI).

Additional file 2: List of Videos SPEEDI Phase 1. Lists the names and length of the videos provided to parents in SPEEDI Phase 1. These videos were available to the parents on an ipad or laptop computer for use during the 21 days of Phase 1 intervention. Parents were asked to watch all the videos at least 1 time, but had access to watch them as often as they wanted.

Additional file 3: SPEEDI Activity Booklet. Includes the text from the SPEEDI activity booklet provided to parents toward the end of phase 1, for implementation in phase 2. Parents used the activity log in this appendix to document which activities were completed each day during Phase 2 of the SPEEDI intervention.

Abbreviations

CP: Cerebral palsy; EI: Early intervention governed by the US individuals with disability educational improvement act; EMR: Electronic medical record; EPSI: Early problem solving indicator; MLM: Mixed linear model; NICU: Neonatal intensive care unit; RMANOVA: A repeated measures analysis of variance; SPEEDI: Supporting play exploration and early development intervention; TIMP: Test of infant motor performance

Acknowledgements

Thank you to Shaaron Brown, Cathy Van Drew, Theresa Izzo, Alison Owens, Hayley Parson and the staff of the Motor Development Lab for your help with data collection, outcome assessment, and behavioral coding for this study. We are grateful to the families who participated in this study for sharing in the growth and development of their infant during a busy time in their lives.

Funding
Funding provided by the Foundation for Physical Therapy and the Children's Hospital of Richmond Foundation. The funding sources had no influence in the study design, implementation, analysis, or publication of the results.

Authors' contributions
SD contributed to all aspect of this project including funding, study design, data collection, interpretation and dissemination. TT contributed to data collection, behavioral coding, interpretation, and dissemination. EM contributed to behavioral coding, interpretation, and dissemination. LT contributed to study design, analysis, interpretation, and dissemination. LB contributed to study design, data collection, interpretation and dissemination, KHM contributed to study design and participant medical status clearance. All authors read and approved the final manuscript.

Competing interests
The authors declare that they have no competing interests.

Author details
[1]Department of Physical Therapy, Motor Development Lab, Virginia Commonwealth University, Office: 1200 E Broad St. B106, PO BOX 980224, Richmond, VA 23298, USA. [2]Rehabilitation and Movement Sciences Program, Virginia Commonwealth University, Richmond, USA. [3]Schools of Nursing and Medicine, Virginia Commonwealth University, Richmond, USA. [4]School of Nursing, Virginia Commonwealth University, Richmond, USA. [5]Children's Hospital of Richmond, Virginia Commonwealth University, Richmond, USA.

References
1. McCormick MC, Litt JS, Smith VC, Zupancic JA. Prematurity: an overview and public health implications. Annu Rev Public Health. 2010;32:367–79.
2. Wocadlo C, Rieger I. Educational and therapeutic resource dependency at early school-age in children who were born very preterm. Early Hum Dev. 2006;82(1):29–37.
3. Kuban KC, Allred EN, O'Shea TM, Paneth N, Pagano M, Dammann O, Leviton A, Du Plessis A, Westra SJ, Miller CR, et al. Cranial ultrasound lesions in the NICU predict cerebral palsy at age 2 years in children born at extremely low gestational age. J Child Neurol. 2009;24(1):63–72.
4. MacKay DF, Smith GC, Dobbie R, Pell JP. Gestational age at delivery and special educational need: retrospective cohort study of 407,503 schoolchildren. PLoS Med. 2010;7(6):e1000289.
5. Wong T, Taylor HG, Klein N, Espy KA, Anselmo MG, Minich N, Hack M. Kindergarten classroom functioning of extremely preterm/extremely low birth weight children. Early Hum Dev. 2014;90(12):907–14.
6. Iwata S, Nakamura T, Hizume E, Kihara H, Takashima S, Matsuishi T, Iwata O. Qualitative brain MRI at term and cognitive outcomes at 9 years after very preterm birth. Pediatrics. 2012;129(5):e1138–47.
7. Allen MC, Cristofalo EA, Kim C. Outcomes of preterm infants: morbidity replaces mortality. Clin Perinatol. 2011;38(3):441–54.
8. Orton J, Spittle A, Doyle L, Anderson P, Boyd R. Do early intervention programmes improve cognitive and motor outcomes for preterm infants after discharge? A systematic review. Dev Med Child Neurol. 2009;51(11):851–9.
9. Johnston MV. Plasticity in the developing brain: implications for rehabilitation. Dev Disabil Res Rev. 2009;15(2):94–101.
10. Nadeau SE, Wu SS, Dobkin BH, Azen SP, Rose DK, Tilson JK, Cen SY, Duncan PW. Effects of task-specific and impairment-based training compared with usual care on functional walking ability after inpatient stroke rehabilitation: LEAPS trial. Neurorehabil Neural Repair. 2013;27(4):370–80.
11. Martin JH, Chakrabarty S, Friel KM. Harnessing activity-dependent plasticity to repair the damaged corticospinal tract in an animal model of cerebral palsy. Dev Med Child Neurol. 2011;53(Suppl 4):9–13.
12. Morgan C, Novak I, Badawi N. Enriched environments and motor outcomes in cerebral palsy: systematic review and meta-analysis. Pediatrics. 2013; 132(3):e735–46.
13. Lobo MA, Harbourne RT, Dusing SC, McCoy SW. Grounding early intervention: physical therapy cannot just be about motor skills anymore. Phys Ther. 2013;93(1):94–103.
14. Marlow N, Hennessy EM, Bracewell MA, Wolke D. Motor and executive function at 6 years of age after extremely preterm birth. Pediatrics. 2007; 120(4):793–804.
15. Korkman M, Mikkola K, Ritari N, Tommiska V, Salokorpi T, Haataja L, Tammela O, Paakkonen L, Olsen P, Fellman V. Neurocognitive test profiles of extremely low birth weight five-year-old children differ according to neuromotor status. Dev Neuropsychol. 2008;33(5):637–55.
16. Kodric J, Sustersic B, Paro-Panjan D. Assessment of general movements and 2.5 year developmental outcomes: pilot results in a diverse preterm group. Eur J Paediatr Neurol. 2010;14(2):131–7.
17. Soska KC, Adolph KE, Johnson SP. Systems in development: motor skill acquisition facilitates three-dimensional object completion. Dev Psychol. 2010;46(1):129–38.
18. Adolph K, Berger S. Motor Development. In: Kuhn D, Siegler R, editors. Handbook of child psychology: Vol 2: Cognition, perception, and language. 6 edn. New York: Wiley; 2006. p. 161–213.
19. James KH, Swain SN. Only self-generated actions create sensori-motor systems in the developing brain. Dev Sci. 2011;14(4):673–8.
20. Von Hofsten C. Action, the foundation for cognitive development. Scand J Psychol. 2009;50(6):617–23.
21. Gibson EJ. Exploratory behavior in the development of perceiving, acting, and the acquiring of knowledge. Annu Rev Psychol. 1988;39(1):1.
22. Harbourne RT, Deffeyes JE, Kyvelidou A, Stergiou N. Complexity of postural control in infants: linear and nonlinear features revealed by principal component analysis. Nonlinear Dynamics Psychol Life Sci. 2009;13(1):123–44.
23. Fallang B, Oien I, Hellem E, Saugstad OD, Hadders-Algra M. Quality of reaching and postural control in young preterm infants is related to neuromotor outcome at 6 years. Pediatr Res. 2005;58(2):347–53.
24. Plantinga Y, Perdock J, de Groot L. Hand function in low-risk preterm infants: its relation to muscle power regulation. Dev Med Child Neurol. 1997;39(1):6–11.
25. Dusing S, Mercer V, Yu B, Reilly M, Thorpe D. Trunk position in supine of infants born preterm and at term: an assessment using a computerized pressure mat. Pediatr Phys Ther. 2005;17(1):2–10.
26. Dusing S, Kyvelidou A, Mercer VS, Stergiou N. Infants born preterm exhibit different patterns of Center of Pressure Movement than Infants Born at term. Phys Ther. 2009;89(12):1354–62.
27. Dusing SC, Harbourne RT. Variability in postural control during infancy: implications for development, assessment, and intervention. Phys Ther. 2010;90(12):1838–49.
28. Spittle A, Orton J, Anderson PJ, Boyd R, Doyle LW. Early developmental intervention programmes provided post hospital discharge to prevent motor and cognitive impairment in preterm infants. Cochrane Database Syst Rev. 2015;11:CD005495.
29. Korner AF, Stevenson DK, Kraemer HC, Spiker D, Scott DT, Constantinou J, Dimiceli S. Prediction of the development of low birth weight preterm infants by a new neonatal medical index. J Dev Behav Pediatr. 1993;14(2):106–11.
30. Individuals with Disabilities Education Improvement Act. In.; 2004. http://www.copyright.gov/legislation/pl108-446.pdf.
31. Als H, Gilkerson L. The role of relationship-based developmentally supportive newborn intensive care in strengthening outcome of preterm infants. Semin Perinatol. 1997;21(3):178–89.
32. Als H. A synactive model of neonatal behavioral organization: framework for the assessment of neurobehavioral development in the premature infant and for support of infants and parents in the neonatal intensive care environment. Physical & Occupational Therapy in Pediatrics. 1986;6(2–3):3–53.
33. Dusing S, Brown S, Van Drew C, Thacker L, Hendricks-Munoz K. Supporting play exploration and early development intervention (SPEEDI) from NICU to home: a feasibility study. Pediatr Phys Ther. 2015;27(3):267–74.
34. Greenwood C, Walker D, Carta JJ, Higgins SK. Developing a general outcome measure of growth in cognitive abilities of children 1 to 4 years old: the early problem solving indicator. Sch Psychol Rev. 2006;35:536–51.

35. Carta J, Greenwood C, Walker D KR, Good R, McConnell S, et al. (2002) .4: 15–28.: Individual growth and development indicators (IGDIs): Assessment that guides intervention for youngchildren. In: *Young Except Child Mono Series.* vol. 4. Denver, CO: Sopris West.; 2002: 15-28.
36. O'Grady MG, Dusing SC. Reliability and validity of play-based assessments of motor and cognitive skills for infants and young children: a systematic review. Phys Ther. 2014. Public Law 108-443, STAT. 2647, 2004 July 15, 2013.
37. Campbell S. The test of infant motor performance: test User's manual version 2.0 vol. 37. Chicago, IL: Infant Motor Performance Scales, LLC; 2005.
38. Campbell SK, Levy P, Zawacki L, Liao P-j: Population-based age standards for interpreting results on the test of motor infant performance. Pediatric Physical Therapy Summer 2006, 18(2):119-125. PMID: 16735859.
39. Wolfinger R. A tutorial on mixed models, TS-260. Cary, NC: SAS Institute, Inc; 1992.
40. Morgan C, Darrah J, Gordon AM, Harbourne R, Spittle A, Johnson R, Fetters L. Effectiveness of motor interventions in infants with cerebral palsy: a systematic review. Dev Med Child Neurol. 2016;58(9):900-9. https://doi.org/10.1111/dmcn.13105.
41. Novak I, McIntyre S, Morgan C, Campbell L, Dark L, Morton N, Stumbles E, Wilson S-A, Goldsmith S. A systematic review of interventions for children with cerebral palsy: state of the evidence. Developmental Medicine & Child Neurology. 2013;55(10):885–910.
42. Valvano J. Activity-focused motor interventions for children with neurological conditions. Phys Occup Ther Pediatr. 2004;24(1–2):79–107.
43. Bhat AN, Galloway JC. Toy-oriented changes during early arm movements: hand kinematics. Infant Behav Dev. 2006;29(3):358–72.
44. Bayley N. Bayley scales of infant and toddler development, 3rd edition. 3rd ed. San Antonio, TX: PsychCorp; 2006.
45. O'Grady MG, Dusing SC. Assessment position affects problem-solving behaviors in a child with motor impairments. Pediatr Phys Ther. 2016;28(2):253–8.
46. Rosenberg SA, Robinson CC, Shaw EF, Ellison MC. Part C early intervention for infants and toddlers: percentage eligible versus served. Pediatrics. 2013; 131(1):38–46.
47. Dusing SC, Murray T, Stern M. Parent preferences for motor development education in the neonatal intensive care unit. Pediatr Phys Ther. 2008;20(4):363–8.

10

Transcapillary fluid flux and inflammatory response during neonatal therapeutic hypothermia

Hans Jørgen Timm Guthe[1,2*], Torbjørn Nedrebø[3,6], Jan Kristian Damås[4,5], Helge Wiig[6] and Ansgar Berg[1,2]

Abstract

Background: Therapeutic hypothermia is neuroprotective in asphyxiated neonates by counteracting mechanisms contributing to brain injury. Although an initial increased permeability is part of an inflammatory reaction and thereby a natural healing process, an excessive endothelial permeability with edema formation may result in impaired hemodynamics. Reduced permeability may, however, benefit healing. Although plasma and interstitial colloid osmotic pressure are accessible and essential parameters for understanding fluid imbalance, the mechanisms of fluid exchange remain poorly understood. The potential influence of therapeutic hypothermia on plasma and interstitial colloid osmotic pressure, and the relationship between inflammatory markers and colloid osmotic pressure in asphyxiated neonates, was investigated.

Methods: Seventeen neonates with moderate to severe hypoxic ischemic encephalopathy, born after 35 weeks gestation, received servo-controlled whole body cooling before 6 h of age, followed by gradual rewarming after 72 h. All infants were treated according to a national hypothermia protocol. Interstitial fluid in the skin was collected at 7, 13, 25, 49, and 73 h after birth by subcutaneous implantation of multifilamentous nylon wicks with 60 min of implantation time. Biomarkers of inflammation and colloid osmotic pressure were measured in serum and interstitial fluid.

Results: A modest decrease in serum and interstitial colloid osmotic pressure was measured, leaving an unaltered difference in colloid osmotic pressure gradient. A decline in mean arterial pressure was observed between 7 and 13 h of life, with a concomitant decrease in positive fluid balance within the same time frame. White blood cell count and leukocyte subclasses dropped significantly throughout treatment, with elevated interstitial interleukin (IL)-1α and decreased serum IL-1RA, IL-6, and IL-10 during treatment time points.

Conclusions: Colloid osmotic pressures measured in serum and interstitial fluid during asphyxia is lower than previously reported, with small alteration of pressure differences across capillaries, reducing vascular filtration. An inherent local and systemic regulation of inflammation together with changes in colloid osmotic pressure may indicate a possible preventive mechanism of edema generation during neonatal asphyxia and therapeutic hypothermia.

Keywords: Neonate, Osmotic pressure, Edema, Asphyxia, Therapeutic hypothermia, Inflammation, Cytokines

* Correspondence: hjgu@helse-bergen.no
[1]Department of Pediatrics and Adolescent Medicine, Haukeland University Hospital, Bergen, Norway
[2]Department of Clinical Science, University of Bergen, Bergen, Norway

Background

Hypoxic ischemic encephalopathy (HIE) due to perinatal asphyxia is an important cause of childhood neurodevelopmental deficits that include loss of motor and cognitive functions [1, 2]. Hypoxic ischemia could be involved in the injuries correlating with HIE by initiating a detrimental inflammatory response, partly through the release of reactive oxygen species and amplified by inflammatory cytokines. Several clinical studies and reports from experimental models have shown that immune pathogenic mechanisms may play an essential role in HIE by affecting both the central nervous system and systemic circulation [3–6]. Therapeutic hypothermia (TH) induces an artificial reduction of core and brain temperature to 33.5 °C. This results in reduced cerebral and whole-body metabolism, followed by attenuation of oxidative stress after hypoxemia [7]. Several studies have shown that TH also provides neuroprotection in neonates with moderate to severe HIE [8, 9], potentially through favorable effects on multiple pathways contributing to brain injury. Thus, TH has been demonstrated to induce an anti-inflammatory response with reduced amounts of circulating leukocytes and chemokines in neonates with HIE, as well as in animal models [5, 10]. This inhibiting effect of the immune system in response to TH may be protective against the over-functioning immune reaction observed in these children [11]. Moreover, hypothermia has been shown to have beneficial effects on capillary integrity, as evidenced by reduced accumulation of interstitial fluid (IF) through decreased endothelial permeability, in rats after hemorrhagic shock [12]. However, increased intravascular hydrostatic pressure, due to TH-induced peripheral vasoconstriction, along with reduced venous return [13], could theoretically result in interstitial accumulation of fluid. Few studies have addressed these mechanisms of fluid imbalance during TH in neonates, and cytokine concentrations in the cellular microenvironment have not been previously measured. Because plasma colloid osmotic pressure (COP_p) and interstitial colloid osmotic pressure (COP_i) are essential determinants of fluid exchange during edema formation [14], we herein examined whether TH influenced these parameters in neonates with HIE, expecting a reduced COP_p as reported in sick neonates [15]. We also explored the association between COP_p and COP_i and inflammatory processes during TH by measuring a wide panel of cytokines in the plasma and IF.

Methods

Ethics

The study was approved by the Regional Committees for Medical and Health Research Ethics, Western Norway, and was conducted at the Neonatal Intensive Care Unit (NICU), Haukeland University Hospital, Bergen, Norway. All patients were included in the study following written informed consent obtained from a parent or guardian after explanation of the study in accordance with the Declaration of Helsinki. The study trial was registered in ClinicalTrials.gov (ClinicalTrials.gov Identifier: NCT01044940).

Study population

The study was an open, longitudinal, observational study, taking place between June 2009 and October 2014. Newborns treated with TH owing to moderate and severe HIE were included after fulfillment of national inclusion criteria for neonatal TH. Inclusion and exclusion criteria are presented in Table 1.

Clinical management

All recruited patients were, as part of the clinical routine, sedated with morphine or fentanyl and intubated after delivery or before transport from referring hospitals at the attending physicians discretion. Rectal temperature was continuously monitored, with a target body temperature between 34 and 36 °C before TH. All patients received prophylactic antibiotics (penicillin and gentamycin) throughout TH, and scheduled clinical and biochemical monitoring was performed by the attending physician discretion.

Neonatal TH protocol

TH was conducted according to the hospital hypothermia protocol. Induction and maintenance of hypothermia was achieved by servo-controlled whole body cooling equipment (Criticool; Mtre, Yavne, Israel) and the core

Table 1 Criteria for inclusion of therapeutic hypothermia

Inclusion criteria	Exclusion Criteria
A: Gestational age ≥ 36 weeks	Expected need for surgical treatment (before 3 days of age)
B: At least one of the following:	Severe birth defects with expected poor prognosis
1. Apgar score ≤ 5 at 10 min after birth	
2. Requires positive pressure ventilation 10 min after birth	
3. pH < 7.00 in umbilical arterial blood or arterial blood within 60 min after birth	
4. Base excess ≤ − 16 in umbilical arterial blood or arterial blood within 60 min after birth	
C: Signs of moderate to severe encephalopathy with at least one of the following:	Age > 6 h before hypothermia could be initiated
1. Hypotonia	
2. Abnormal reflexes or constricted/ deviated, dilated, nonreactive to light pupils	
3. Weak or absent sucking reflex	
4. Presence of seizures	

temperature was reduced to 33.5 °C before 6 h of age and maintained until 72 h after birth. The rectal temperature was not allowed to increase more than 0.3 °C per hour during rewarming. After rewarming, rectal temperature was monitored for 24 h to prevent rebound hyperthermia. Patients with the expected poorest prognosis (in extremis) underwent magnetic resonance imaging (MRI) during cooling (second or third day of TH). Otherwise, imaging took place at day 4 to 7. Cerebral ultrasound was conducted during the first 3 days and before discharge.

Intensive care monitoring and treatment

Patients were treated in an open-radiant infant warmer incubator (Dräger Babytherm 8010, Dräger Medical, Lübeck, Germany) with the heating blanket and radiant warmer turned off. TH data were recorded according to local protocols and monitoring was performed (Intellivue MP70 Neonatal, Philips, Eidhoven, Nederland) with continuous arterial pressure, oxygen saturation, heart rate, and respiration registration. All patients were monitored with an amplitude-integrated electroencephalogram to assess cerebral function within 3–6 h after TH initiation. From January 2011 onward, ventilation therapy was provided by Dräger Babylog® VN500 (Dräger Medical, Lübeck, Germany) with the pressure- and assist-controlled, volume-guaranty mode. Prior to 2011, the Stephanie Neonatal and Paediatric ventilator (Stephan, Gackenback, Germany) was utilized, with the pressure-controlled synchronized intermittent mandatory ventilation mode. Morphine sedation was administered throughout treatment if the patient showed signs of improvement during TH. Otherwise, if expected poor prognosis, sedation was halted and early MRI was performed. All neonates received the recommended reduced fluid intake [16] of approximately 40 ml/kg/day adjusted to weight, urine output, and serum sodium levels. Intravenously administered fluids consisted of isotonic saline (NaCl 9 mg/ml), glucose (concentration range of 100 mg/ml to 300 mg/ml, adjusted to a calculated need of 6 mg/kg/min), and blood products according to the patients' requirements. Enteral feeding was not established during TH. The calculation of fluid balance was based on the total amount of fluid intravenously administered and measurements of hourly diuresis (urinary catheter) and gastric aspiration. Daily weight was not measured due to attached technical equipment, and fluid loss from respiratory evaporation or obvious fluid accumulation during TH was deemed not feasible due to the clinical setting. If the mean arterial pressure (MAP) was < 40 mmHg, and a fluid load of 9 mg/ml NaCl (10–20 ml/kg) proved ineffective, dopamine was administered. In the case of no clinical improvement, treatment was followed by adrenaline. Seizures during TH were treated with phenobarbital/phenytoin, and hypothermia was prolonged if the seizures appeared during rewarming.

Sampling of interstitial fluid and blood

Sterile, nylon, multifilament wicks soaked in 9 mg/ml NaCl were subcutaneously implanted 4 cm in length into either the arm or the leg for 60 min in accordance with previous studies [14, 17]. The wicks were implanted at 6, 12, 24, 48, and 72 h after birth. Retracted wicks were placed into 1.5-ml Eppendorf centrifuge tubes with funnel (Sarstedt, Nümbrecht, Germany) containing mineral oil. Following centrifugation of the wicks, IF was extracted and frozen at – 20 °C for later analysis. Colloid osmotic pressure (COP) was measured using a colloid osmometer designed for small samples [18] equipped with a membrane impermeable for molecules > 30 kDa (PM-30, Amicron, Lexington, MA, USA). COP was amplified and recorded with Easy Graph P930 (Gould Inc., Ohio, USA). Blood samples were collected from an arterial line both before installation and retraction of the wick. The blood samples were allowed to clot and serum was subsequently isolated, frozen at – 20 °C. COP determined from either plasma or serum is equivalent [19], and patient serum, a surrogate for patient circulating plasma, was later analyzed in the above-mentioned colloid osmometer and is denoted in the manuscript as COP_p. Additional blood analyses, such as serum albumin and hemoglobin concentrations, were performed at the Laboratory of Clinical Biochemistry at Haukeland University Hospital. The concentrations of 15 cytokines were analyzed in serum and IF using a multiplex bead immunoassay (Milliplex HCYTMAG-60; Merck Millipore, Darmstadt, Germany): interferon gamma, interleukin (IL)-1α, IL-1β, interleukin-1 receptor antagonist (IL-1RA), IL-2, IL-6, IL-8, IL-10, IL-12p40, monocyte chemoattractant protein-1, macrophage inflammatory protein-1α, transforming growth factor-α, tumor necrosis factor (TNF)-α, TNF-β, and vascular endothelial growth factor. The procedure was performed as recommended by the manufacturer, measured in a 1:12.5 dilution, and analyzed, with a Luminex 100™ instrument (Luminex Corp.; Austin, USA) and StarStation software (Applied Cytometry Systems; Dinnington, UK) at the Broegelmann Research Laboratory, Department of Clinical Sciences, University of Bergen, Norway. Values were reported as picograms per milliliter (pg/ml). Because of scarce amounts of material, we were not able to verify cytokine results by running the tests in parallel.

Statistical analysis

Data and analysis were evaluated using SigmaStat 11 (Sy Stat Software Inc.; California, USA). One-way analysis of variance was used to evaluate COP_p, COP_i, cytokines, MAP and fluid balance between different treatment time points. If there was a significant difference between the mean values of the groups, an all pairwise multiple comparison procedure (Holm-Sidak or Dunn's methods) was used to isolate the specific groups. Nonparametric tests for correlation calculations of continuous variables were performed by Spearman's rank correlation test, and categorical variables were analyzed by the Mann–Whitney U-test. Continuous variables are expressed as mean ± SD, and categorical variables are expressed as counts and percentages. A *P*-value < 0.05 was considered statistically significant.

Results

Demographics

Twenty-nine neonates had moderate to severe HIE and were treated with hypothermia in the NICU during the study period. Seventeen of these patients (58%), 8 (47%) female, were included in the study. Twelve neonates could not be included due to lack of study personnel available for implanting wicks. A total of 13 out of 17 participating infants survived after 3 days of TH, and one infant developed necrotizing enterocolitis (NEC). One non-survivor had a congenital diaphragmatic hernia. The included patients did not have known septicemia, genetic or neuromuscular abnormalities and were not influenced by maternal chorioamnionitis. No patients were clinically characterized as edematous throughout TH. Gestational age (GA) varied from 35^{+4} to 42^{+3} weeks (mean GA of 39^{+6} weeks eq. 279 days), and average weight was 3464 g (range 2483–4710 g). One patient received TH despite having a GA below 36 weeks. There were no sex-related responses in included patients, and additional clinical characteristics are presented in Table 2.

Table 2 Study group characteristics of enrolled patients

Characteristics	*N* = 17
Gender: male, *n* (%)	9 (53)
Apgar score at 1 min, mean (range)	1 (0–5)
Apgar score at 5 min, mean (range)	2 (0–6)
Apgar score at 10 min, mean (range)	2 (0–6)
PROM, n (%)	3 (18)
Delivery mode, *n* (%)	
Emergency cesarean	9 (53)
Vaginal	8 (47)
SGA, n (%)	4 (26)
Seizures, requires anticonvulsant drug, *n* (%)	7 (41)
Referred from other hospitals, *n* (%)	6 (35)

PROM Premature rupture of membranes > 24 h, *SGA* Small for gestational age, indicates birth weight below 10th percentile for gestational age

Fluid calculations, hemodynamic and laboratory variables during TH

Seven patients received inotropic support with dopamine as the primary vasopressor. MAP demonstrated a significant drop ($P < 0.05$) from 47.3 ± 6.9 mmHg at 7 h to 42.9 ± 8.2 mmHg at 25 h of life, but increased to 50.7 ± 5.3 when rewarming was initiated. A positive fluid balance of 4.1 ± 2.4 ml/kg/h 7 h after birth decreased significantly ($P < 0.001$) to 1.6 ± 1.9 ml/kg/h 13 h after birth and declined further to 1.0 ± 1.0 ml/kg/h until TH was completed. Urine output increased fourfold ($P < 0.05$) and nearly sevenfold ($P < 0.05$) from 7 to 25 and 73 h after birth (0.19 ml/kg/h to 0.85 ml/kg/h and 1.28 ml/kg/h respectively). Following TH, hemoglobin levels also decreased together with a transient decline in serum sodium levels between 7 and 25 h, whereas potassium and creatinine levels remained stable throughout the period. Serum glucose levels were reduced to approximately 50% during the first 24 h after birth. Albumin remained within the reference range [20], although levels significantly declined from 29 g/l to 26 g/l ($P < 0.05$) from the first 24 h to the 25–97-h period. Laboratory variables during TH and the first 24 h of rewarming are presented in Table 3.

Effect of TH on inflammatory markers

C-reactive protein showed a marginal increase from 16 mg/l to 24 mg/l between 49 and 73 h after birth (Table 3). Circulating total white blood cells (WBC) decreased significantly within the time points (7, 13, 25, 49, 73, and 97 h), as well as leukocyte subclasses, such as neutrophils, lymphocytes, and monocytes. There was a minor decline in the number of thrombocytes throughout TH (defined by platelet count $< 150 \times 10^9$/l).

Effect of TH on COP

An initial power-sample size evaluation based on $n = (2 * (SD/delta))^{2*k}$ calculated $n = 13$ if a change in COP_p of 2.5 mmHg with 90% test strength and 5% level of significance was to be achieved. Similarly, a COP_p change of 1 mmHg or 2 mmHg need $n = 40$ and 20 respectively.

Therefore, n between 12 and 20 should be adequate to detect a 2–2.5 mmHg change of COP_p.

A total of 22/68 wicks (32%) were discarded owing to blood contamination. Mean wick implantation time was 61 min. Mean COP_p and COP_i during TH were 14.5 ± 2.6 mmHg and 8.9 ± 1.9 mmHg, respectively. For COP_p, we observed a decrease from 15.6 ± 1.9 mmHg at 7 h after birth to 13.8 ± 2.4 mmHg at 49 h of life, followed by a modest increase to 14.5 ± 2.6 mmHg at 73 h. For COP_i, there was a small decline throughout TH from 9.2 ± 0.8 mmHg at 7 h to 7.8 ± 1.7 mmHg at 73 h (Fig. 1). However, none of the changes in COP_p or COP_i during TH were significant ($P = 0.12$ and 0.954, respectively).

Table 3 Biological data during therapeutic hypothermia and rewarming

Biological parameters	Therapeutic hypothermia, hours after birth					Rewarming
	7 h	13 h	25 h	49 h	73 h	97 h
pH	7.1 ± 0.2	7.3 ± 0.1	7.3 ± 0.1	7.3 ± 0.1	7.3 ± 0.1	7.3 ± 0.1
pCO_2 (kPa)	6.5 ± 2.7	5.8 ± 1.7	5.5 ± 1.0	5.7 ± 1.0	6.0 ± 1.1	6.1 ± 1.2
BE (mmol/l) (–)	12.4 ± 5.1	6.5 ± 3.7	6.7 ± 3.2	5.8 ± 4.1	4.6 ± 2.9	3.5 ± 1.7
Hemoglobin (g/dl)	15.6 ± 2.2	15.4 ± 1.3	15.8 ± 1.8	15.1 ± 1.8	14.4 ± 1.6	13.5 ± 1.7
WBC ($\times 10^9$/l)	23.7 ± 13.2[1, 2]	24.8 ± 12.7[3, 4]	19.0 ± 7.9	14.9 ± 6.1	11.6 ± 5.5	10.7 ± 3.5
ANC ($\times 10^9$/l)	12.8 ± 10.4	15.5 ± 7.2[3, 4]	13.8 ± 6.3[5, 6]	10.1 ± 4.8	6.4 ± 2.2	6.9 ± 2.8
Lymph. ($\times 10^9$/l)	8.7 ± 5.5[1]	4.1 ± 2.7	3.3 ± 1.7	3.4 ± 1.5	2.9 ± 0.7	2.6 ± 0.7
Mono. ($\times 10^9$/l)	1.5 ± 1.2	2.1 ± 1.2[3, 4]	1.6 ± 0.9[6]	1.0 ± 0.6	0.7 ± 0.4	0.7 ± 0.4
Thrombocytes ($\times 10^9$/l)	217.0 ± 78.9	178.1 ± 57.8	158.9 ± 63.7	165.2 ± 80.3	143.3 ± 75.6	148.2 ± 75.5
CRP (mg/l)	15.6 ± 13.5	11.0 ± 13.5	10.7 ± 10.7	15.0 ± 12.4	23.6 ± 21.6	23.0 ± 28.7
s-glucose (mmol/l)	11.0 ± 4.8	10.1 ± 6.1	8.1 ± 6.6	5.7 ± 1.0	5.8 ± 2.3	5.3 ± 0.9
s-creatine (mcmol/l)	78.1 ± 16.1	86.9 ± 21.2	81.7 ± 32.1	86.5 ± 46.3	91.3 ± 67.9	85.0 ± 80.7
s-sodium (mmol/l)	135.8 ± 3.2	126.4 ± 32.2	133.9 ± 3.0	134.7 ± 4.0	135.2 ± 5.1	135.9 ± 6.2
s-potassium (mmol/l)	4.3 ± 0.7	4.2 ± 0.7	4.1 ± 0.8	4.0 ± 0.5	4.0 ± 0.6	4.2 ± 0.7
s-albumin (g/l)		28.8 ± 3.6[7]			25.7 ± 3.8	

All values represent the mean ± SD. *WBC* White blood cell count, *ANC* Absolute neutrophil count, *Lymph* Lymphocytes, *Mono* Monocytes, *CRP* C-reactive protein, [1]$P < 0.05$ at 0–7 h vs. at 73–97 h, [2]$P < 0.05$ at 0–7 h vs. at 49–73 h, [3]$P < 0.05$ at 7–13 h vs. at 74–97 h, [4]$P < 0.05$ at 7–13 h vs. at 49–73 h, [5]$P < 0.05$ at 13–25 h vs. at 74–97 h, [6]$P < 0.05$ at 13–25 h vs. at 49–73 h, [7]$P = 0.049$ at 0–25 h vs. at 49–97 h

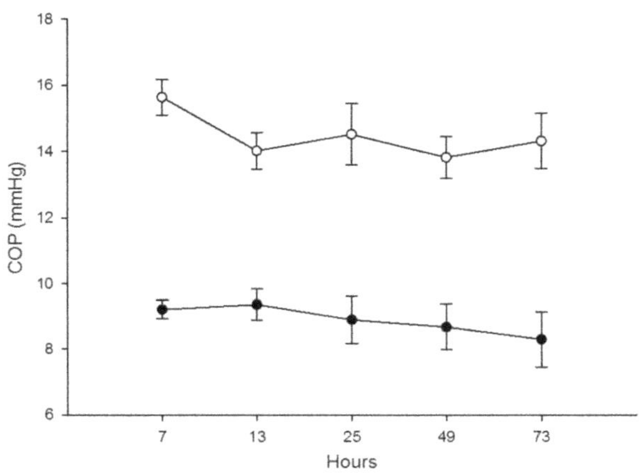

Fig. 1 Colloid osmotic pressure and therapeutic hypothermia. Measured colloid osmotic pressure in serum (○) and interstitial fluid (●) plotted against duration of therapeutic hypothermia

The pressure gradient, ΔCOP, between plasma and interstitium remained unchanged, although there was a tendency to increase during TH.

Effect of TH on IF and serum levels of growth factors, cytokines, and chemokines

In contrast to the minimal changes in COP, there were several alterations in levels of inflammatory mediators during TH. Compared with the measured values at 7 h, the serum IL-1RA levels significantly decreased between 49 and 73 h ($P < 0.05$). IL-6 levels were significantly decreased at 73 compared with levels at 7 h ($P < 0.05$), and IL-10 levels were significantly decreased at 25, 49, and 73 h compared with levels at 7 h ($P < 0.05$). The changes in these IF inflammatory parameters were very different from what we observed in the serum levels. IL-1α was the only IF cytokine with a significant ($P < 0.05$) increase throughout TH, with a rapid rise after 49 h. Conversely, IL-1RA levels were significantly decreased after 7 and 25 h of TH ($P < 0.05$). Additionally, higher serum IL-6 and IL-8 levels, compared with IF, were observed throughout TH. Changes in the remaining cytokine levels were small and non-significant. The mean levels of measurable cytokine concentrations in IF and serum at various time points during TH are presented in Table 4 and selected cytokines in Fig. 2.

Correlations between changes in IF and serum cytokine levels, and clinical and imaging parameters

We found a significant correlation between decreased MAP and increased IL-1α in the IF between 7 and 49 h, and a non-correlating rapid rise in interstitial IL-1α and elevated MAP from 49 to 73 h. We also observed significant negative correlations between IF IL-1α levels at 7 h and later measurements of COP_p (12, 24, and 72 h) and COP_i (48 h). Additionally, the IF IL-1α levels at 13 and 25 h were associated with COP_p at 73 h. Although serum levels of IL-1RA and IL-10 significantly decreased during TH, there were no significant correlations with MAP, COP_p, COP_i, or fluid balance for these cytokines. For all other cytokines, there was no association with MAP, COP_p, COP_i, or fluid balance, as well as no correlations between cytokine levels and clinical variables.

Discussion

In the present study, HIE neonates were treated with TH and experienced a reduced COP_p similar to previously reported in asphyxiated newborns [21]. The interstitial COP from TH treated neonates was nearly halved compared to previous reports from healthy children [14], and during TH a non-significant decrease was found in both COP_p and COP_i throughout the various treatment time points. In the IF, the pro-inflammatory IL-1α showed increased levels during hypothermic treatment, which coincided with decreased total WBC count and no clinical or laboratory signs of edema formation.

Neonates that experience scarce spontaneous ventilation, inadequate heart rates, and low Apgar scores at 1–5 and 10 min after birth are often resuscitated and in need of intensive care treatment. In addition to respiratory support, great care is taken to regulate circulatory homeostasis with adequate intravascular volume and efficient organ perfusion. Although a clinician may control the volume of administered fluid, the ability to dictate its pathways is challenging owing to deviation in blood pressure, circulating blood volume, interstitial accumulation of fluid and capillary permeability. Among the forces that alter passage of fluid from blood vessels to the interstitium, COP_p and COP_i are most easily examined in the plasma (equal to serum) and by extracting IF from subcutaneously implanted wicks. The endothelial glycocalyx, a multicomponent luminal network of membrane bound proteoglycans and glycoproteins covering the endothelial cells, creates a COP gradient close to the barrier of filtration. COP_i, a marker of glycocalyx COP (COP_g), works close to the endothelium border and is thought to mirror COP_g under normal filtration rates [22]. COP_p in healthy adults (25 mmHg) [17, 23] is reported equal to children [14] but higher than in term [24]- and pre-term neonates [15] (20 mmHg and 15 mmHg, respectively). Sick neonates, regardless of maturity, have an even more decreased COP_p [15, 24, 25]. Sussmane et al. showed that COP_p in healthy infants from 1 to 11 months is in proportion to adult values, with an anticipated COP_p increase during the first month of life [26]. Throughout TH treatment in the present study, the mean COP_p (14.3 ± 2.6 mmHg) coincides with earlier observations of lowered plasma COP in sick newborns [15]. Although there were no significant changes in COP in serum during TH, the decline in COP_p

Table 4 Measured cytokines in serum and interstitial fluid throughout therapeutic hypothermia

Cytokines		Therapeutic Hypothermia, hours after birth					
		7 h	13 h	25 h	49 h	73 h	Significance
IFN-γ (pg/ml)	Serum	26 ± 25	5 ± 65	NM	NM	NM	
	IF	24 ± 18	3 ± 25	39 ± 36	47 ± 59	28 ± 25	NS
IL-1α (pg/ml)	Serum	119 ± 41	287 ± 501	300 ± 280	246 ± 262	958 ± 945	NS
	IF	1840 ± 2034	2387 ± 2719	2652 ± 2682	2562 ± 3006	8845 ± 7055	$P < 0.05$[1]
IL-1RA (pg/ml)	Serum	38,845 ± 29,946	18,663 ± 17,076	8226 ± 9959	7917 ± 10,524	3069 ± 4132	$P < 0.05$[2]
	IF	1966 ± 1219	1141 ± 787	849 ± 1338	751 ± 421	2033 ± 2047	$P < 0.05$[3]
IL-6 (pg/ml)	Serum	6441 ± 6935	3343 ± 4747	9419 ± 4747	4204 ± 11,622	4297 ± 11,622	$P < 0.05$[4]
	IF	1646 ± 2663	742 ± 1098	868 ± 1325	964 ± 232	134 ± 104	NS
IL-8 (pg/ml)	Serum	3733 ± 2641	3025 ± 3590	2648 ± 4248	2059 ± 2567	1940 ± 2570	NS
	IF	678 ± 904	642 ± 904	1192 ± 2628	669 ± 1022	366 ± 534	NS
IL-10 (pg/ml)	Serum	12,519 ± 11,403	5059 ± 9073	557 ± 664	647 ± 1468	327 ± 665	$P < 0.05$[5]
	IF	NM	NM	NM	NM	NM	
IL-12p40 (pg/ml)	Serum	1018 ± 930	1064 ± 1088	1132 ± 1224	836 ± 875	NM	NS
	IF	NM	NM	NM	NM	NM	
MCP-1α (pg/ml)	Serum	51,752 ± 36,294	52,073 ± 43,265	63,297 ± 49,865	71,682 ± 42,825	54,762 ± 41,092	NS
	IF	3369 ± 2900	4367 ± 5604	6260 ± 8353	4381 ± 4062	5955 ± 3863	NS
TGFα (pg/ml)	Serum	64 ± 84	74 ± 98	53 ± 59	95 ± 114	73 ± 73	NS
	IF	NM	NM	NM	NM	NM	
TNFα (pg/ml)	Serum	503 ± 267	444 ± 246	449 ± 233	418 ± 213	505 ± 199	NS
	IF	19 ± 11	24 ± 19	24 ± 16	24.3 ± 18	37 ± 17	NS
VEGF (pg/ml)	Serum	4282 ± 3168	5103 ± 3309	1597 ± 1055	2514 ± 1545	3663 ± 1391	NS
	IF	1597 ± 1631	2654 ± 3044	717 ± 1071	1465 ± 2305	NM	NS

All values represent mean ± SD. *IF* Interstitial fluid, *NM* not measurable, *NS* no statistical significant difference. [1]Significance between 73 h and all other time points; [2]significance between 73 and 49 h and 7 h; [3]significance between 25 and 7 h; [4]significance between 73 and 7 h; [5]significance between 73, 49, and 25 h and 7 h

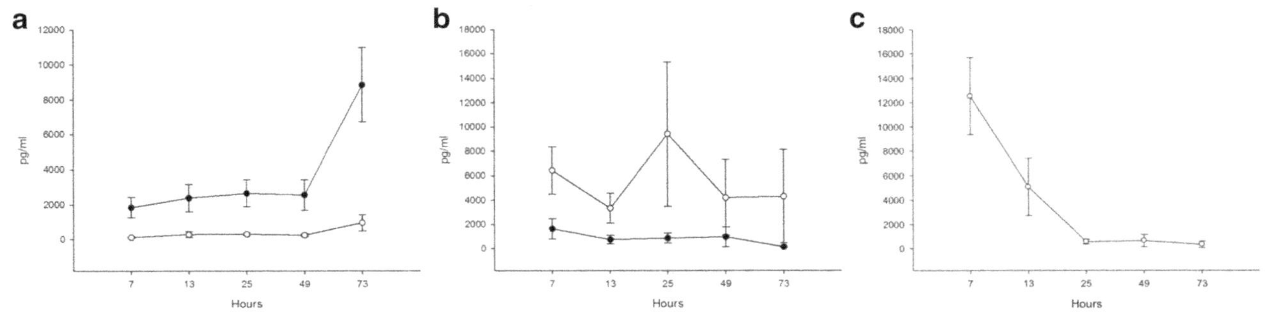

Fig. 2 Cytokines and neonatal asphyxia. Median cytokines levels over time in serum (○) and interstitial fluid (●) during therapeutic hypothermia. X-axis refers to hours after initiation of therapeutic hypothermia, y-axis refers to concentration, pg/ml. **a**, Interleukin (IL)-1α **b**, IL-6. **c**, IL-10 (IF IL-10 not detectable)

during the first 13 h was most likely due to simple dilution of plasma proteins. A possible explanation is the initial treatment with intravenous fluid resuscitation and subsequent stabilization in the NICU. The following fluid restriction will result in a more constant COP_p (Fig. 1). These results correspond with the significantly increased positive fluid balance during the first 7 h after birth compared with the remaining TH period ($P < 0.01$) and a transient hyponatremia of 126 mmol/l serum sodium at 13 h after birth. Skin vasoconstriction due to whole body cooling, as well as reduced urine output, elevated serum creatinine, and mechanical ventilation, are potential reasons for excess fluid. Such fluid accumulation occurred despite our adherence to the recommended reduced daily fluid intake. More novel is the finding of a reduced COP_i of 8.9 ± 1.9 mmHg compared with COP_i from children between 2 and 10 years (13.9 ± 3.5 mmHg) [14], and a corresponding ΔCOP (i.e., $COP_p - COP_i$) nearly constant during TH. A relatively balanced COP gradient together with a reduced serum albumin, suggests that other plasma proteins compensate in maintaining COP_p since the patients were only, to a small extent, administered crystalloids and blood products. Unfortunately, there was not enough material to measure total protein and albumin concentration in the IF owing to protocol restrictions. The significant decline ($P < 0.05$) in serum albumin from 29 to 26 g/l with stable COP_p between the first day and the last 2 days of TH may indicate capillary hyperpermeability propelled by the asphyxia event inducing an inflammatory cascade [11]. Other macromolecules that replace plasma albumin or reduced circulatory fluid would maintain an unaltered COP_p. Conversely, reduced liver function with less synthesized albumin and restricted fluid access would produce a similar situation.

The present results showing albumin within the reference range, although reduced during TH, may be due to a reduced inflammatory stimulus as a result of hypothermia [27] or increased lymphatic fluid removal, although the latter was shown to be less likely in sedated and immobilized dogs [28].

According to the Starling equation, increased capillary filtration coefficient (CFC) (proportional to hydraulic conductivity (L_p) and the capillary area accessible for fluid shift) and/or elevated capillary hydrostatic pressure (Pc), as well as a decline in the reflection coefficient (σ), may increase fluid extravasation. Capillary pressure is dependent on arterial pressure and venous pressure, together with pre- and post-capillary resistance [29]. Michel et al. demonstrated increased permeability due to elevated L_p after mild thermal injury, which expressed a biphasic course and diminished after several hours [30], whereas Lundblad et al. showed that endotoxemia in cat skeletal muscle resulted in reduced σ and significantly increased CFC [31]. Whether asphyxia and inflammation stimulates changes triggering barrier disruption owing to altered L_p or σ is uncertain, as well as how TH affects these parameters.

MAP, which decreased during the first 25 h of TH, is dependent on peripheral resistance and cardiac output, the latter known to be reduced during asphyxia and TH [32]. Consequently, an expected increased peripheral resistance, primarily post-capillary, takes place after TH initiation and results in increased Pc (given unaltered CFC and σ), thereby forcing extravasation to the interstitium. A small, but detectable, fall in COP_i compared with COP_p is maintained by removal of albumin or other proteins comparable in size from the interstitium. The reduced COP_i and COP_p during TH in asphyxiated neonates and the ability of TH to oppose changes in capillary filtration by COP in IF is an edema preventive mechanism demonstrated in animal [33] and human [34] studies.

Two thirds of patients in the present study developed mild thrombocytopenia, which is associated with birth asphyxia [35] as well as TH activation and aggregation of platelets with potential thrombus formation [13]. The reduced platelet count as a result of hypothermia is thought to be protective from microvascular slugging and related to increased blood viscosity and vasoconstriction; the patients in the present study exhibited no vascular incidents, with exception of one patient who required platelet transfusion and surgery owing to NEC during TH.

Results from the present study showed decreased levels of IL-6, a pleotropic cytokine, in IF compared with serum, which could be due to negligible tissue damage and subsequent inflammation; this supports the validity of the wick technique as a less traumatic method for sampling of IF. A significant reduction in WBC count with neutropenia was also observed along with a delayed initiation of CRP response. This was in accordance with recent observations of non-sepsis-risk neonates treated with TH [36]. Leukopenia with reduced IL-10 is associated with better outcome in animal models of brain injury and in human adult stroke patients; the observed functional immune compromise may be due to bone marrow suppression and reduced leucocyte release [10]. Conversely, a prolonged leukopenia that does not recover after rewarming, as we observed, is associated with a poor prognosis at 12 months [37], although treatment outcome was beyond the scope of this trial to measure.

Endothelial dysfunction is associated with perinatal asphyxia [38], and the concomitant acute inflammation from ischemia-reperfusion injury triggers a compulsory formation of intracellular gaps owing to activation of the actin-myosin system with increased permeability. To the best of our knowledge, increased levels of IL-1α in IF from skin, which suggests local cytokine production, has never been measured in neonates. The finding of an amplified IL-1α in the IF throughout TH treatment, suggests an upregulation from keratinocytes and other cells in the subcutis [39]. Whether IL-1RA, which decreased during the first 49 h of TH, antagonized IL-1α initially is uncertain. Although recombinant IL-1α injected intravenously into rabbits exerts a rise in temperature [39], it remains unclear whether the increased IL-1α in IF was due to asphyxia or potentiated by the hypothermic environment. The correlation between increased IL-1α and decreased MAP was not obvious, although TH-increased post-capillary resistance may be influenced by inflammation-affected endothelium and the resulting increased extravasation resulting in a lowered COP_i. Mild hypothermia can be demonstrated by a lowered secretion of IL-10 in cell culture [40], as well as by interleukin expression in hypothermic neonates, although levels are initially higher during TH [37]. This was in line with the findings from the present study. The anti-inflammatory effects of TH on the vascular endothelium remain uncertain and not well studied, although a recent report showed better outcomes in neonates treated with shortened TH for 49 h, as well as down-regulation of serum IL-6, IL-8, and IL-10 [37].

The present study has some limitations. The most important of these limitations is that an unusually high number of wicks had to be discarded due to blood contamination, thus limiting the aggregate of measurements with each time-period during TH and thereby the power of the analysis at some data points. Unusable wicks represented nearly 50% of extracted wicks at 7 and 73 h after birth. Time from birth to initiation of TH was not identical within the group and may have influenced the relationship between biological parameters and time periods of TH, although less likely since body temperature were kept between 34 and 36 °C after initial stabilization. Also, the results presented are limited to the experience of one tertiary NICU and may not be generalizable. The osmolality of fluids intravenously administered during TH was not calculated, although it is less likely that crystalloids have a major impact on intravascular tonicity. Daily weight was not measured owing to the attached technical equipment. Therefore, potential fluid loss from respiratory evaporation or obvious fluid accumulation during TH was undetected. The clinical evaluation of edematous skin, together with fluid calculations and measurements of vascular tonicity, was performed by the attending physician and variations in fluid treatment may have occurred. Furthermore, the degree of asphyxia is difficult to interpret with altered physiology in response to both hypoxic ischemia and TH.

Conclusions

Neonates treated with TH have a decreased, but stable, COP_p and a compensatory low COP_i. This results in reduced vascular filtration with a COP gradient counteracting fluid flux from the capillaries to the interstitium, which likely functions as an edema-preventing mechanism. The decrease in MAP and reduced positive fluid balance during the first 24 h of TH, as well as no observed clinical edema, supports this assumption. Furthermore, hypothermia induces an expected low WBC and platelet count in neonates without any risk factors for infection. This is likely part of an inherent asphyxia protection system together with a fairly balanced local and systemic cytokine production. The results presented in this study provide novel and valuable information concerning tissue cytokine production during TH.

Abbreviations

CFC: Capillary filtration coefficient; COP: Colloid osmotic pressure; COP_i: Interstitial colloid osmotic pressure; COP_p: Plasma colloid osmotic pressure; GA: Gestational age; HIE: Hypoxic ischemic encephalopathy; IF: Interstitial fluid; IL: Interleukin; L_p: Hydraulic conductivity; MAP: Mean arterial pressure; MRI: Magnetic resonance imaging; NEC: Necrotizing enterocolitis; NICU: Neonatal Intensive Care Unit; Pc: Capillary hydrostatic pressure; TH: Therapeutic hypothermia; WBC: White blood cells

Acknowledgments
We would like to thank Jan Magnus Aase for help with technical work and Karl Albert Brokstad and Marianne Eidsheim at the Broegelmann Research Laboratory, Department of Clinical Sciences, University of Bergen, for technical assistance with cytokine assays.

Funding
This work was supported by research grants (HJTG received funding) from West Norway Regional Health Authority (Helse Vest); grant number 911441. The funder had no role in study design, data collection and analysis, decision to publish, or preparation of the manuscript.

Authors' contributions
HJTG and AB conceptualized and designed the study. HJTG, TN, HW, and AB performed data collection and initial analyses. HJTG, TN, JKD, HW, and AB interpreted data. HJTG, TN, JKD, HW, and AB drafted the manuscript. HJTG, TN, JKD, HW, and AB approved the final manuscript as submitted and agree to be accountable for all aspects of the work, as well as ensuring that questions related to the accuracy or integrity of any part of the work are appropriately investigated and resolved. All authors read and approved the final manuscript.

Ethics approval and consent to participate
The study was approved by the Regional Committee for Medical and Health Research Ethics, Western Norway (ref 2009/3137-CAG) and was conducted at the Neonatal Intensive Care Unit (NICU), Haukeland University Hospital, Bergen, Norway. All patients were included in the study following written informed consent obtained from a parent or guardian after explanation of the study in accordance with the Declaration of Helsinki. The study trial was registered in ClinicalTrials.gov (ClinicalTrials.gov Identifier: NCT01044940).

Competing interests
The authors declare that they have no competing interest.

Author details
[1]Department of Pediatrics and Adolescent Medicine, Haukeland University Hospital, Bergen, Norway. [2]Department of Clinical Science, University of Bergen, Bergen, Norway. [3]Surgical Department, Haraldsplass Deaconess Hospital, Bergen, Norway. [4]Centre of Molecular Inflammation Research, Department of Cancer Research and Molecular Medicine, Norwegian University of Science and Technology, Trondheim, Norway. [5]Department of Infectious Diseases, St. Olav's Hospital, Trondheim, Norway. [6]Department of Biomedicine, University of Bergen, Bergen, Norway.

References

1. van Handel M, Swaab H, de Vries LS, Jongmans MJ. Long-term cognitive and behavioral consequences of neonatal encephalopathy following perinatal asphyxia: a review. Eur J Pediatr. 2007;166(7):645–54.
2. Gonzalez FF, Miller SP. Does perinatal asphyxia impair cognitive function without cerebral palsy? Arch Dis Child Fetal Neonatal Ed. 2006;91(6):F454–9.
3. Bhalala US, Koehler RC, Kannan S. Neuroinflammation and neuroimmune dysregulation after acute hypoxic-ischemic injury of developing brain. Front pediatr. 2014;2:144.
4. Weston RM, Jones NM, Jarrott B, Callaway JK. Inflammatory cell infiltration after endothelin-1-induced cerebral ischemia: histochemical and myeloperoxidase correlation with temporal changes in brain injury. J Cereb Blood Flow Metab. 2007;27(1):100–14.
5. Gu LJ, Xiong XX, Ito T, Lee J, Xu BH, Krams S, et al. Moderate hypothermia inhibits brain inflammation and attenuates stroke-induced immunodepression in rats. CNS neurosci ther. 2014;20(1):67–75.
6. Wei X, Wan X, Zhao B, Hou J, Liu M, Cheng B. Propofol inhibits inflammation and lipid peroxidation following cerebral ischemia/reperfusion in rabbits. Neural Regen Res. 2012;7(11):837–41.
7. Kakita H, Hussein MH, Kato S, Yamada Y, Nagaya Y, Asai H, et al. Hypothermia attenuates the severity of oxidative stress development in asphyxiated newborns. J Crit Care. 2012;27(5):469–73.
8. Tagin MA, Woolcott CG, Vincer MJ, Whyte RK, Stinson DA. Hypothermia for neonatal hypoxic ischemic encephalopathy: an updated systematic review and meta-analysis. Arch Pediatr Adolesc Med. 2012;166(6):558–66.
9. Jacobs SE, Berg M, Hunt R, Tarnow-Mordi WO, Inder TE, Davis PG. Cooling for newborns with hypoxic ischaemic encephalopathy. Cochrane Database Syst Rev. 2013; https://doi.org/10.1002/14651858.CD003311.pub3.
10. Jenkins DD, Lee T, Chiuzan C, Perkel JK, Rollins LG, Wagner CL, et al. Altered circulating leukocytes and their chemokines in a clinical trial of therapeutic hypothermia for neonatal hypoxic ischemic encephalopathy. Pediatr Crit Care Med. 2013;14(8):786–95.
11. Wood T, Thoresen M. Physiological responses to hypothermia. Semin fetal neonatal med. 2015;20(2):87–96.
12. Childs EW, Udobi KF, Hunter FA. Hypothermia reduces microvascular permeability and reactive oxygen species expression after hemorrhagic shock. J Trauma. 2005;58(2):271–7.
13. Zanelli S, Buck M, Fairchild K. Physiologic and pharmacologic considerations for hypothermia therapy in neonates. J Perinatol. 2011;31(6):377–86.
14. Guthe HJ, Indrebo M, Nedrebo T, Norgard G, Wiig H, Berg A. Interstitial fluid colloid osmotic pressure in healthy children. PLoS One. 2015; https://doi.org/10.1371/journal.phone0122779.
15. Bhat R, Javed S, Malalis L, Vidyasagar D. Critical care problems in neonates. Colloid osmotic pressure in healthy and sick neonates. Crit Care Med. 1981;9(8):563–7.
16. Azzopardi D. Clinical management of the baby with hypoxic ischaemic encephalopathy. Early Hum Dev. 2010;86(6):345–50.
17. Guthe HJ, Nedrebo T, Tenstad O, Wiig H, Berg A. Effect of topical anaesthetics on interstitial colloid osmotic pressure in human subcutaneous tissue sampled by wick technique. PLoS One. 2012; https://doi.org/10.1371/journal.phone.0031332.
18. Wiig H, Halleland EG, Fjaertoft M, Aukland K. Measurement of colloid osmotic pressure in submicrolitre samples. Acta Physiol Scand. 1988; 132(4):445–52.
19. Noddeland H. Colloid osmotic pressure of human subcutaneous interstitial fluid sampled by nylon wicks: evaluation of the method. Scand J Clin Lab Invest. 1982;42(2):123–30.
20. Ghoshal AK, Soldin SJ. Evaluation of the Dade Behring dimension RxL: integrated chemistry system-pediatric reference ranges. Clin Chim Acta. 2003;331(1–2):135–46.
21. Wu PY. Colloid oncotic pressure: current status and clinical applications in neonatal medicine. Clin Perinatol. 1982;9(3):645–57.
22. Wiig H, Swartz MA. Interstitial fluid and lymph formation and transport: physiological regulation and roles in inflammation and cancer. Physiol Rev. 2012;92(3):1005–60.
23. Weil MH, Morissette M, Michaels S, Bisera J, Boycks E, Shubin H, et al. Routine plasma colloid osmotic pressure measurements. Crit Care Med. 1974;2(5):229–34.
24. Sola A, Gregory GA. Colloid osmotic pressure of normal newborns and premature infants. Crit Care Med. 1981;9(8):568–72.
25. Zimmermann B, Francoise M, Germain JF, Lallemant C, Gouyon JB. Colloid osmotic pressure and neonatal respiratory distress syndrome. Archives de pediatrie. 1997;4(10):952–8.
26. Sussmane JB, de Soto M, Torbati D. Plasma colloid osmotic pressure in healthy infants. Crit Care. 2001;5(5):261–4.
27. Gunn AJ, Thoresen M. Hypothermic neuroprotection. NeuroRx. 2006;3(2): 154–69.
28. Schad H, Brechtelsbauer H. Thoracic duct lymph flow and composition in conscious dogs and the influence of anaesthesia and passive limb movement. Eur J Phys. 1977;371(1–2):25–31.
29. Levick JR. Circulation of fluid between plasma, interstitium and lymph. In: An introduction to cardiovascular physiology. 5th ed: Taylor &Francis Group, London, Great Britain; 2010. p. 189–219.
30. Michel CC, Curry FE. Microvascular permeability. Physiol Rev. 1999;79(3):703–61.
31. Lundblad C, Bentzer P, Grande PO. The permeability-reducing effects of prostacyclin and inhibition of rho kinase do not counteract endotoxin-

induced increase in permeability in cat skeletal muscle. Microvasc Res. 2004; 68(3):286–94.
32. Sehgal A, Wong F, Mehta S. Reduced cardiac output and its correlation with coronary blood flow and troponin in asphyxiated infants treated with therapeutic hypothermia. Eur J Pediatr. 2012;171(10):1511–7.
33. Fadnes HO. Effect of increased venous pressure on the hydrostatic and colloid osmotic pressure in subcutaneous interstitial fluid in rats: edema-preventing mechanisms. Scand J Clin Lab Invest. 1976;36(4):371–7.
34. Oian P, Maltau JM, Noddeland H, Fadnes HO. Oedema-preventing mechanisms in subcutaneous tissue of normal pregnant women. Br J Obstet Gynaecol. 1985;92(11):1113–9.
35. Castle V, Andrew M, Kelton J, Giron D, Johnston M, Carter C. Frequency and mechanism of neonatal thrombocytopenia. J Pediatr. 1986;108(5):749–55.
36. Chakkarapani E, Davis J, Thoresen M. Therapeutic hypothermia delays the C-reactive protein response and suppresses white blood cell and platelet count in infants with neonatal encephalopathy. Arch Dis Child Fetal Neonatal Ed. 2014;99(6):F458–63.
37. Jenkins DD, Rollins LG, Perkel JK, Wagner CL, Katikaneni LP, Bass WT, et al. Serum cytokines in a clinical trial of hypothermia for neonatal hypoxic-ischemic encephalopathy. J Cereb Blood Flow Metab. 2012;32(10):1888–96.
38. Nako Y, Tomomasa T, Morikawa A. Plasma thrombomodulin level in newborn infants with and without perinatal asphyxia. Acta Paediatr. 1997; 86(1):91–5.
39. Akdis M, Burgler S, Crameri R, Eiwegger T, Fujita H, Gomez E, et al. Interleukins, from 1 to 37, and interferon-gamma: receptors, functions, and roles in diseases. J Allergy Clin Immunol. 2011;127(3):701–21.
40. Russwurm S, Stonans I, Schwerter K, Stonane E, Meissner W, Reinhart K. Direct influence of mild hypothermia on cytokine expression and release in cultures of human peripheral blood mononuclear cells. J Interf Cytokine Res. 2002;22(2):215–21.

11

The minimally effective dose of sucrose for procedural pain relief in neonates

Bonnie Stevens[1*], Janet Yamada[2], Marsha Campbell-Yeo[3], Sharyn Gibbins[4], Denise Harrison[5], Kimberley Dionne[6], Anna Taddio[7], Carol McNair[8], Andrew Willan[9], Marilyn Ballantyne[10], Kimberley Widger[11], Souraya Sidani[12], Carole Estabrooks[13], Anne Synnes[14], Janet Squires[15], Charles Victor[16] and Shirine Riahi[17]

Abstract

Background: Orally administered sucrose is effective and safe in reducing pain intensity during single, tissue-damaging procedures in neonates, and is commonly recommended in neonatal pain guidelines. However, there is wide variability in sucrose doses examined in research, and more than a 20-fold variation across neonatal care settings. The aim of this study was to determine the minimally effective dose of 24% sucrose for reducing pain in hospitalized neonates undergoing a single skin-breaking heel lance procedure.

Methods: A total of 245 neonates from 4 Canadian tertiary neonatal intensive care units (NICUs), born between 24 and 42 weeks gestational age (GA), were prospectively randomized to receive one of three doses of 24% sucrose, plus non-nutritive sucking/pacifier, 2 min before a routine heel lance: 0.1 ml (Group 1; $n = 81$), 0.5 ml (Group 2; $n = 81$), or 1.0 ml (Group 3; $n = 83$). The primary outcome was pain intensity measured at 30 and 60 s following the heel lance, using the Premature Infant Pain Profile-Revised (PIPP-R). The secondary outcome was the incidence of adverse events. Analysis of covariance models, adjusting for GA and study site examined between group differences in pain intensity across intervention groups.

Results: There was no difference in mean pain intensity PIPP-R scores between treatment groups at 30 s ($P = .97$) and 60 s ($P = .93$); however, pain was not fully eliminated during the heel lance procedure. There were 5 reported adverse events among 5/245 (2.0%) neonates, with no significant differences in the proportion of events by sucrose dose ($P = .62$). All events resolved spontaneously without medical intervention.

Conclusions: The minimally effective dose of 24% sucrose required to treat pain associated with a single heel lance in neonates was 0.1 ml. Further evaluation regarding the sustained effectiveness of this dose in reducing pain intensity in neonates for repeated painful procedures is warranted.

Keywords: Adverse event, Analgesia, Heel lance, Neonates, NICU, Pain, PIPP-R, Preterm infants, Sucrose

* Correspondence: bonnie.stevens@sickkids.ca
[1]The Hospital for Sick Children, Lawrence S. Bloomberg Faculty of Nursing, University of Toronto, 686 Bay Street, Toronto, Ontario M5G 0A4, Canada
Full list of author information is available at the end of the article

Background

Multiple trials and recent systematic reviews with meta-analyses have shown that sweet solutions, including orally administered sucrose, are effective and safe in reducing pain intensity (using clinical observational or composite measures) during single, tissue-damaging procedures in neonates [1, 2]. These solutions are commonly recommended in neonatal pain guidelines [3]. However, there is wide variability in sucrose doses examined in research, and more than a 20-fold variation across neonatal care settings [4]. Despite the large number of randomized controlled trials in the 2016 Cochrane review [2], an optimal dose of sucrose could not be determined due to the wide range of volumes and concentrations (0.05 ml of 24% to 2.0 ml of 50% solution) studied, and due to variation in study methods (e.g., administration techniques, types of painful procedures, outcome measures, and co-interventions). There are no definitive conclusions about the minimally effective dose of sucrose associated with a clinically significant reduction in pain intensity scores in neonates.

To our knowledge, there have been no direct comparisons of different volumes of sucrose at the same concentration. In this study, we evaluated the three smallest doses of sucrose most commonly reported to be effective in previous research (i.e., 0.1 ml, 0.5 ml, and 1.0 ml of 24% sucrose) [2] to determine the minimally effective dose for neonates undergoing a skin-breaking heel lance procedure while in the neonatal intensive care unit (NICU). Doses smaller than 0.1 ml were not included in the study due to challenges posed by accurate measurement and delivery. All neonates received sucrose for procedural pain (i.e., there was no placebo or no-treatment group), which was consistent with neonatal pain guidelines and in keeping with the ethical conduct of clinical trials in newborns [5–7]. We hypothesized that (a) there was no difference in pain intensity between the sucrose doses, measured at 30 and 60 s following the heel lance using the Premature Infant Pain Profile-Revised (PIPP-R), and (b) adverse events would be minimal.

Methods

A prospective multi-centered single-blind randomized controlled trial was conducted from July 2013–April 2015 at 4 Canadian tertiary NICUs following research ethics approval. The inclusion criteria were neonates 24 to 42 weeks gestational age (GA) at birth and less than 30 days of life/or less than 44 weeks GA at the time of the intervention, scheduled to receive a heel lance, and who had not received opioids within 24 h prior to the heel lance. The exclusion criteria were neonates with a contraindication for sucrose administration (e.g., were too ill or unstable as per neonatologist's assessment, unable to swallow, pharmacologically muscle relaxed) and/or inability to assess behavioral responses to pain accurately (e.g., the neonate's face was blocked with taping). We did not use the diagnosis of neurological impairment as an exclusion criterion because the timing of diagnosis and determining the severity of impairment can be very difficult in this population. However, inability to swallow had the effect of excluding neonates with severe neurologic impairment from hypoxic-ischemic encephalopathy. Observation of the procedure was timed to ensure that no additional sucrose doses were provided within the previous 4 h. All parents or legal guardians provided informed consent.

Randomization was performed using a web-based privacy protected randomization service [8]. Randomization was block stratified by GA at birth (< 29 weeks or 29–42 weeks) to enhance balanced intervention groups. A research nurse, aware of group allocation, drew up the assigned sucrose dose into an amber colored syringe. The dose was double-checked by a second nurse, not involved with the study, and documented on the medication administration record as per unit protocol. The research nurse followed a standard dose administration time to blind the bedside nurse performing the heel lance to the sucrose volume. The syringes used to administer sucrose were also shielded from view by the research nurse from the bedside nurse and video recording. No other study personnel had access to the treatment allocation.

The treatment intervention was videotaped and included 4 phases. (a) Baseline observation of the neonate for 2 min prior to the heel lance. (b) Administering the total volume of 24% sucrose [0.1 ml(Group 1), 0.5 ml (Group 2), or 1.0 ml (Group 3)] drop-by-drop via syringe over the anterior surface of the tongue, allowing for individual neonate swallowing rates over a period of 1–2 min (for the largest dose). A pacifier was offered to all neonates immediately following sucrose administration to facilitate non-nutritive sucking, which has been shown to enhance sucrose efficacy in a synergistic way [9]. (c) Conducting the heel lance procedure with an automated lancet approximately 2 min after the sucrose administration, to allow for peak effects [10]. (d) Observation of return-to-baseline pain indicator values over 30 s to several minutes. The bedside nurse conducted the heel lance according to the specific unit policy, while the research nurse experienced in NICU care ensured complete data collection.

We did not limit participating neonates from receiving other pain-relieving parent-initiated interventions (e.g., skin-to-skin/kangaroo care and breastfeeding) [11] as per unit protocols. These were documented by the research nurse, so any group differences could be controlled for in the analysis. Pharmacological interventions shown to be ineffective in reducing heel lance pain (e.g., acetaminophen) [12] were not administered.

Outcome measures

The primary outcome was pain intensity measured with the PIPP-R [13, 14], which has demonstrated construct validity in neonates of varying GA [13–15]. The PIPP-R includes 2 physiological (heart rate, oxygen saturation), 3 behavioral (brow bulge, eye squeeze, nasolabial furrow) and 2 contextual (GA, behavioral state) variables known to modify pain responses. Throughout the treatment intervention, physiological and behavioral/facial indicators of pain intensity were collected using an infant monitoring system developed and used extensively by the research team over the past decade. The research nurse placed pulse oximetry probes on the neonate to record heart rate and oxygen saturation continuously, and positioned a digital video recorder to capture facial movements. Electronic event markers synchronized all physiological and behavioral data, and demarcated the 4 phases of the treatment intervention.

Two trained coders, blinded to group allocation and study purpose, viewed the physiological and behavioral data captured by the infant monitoring system, and coded neonates' pain intensity using the PIPP-R. An inter-rater reliability > 0.9 was achieved on a random sample of 5 neonates, early in the study and with each 25% of data collected.

The secondary outcome was frequency of a priori specified adverse event/tolerance criteria (heart rate > 240 beats/min or heart rate < 80 beats/min for > 20 s; oxygen saturation < 80% for > 20 s; no spontaneous respirations for > 20 s; and choking/gagging). Adverse event data were collected by the research nurse during the intervention. The research nurse kept a record of 'rescue doses' administered (i.e., additional doses of sucrose given on direction of the nurse caring for the neonate, if the neonate became overly distressed during the procedure).

Statistical analyses

We estimated a sample size of 71 neonates per group (total sample size of 213). The sample size calculation accounts for multiple testing due to 3 intervention groups, and is based on a type I error probability of 5%, a power of 80%, and a smallest minimally clinically significant difference of 1 on the PIPP-R with a standard deviation (SD) of 2. Consistent with previous research, this minimally clinically significant difference was justifiable given the lack of a treatment control in this study versus preceding studies [16]. To account for potential missing data (e.g., equipment failure), we increased the sample size by 15% to 245. Analysis of covariance models adjusting for GA and study site examined between group differences in PIPP-R scores.

Results

Randomization and demographic characteristics

The trial profile is presented in Fig. 1. Of the 4172 neonates screened for eligibility, 248 were enrolled and randomly allocated to Group 1, 2 or 3. Three neonates were excluded following randomization, as they did not undergo a heel lance, leaving 245 for the outcomes analyses. Demographic characteristics in all 3 groups were adequately matched (Table 1). These included GA at birth, days since birth, birth weight, sex, severity of illness assessed using the Score for Neonatal Acute Physiology Perinatal Extension-II (SNAPPE-II) [17, 18], number of prior painful procedures, number of previous doses of sucrose, and concurrent use of non-pharmacologic pain strategies. As standard care in each unit included parent-initiated non-pharmacologic strategies (e.g., swaddling, skin-to-skin/kangaroo care, and breastfeeding) we could not ethically disallow these interventions during the painful procedure. However, there was no difference in the use of parent-initiated pain strategies across groups (Table 1). All neonates were offered a pacifier for non-nutritive sucking following sucrose administration. Overall 204/ 245 (83.2%) sucked on the pacifier, while the remainder refused or did not receive the pacifier due to medical considerations (e.g., intubated, or not tolerated well). We noted a discrepancy between the number of painful procedures documented and the number of sucrose doses documented since birth. Information on non-pharmacologic interventions was often not available in the neonates' medical records; therefore, it was difficult to discern if the discrepancy was an administration or documentation issue.

Pain intensity

The mean pain intensity [SD] PIPP-R scores at 30 s post heel lance (Group 1 6.8[3.5]; Group 2 6.8[3.2]; Group 3 6.7[3.4]) were not statistically different after adjusting for GA and research site ($F[6233] = 0.01$, $P = .97$; Table 2). Similarly, there were no significant differences in mean PIPP-R scores between groups at 60 s ($F\ [2229] = 0.10$, $P = .93$; Table 2). Mean pain intensity PIPP-R scores at 30 and 60 s were inversely associated with GA ($P < .001$) and significantly different when stratified by site ($P < .001$; Table 3); therefore both factors were controlled for in the analysis. Mean PIPP-R scores ranged from 6.03 (3.37) for neonates > 36 weeks GA to 9.07 (4.00) for neonates < 28 weeks GA at 30 s and 5.70 (3.31) for neonates > 36 weeks GA to 9.43 (4.04) for neonates < 28 weeks GA. No associations were found between pain intensity scores and other demographic characteristics [i.e., SNAPPE-II/ severity of illness on admission, gender, concurrent use of non-pharmacologic pain strategies (e.g. breastfeeding and skin-to-skin care), and number

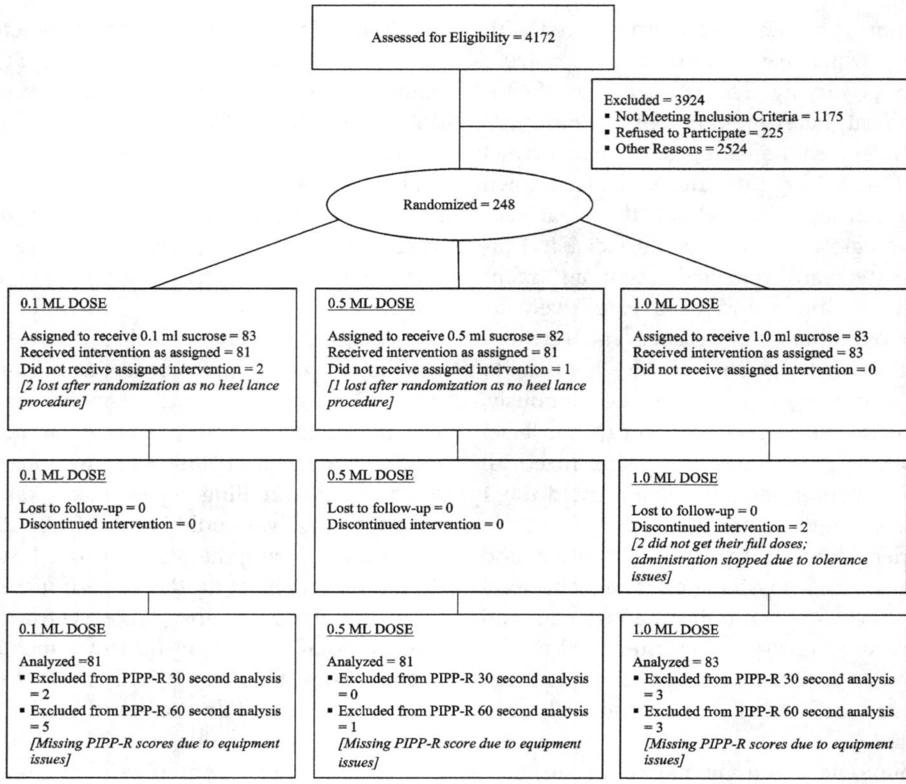

Fig. 1 Consort flow diagram of all neonates in participating NICUs screened for eligibility and randomized to sucrose intervention groups. Reasons for exclusion included not meeting inclusion criteria, refusals to participate, and other reasons [e.g., exclusion criteria, medical refusal (palliative care, social issues, and multiple research studies), isolation precautions, and researcher or parents unavailable for consent discussion]

Table 1 Demographic characteristics of the sucrose intervention groups

	Intervention		
	0.1 ml n = 81	0.5 ml *n* = 81	1.0 ml *n* = 83
Sex, n (%)			
-Female	44 (54.3)	32 (39.5)	41 (49.4)
-Male	37 (45.7)	49 (60.5)	42 (50.6)
Gestational age in weeks, mean (SD)	32.6 (4.2)	32.5 (4.1)	32.7 (4.1)
Weight in grams, mean (SD)	2002.3 (859.5)	1933.0 (927.0)	2055.5 (886.0)
Day of life, median (interquartile range)	6 (4 to 9)	7 (4 to 10)	6 (4 to 9)
Birthplace, n (%) (55 missing)			
-Inborn	31 (52.5)	33 (51.6)	40 (59.7)
-Outborn	28 (47.5)	31 (48.4)	27 (40.2)
SNAPPE-II score on admission, median (interquartile range)	5.0 (0 to 19)	5.0 (0 to 18)	8.0 (0 to 18)
Number of painful procedures since birth, median (interquartile range)	22 (14 to 34)	23 (15 to 37)	23 (13 to 40)
Number of sucrose doses since birth, median (interquartile range)	5 (2 to 8)	5 (3 to 9)	6 (3 to 9)
Use of concurrent non-pharmacologic pain strategies, n (%)	27 (33.3)	31 (35.2)	30 (34.1)

SNAPPE-II scores range from 0 to 158. Higher scores indicate greater severity of illness

Table 2 Mean pain intensity scores at 30s and 60s post heel lance

	Intervention			*P*
	0.1 ml	0.5 ml	1.0 ml	
PIPP-R 30s	*n = 79*	*n = 81*	*n = 80*	
	Mean (SD): 6.8 (3.5)	Mean (SD): 6.8 (3.2)	Mean (SD): 6.7 (3.4)	0.97
	Min: 0	Min: 1.0	Min: 0	
	Max: 17.5	Max: 16.3	Max: 18.7	
PIPP-R 60s	*n = 76*	*n = 80*	*n = 80*	
	Mean (SD): 7.0 (3.3)	Mean (SD): 6.9 (3.6)	Mean (SD): 6.7 (3.4)	0.93
	Min: 0	Min: 0	Min: 0	
	Max: 17.0	Max: 18.0	Max: 18.7	

PIPP-R scores range from 0 to 21. Higher scores indicate greater pain intensity

of painful procedures and sucrose doses since birth; Table 3]. Pain intensity scores across the 3 groups equated to mild pain for the majority of neonates (scores of < 7 on the PIPP-R; Table 4).

Adverse events and rescue doses

There were 5 reported adverse events among 5/245 (2.0%) neonates as defined by the a priori criteria. These events included 3 neonates who gagged/choked, 1 with heart rate < 80 bpm and 1 with oxygen saturation < 80% following sucrose administration. All events resolved spontaneously without medical intervention. The neonate who experienced oxygen saturation < 80%, was repositioned and recovered quickly. There were no significant differences in the proportion of adverse events by sucrose group ($P = .62$); however, a higher proportion of younger neonates experienced an adverse event (6.7% < 29 weeks versus 1.0% 29–42 weeks; $P = .044$).

In 13/245 (5.3%) neonates, the bedside nurse perceived that the intervention was not effective in minimizing pain during the procedure, and the research nurse (at the discretion of the bedside nurse) administered a "rescue" dose of sucrose (amount determined by the unit standard/policy). There was no significant difference in the number of rescue doses by sucrose group ($P = .33$), site ($P = .070$), or GA ($P = .47$).

Discussion

Oral administration of a very small dose of sucrose (0.1 ml) appears to be equally effective at reducing pain in neonates during a single painful procedure as larger doses. Sucrose administration in the clinical setting was associated with very few adverse events. This trial was

Table 3 Association of mean pain intensity scores with site and demographic characteristics

	PIPP-R 30 seconds		PIPP-R 60 seconds	
	Mean (SD)	*P*	Mean (SD)	*P*
Site		< 0.001		< 0.001
1	5.68 (3.31)		5.66 (3.26)	
2	7.55 (3.58)		8.09 (4.16)	
3	6.13 (2.31)		6.05 (2.54)	
4	8.21 (3.87)		8.23 (3.55)	
SNAPPE-II score on admission		0.087		0.058
-Median or below (0 to 5)	6.35 (3.06)		6.38 (3.22)	
-Above Median (6+)	7.03 (3.53)		7.17 (3.70)	
Gender	0.31 (3.32)	0.44	−0.05 (3.49)	0.90
Concurrent use of non-pharmacologic pain strategies during heel lance	0.38 (3.31)	0.33	0.10 (3.49)	0.82
	Spearman's correlation (r_s)	*P*	Spearman's correlation (r_s)	*P*
Gestational age	−0.26	< 0.001	− 0.30	< 0.001
Number of painful procedures	0.07	0.24	0.03	0.61
Number of sucrose doses since birth	0.004	0.95	−0.02	0.74

PIPP-R scores range from 0 to 21. Higher scores indicate greater pain intensity. SNAPPE-II scores range from 0 to 158. Higher scores indicate greater severity of illness

Table 4 Frequency of pain intensity scores by severity at 30s and 60s post heel lance

	Intervention			P
	0.1 ml	0.5 ml	1.0 ml	
PIPP-R at 30s, n (%)	*n* = 79	*n* = 81	*n* = 80	0.74
-None (0)	2 (2.5)	0 (0.0)	2 (2.5)	
-Mild (1 to 6.9)	40 (50.6)	46 (56.8)	39 (48.8)	
-Moderate (7 to 11.9)	30 (38.0)	27 (33.3)	33 (41.3)	
-Severe (12+)	7 (8.9)	8 (9.9)	6 (7.5)	
PIPP-R at 60s, n (%)	*n* = 76	*n* = 80	*n* = 80	0.97
-None (0)	1 (1.3)	1 (1.3)	2 (2.5)	
-Mild (1 to 6.9)	38 (50.0)	44 (55.0)	41 (51.3)	
-Moderate (7 to 11.9)	29 (38.2)	26 (32.5)	30 (37.5)	
-Severe (12+)	8 (10.5)	9 (11.3)	7 (8.8)	

PIPP-R scores range from 0 to 21. Higher scores indicate greater pain intensity

more closely aligned with a pragmatic design on the continuum between pragmatic and exploratory trials [19]. Unlike explanatory trials that test interventions under optimal conditions, pragmatic trials are more generalizable; however, they are also more prone to co-intervention.

Although site was controlled for in the primary outcome analyses, there was a difference in PIPP-R scores across sites (Table 3) that may be partially explained by organizational contextual factors that were not controlled for or assessed in the analyses. For example, although we enrolled neonates in the first 30 of days of life and collected information on exposure to painful procedures and sucrose received since birth, it is possible that sucrose administration and documentation practices differed due to clinical practice guidelines or organizational contextual factors (e.g., workload/staff ratios, unit culture, and the research or clinical experience of the bedside nurses) [20]. We also found higher pain scores were associated with more preterm neonates ($P < .001$; Table 3) and they experienced a slightly greater proportion of adverse events (3 versus 2 in neonates > 29 weeks GA), although total numbers were very small. Despite higher pain scores with lower GA, there was no difference in the number of rescue doses across GA, which might be explained by site differences in sucrose administration practices.

We could think of two possible explanations for why PIPP-R scores were significantly higher in the least mature group of neonates: (a) the PIPP-R measure inherently scores younger GA higher, or b) sucrose is less effective in these babies (e.g., they are less able to mount an endogenous opioid response that is the underlying mechanism of action of sweet taste [21]). Differences seen in mean pain intensity were not thought to be due to additional weighting in the PIPP-R measure by GA [< 28 weeks (+ 3), 28–31 weeks and 6 days (+ 2), 32 weeks to 35 weeks and 6 days (+ 1), and ≥ 36 weeks (0)], as there were no corresponding incremental differences seen by GA group. In terms of the latter explanation (b), this needs to be further researched with an adequate sample size of extremely premature neonates (< 28 weeks GA).

Our findings are consistent with past research (primarily in animals) that demonstrated that the analgesic effects of sucrose were primarily mediated by exposure and not dose [10, 22]. Although there was no difference in pain intensity at 30 and 60 s, pain was not fully eliminated during the heel lance procedure. Mean pain intensity scores equated to mild pain (Table 2), or approximately 3/10 if converted to the more common 10-point scale metric. As pain intensity was measured on a continuum, and treatment failure was not defined, the incidence of treatment failure was not determined. However, severe pain could definitely be considered a treatment failure and this occurred in 7.5 to 11.3% of neonates (Table 4) across sucrose doses. These results are similar to systematic reviews of other behavioral interventions, including breastfeeding [23] and skin-to-skin care [24]. Given that the majority of previous studies have used a single procedure, it is uncertain if the wide variably in neonatal pain response is attributed to the intervention or other factors which remain unknown [25]. Future work in the repeated use of interventions is warranted. In the meantime, we would recommend that if the initial dose of sucrose does not appear to be ameliorating the pain that additional rescue doses be provided during the procedure up to a specified amount. We would also recommend that multiple non-pharmacologic strategies be implemented simultaneously including swaddling, facilitated tucking, skin-to-skin/ kangaroo care, breastfeeding, and/ or pacifiers.

Knowledge is lacking on the long-term effects of sucrose with repeated administration. Of the studies that have evaluated repeated doses of sucrose [26–30], none have evaluated long-term outcomes of using sucrose for all painful procedures performed throughout the neonate's stay in the NICU. Johnston [26, 31] reported that 107 preterm infants < 31 weeks GA who were exposed to > 10 doses of sucrose per day in the first 7 days of life, after which time no pain relief was used, were more likely to exhibit poorer attention and motor development on the Neurobehavioral Assessment of Preterm Infants (NAPI) scale in the early months of life. Conversely, Banga [32] reported that of 93 neonates randomized to either repeated doses of sucrose or water for painful procedures for 7 consecutive days, there were no significant differences in NAPI scores or adverse events. Stevens [27] found no statistically significant differences between sucrose plus pacifier, water plus pacifier, or the standard care group on neurobiological risk status outcomes. Future research needs to address the repeated use of minimally effective doses of sucrose on the neurodevelopment of neonates and effectiveness over time.

Approximately 2% of neonates suffered adverse events. These all resolved spontaneously without medical intervention or with minimal caregiver intervention (e.g. positioning). Most adverse events occurred at one site, where the highest proportion of the sickest neonates is cared for, although this is not represented in the study sample. This adverse event rate is consistent with the 2016 Cochrane sucrose review [2]. Although researchers are becoming more vigilant in observing and reporting adverse events, it remains unclear how adverse events are reported (i.e., chart review is considerably different from careful direct observation of every newborn infant who is receiving the intervention).

A few study limitations need mention. Pain intensity did not differ significantly between the 30 and 60-s time points. Although these time intervals have been used in multiple research studies of acute procedural pain, they are arbitrary and designed based on mean behavioral response time; observing neonates for longer periods of time may demonstrate additional responses of less typical responders or other types of responses (e.g. physiologic, cortical). Although there has been significant validation and updating of the PIPP-R measure, there remains no gold standard for measuring pain in infants that may influence the determination of the effectiveness (or lack thereof) of pain relieving interventions. The future, which includes novel strategies for better understanding of the developing cortical pain circuitry, will pave the way for better prevention and treatment of pain in this vulnerable population.

Finally, we were limited by the documentation in the medical records, which may not have included all pain relieving strategies such as sucrose and non-pharmacologic interventions. Although we believe infants should receive some form of intervention for all painful procedures, it is difficult to speculate on whether the discrepancy between number of documented painful procedures and pain-relieving interventions is an administration or documentation issue. As the number of painful procedures included since birth was extensive (e.g., tape removals, bloodwork, injections, vascular access attempts/insertions, NG/OG tube insertions and suctioning, chest tube attempts/insertions, lumbar punctures, eye exams, and urinary catheterizations), it is possible oral sucrose is not routinely administered for each of these types of procedures, depending on unit standards/practices.

Conclusions

No difference in pain intensity was shown among 3 doses of sucrose during an acute tissue-damaging procedure in hospitalized neonates. The 0.1 ml of 24% sucrose dose was the minimally effective dose that can be recommended for use out of the 3 doses most commonly reported to be effective in previous research. Subsequent study is required to determine the sustained effectiveness of this dose in reducing pain intensity during painful procedures neonates experience in the NICU over time and across GA, and the long-term effects of cumulative sucrose use.

Abbreviations

GA: Gestational age; NAPI: Neurobehavioral assessment of preterm infants; NICU: Neonatal intensive care unit; PIPP-R: Premature infant pain profile-revised; SD: Standard deviation; SNAPPE-II: Score for neonatal acute physiology perinatal extension- II

Acknowledgements

Thank you to the research nurses who collected data at each site: KC, BG, MP, JR and JW; the research database manager: VK; and the neonatal intensive care units that agreed to participate.

Funding

Supported by the Canadian Institutes of Health Research (MOP-126167). All study sucrose and supplies were purchased through grant funds. The funder had no role in the design and conduct of the study; collection, management, analysis, and interpretation of the data; preparation, review, or approval of the manuscript; and decision to submit the manuscript for publication.

Authors' contributions

The authors have read and given final approval for this version to be published, and take full responsibility for the work. Each meets the criteria set out by ICMJE for authorship. BS and CV had full access to all of the data in the study and take responsibility for the integrity of the data and the accuracy of the data analysis. *Study design and concept:* BS, MB, MCY, KD, CE, SG, DH, CM, SS, JS, AS, AT, CV, KW, AW, and JY. *Management, analysis, and interpretation of data:* BS, MCY, SG, DH, CM, SR, AT, CV, KW, and JY. *Preparation, review, or approval of the final manuscript:* BS, MB, MCY, KD, CE, SG, DH, CM, SR, SS, JS, AS, AT, CV, KW, AW, and JY. *Statistical analysis:* CV. *Obtained funding:* BS, MB, MCY, KD, CE, SG, DH, CM, SS, JS, AS, AT, CV, KW, AW, and JY. *Administrative, technical, or material support:* BS and CV. *Study supervision:* BS, MCY, KD, SG, DH, and JY. All authors read and approved the final manuscript.

Competing interests

The authors declare that they have no competing interests.

Author details

[1]The Hospital for Sick Children, Lawrence S. Bloomberg Faculty of Nursing, University of Toronto, 686 Bay Street, Toronto, Ontario M5G 0A4, Canada. [2]Daphne Cockwell School of Nursing, Ryerson University, 350 Victoria Street, Toronto, Ontario M5B 2K3, Canada. [3]School of Nursing and Departments of Pediatrics, Psychology, and Neuroscience, Dalhousie University, IWK Health Centre, Forrest Building, P.O. Box 15000, Halifax, Nova Scotia B3H 4R2, Canada. [4]Trillium Health Partners, 100 Queensway West, Mississauga, Ontario L5B 1B8, Canada. [5]Faculty of Health Sciences, School of Nursing, University of Ottawa, Children's Hospital of Eastern Ontario, Research Institute, 451 Smyth Road, Ottawa, Ontario K1H 8M5, Canada. [6]The Hospital for Sick Children, 686 Bay Street, Toronto, Ontario M5G 0A4, Canada. [7]The Hospital for Sick

Children, Leslie Dan Faculty of Pharmacy, University of Toronto, 686 Bay Street, Toronto, Ontario M5G 0A4, Canada. [8]The Hospital for Sick Children, 686 Bay Street, Toronto, Ontario M5G 0A4, Canada. [9]The Hospital for Sick Children, Dalla Lana School of Public Health, University of Toronto, 686 Bay Street, Toronto, Ontario M5G 0A4, Canada. [10]Holland Bloorview Kids Rehabilitation Hospital, Lawrence S. Bloomberg Faculty of Nursing, University of Toronto, 150 Kilgour Road, Toronto, Ontario M4G 1R8, Canada. [11]The Hospital for Sick Children, Lawrence S. Bloomberg Faculty of Nursing, University of Toronto, 155 College Street, Suite 130, Toronto, Ontario M5T 1P8, Canada. [12]Daphne Cockwell School of Nursing, Ryerson University, 350 Victoria Street, Toronto, Ontario M5B 2K3, Canada. [13]Faculty of Nursing, University of Alberta, 3-141 Edmonton Clinic Health Academy, 11405 87 Avenue, Edmonton, Alberta T6G 1C9, Canada. [14]Division of Neonatology, Department of Pediatrics, University of British Columbia, 2D19-4480 Oak Street, Vancouver, British Columbia V6H 4V4, Canada. [15]Faculty of Health Sciences, School of Nursing, University of Ottawa, Ottawa Hospital Research Institute, 451 Smyth Road, Ottawa, Ontario K1H 8M5, Canada. [16]Institute for Clinical Evaluative Sciences (ICES), The Institute of Health Policy, Management and Evaluation, University of Toronto, Veterans Hill Trail, 2075 Bayview Avenue G1 06, Toronto, Ontario M4N 3M5, Canada. [17]The Hospital for Sick Children, 686 Bay Street, Toronto, Ontario M5G 0A4, Canada.

References

1. Bueno M, Yamada J, Harrison D, Khan S, Ohlsson A, Adams-Webber T, et al. A systematic review and meta-analyses of nonsucrose sweet solutions for pain relief in neonates. Pain Res Manage. 2013;18(3):153–61.
2. Stevens B, Yamada J, Ohlsson A, Haliburton S, Shorkey A. Sucrose for analgesia in newborn infants undergoing painful procedures. Cochrane Database Syst Rev. 2016;7(7):CD001069.
3. Lee GY, Yamada J, Kyololo O, Shorkey A, Stevens B. Pediatric clinical practice guidelines for acute procedural pain: a systematic review. Pediatrics. 2014; 133(3):500–15.
4. Taddio A, Yiu A, Smith RW, Katz J, McNair C, Shah V. Variability in clinical practice guidelines for sweetening agents in newborn infants undergoing painful procedures. Clin J Pain. 2009;25(2):153–5.
5. Bellieni CV, Johnston CC. Analgesia, nil or placebo to babies, in trials that test new analgesic treatments for procedural pain. Acta Paediatr. 2016;105(2):129–36.
6. Campbell-Yeo M. 'First, do no harm'–the use of analgesia or placebo as control for babies in painful clinical trials. Acta Paediatr. 2016;105(2):119–20.
7. Harrison D, Bueno M, Yamada J, Adams-Webber T, Stevens B. Analgesic effects of sweet-tasting solutions for infants: current state of equipoise. Pediatrics. 2010;126(5):894–902.
8. Randomize.net. A comprehensive internet-based randomization service for clinical trials. http://www.randomize.net (2015). Accessed 11 Apr 2017.
9. Stevens B, Johnston C, Franck L, Petryshen P, Jack A, Foster G. The efficacy of developmentally sensitive interventions and sucrose for relieving procedural pain in very low birth weight neonates. Nurs Res. 1999;48(1):35–43.
10. Blass EM, Shide DJ. Some comparisons among the calming and pain-relieving effects of sucrose, glucose, fructose and lactose in infant rats. Chem Senses. 1994;19(3):239–49.
11. Pillai Riddell RR, Racine NM, Gennis HG, Turcotte K, Uman LS, Horton RE, et al. Non-pharmacological management of infant and young child procedural pain. Cochrane Database Syst Rev. 2015;(12):Cd006275.
12. Ohlsson A, Shah PS. Paracetamol (acetaminophen) for prevention or treatment of pain in newborns. Cochrane Database Syst Rev. 2015;(6): Cd011219.
13. Gibbins S, Stevens BJ, Yamada J, Dionne K, Campbell-Yeo M, Lee G, et al. Validation of the premature infant pain profile-revised (PIPP-R). Early Hum Dev. 2014;90(4):189–93.
14. Stevens BJRNP, Gibbins SRNP, Yamada JRNP, Dionne KRNMN, Lee GRNM, Johnston CRNDF, et al. The premature infant pain profile-revised (PIPP-R): initial validation and feasibility. Clin J Pain. 2014;30(3):238–43.
15. Lee GY, Stevens BJ. Neonatal and infant pain assessment. In: McGrath PJ, Stevens BJ, Walker SM, Zempsky WT, editors. Oxford textbook of paediatric pain. 1st ed. Oxford: Oxford University Press; 2014. p. 353–69.
16. Campbell-Yeo ML, Johnston CC, Joseph KS, Feeley N, Chambers CT, Barrington KJ. Cobedding and recovery time after heel lance in preterm twins: results of a randomized trial. Pediatrics. 2012;130(3):500–6.
17. Harsha SS, Archana BR. SNAPPE-II (score for neonatal acute physiology with Perinatal extension-II) in predicting mortality and morbidity in NICU. J Clin Diagn Res. 2015;9(10):Sc10–2.
18. Richardson DK, Corcoran JD, Escobar GJ, Lee SK. SNAP-II and SNAPPE-II: simplified newborn illness severity and mortality risk scores. J Pediat. 2001; 138(1):92–100.
19. Patsopoulos NA. A pragmatic view on pragmatic trials. Dialogues Clin Neurosci. 2011;13(2):217–24.
20. Estabrooks CA, Squires JE, Hutchinson AM, Scott S, Cummings GG, Kang SH, et al. Assessment of variation in the Alberta context tool: the contribution of unit level contextual factors and specialty in Canadian pediatric acute care settings. BMC Health Ser Res. 2011;11(1):1.
21. Johnston CC, Fillion F, Campbell-Yeo M, Goulet C, Bell L, McNaughton K, Byron J, Aita M, Finley GA, Walker CD. Kangaroo mothercare diminishes pain from heel lance in very preterm neonates: a crossover trial. BMC Pediatr. 2008;8(1):13.
22. Anseloni VC, Weng HR, Terayama R, Letizia D, Davis BJ, Ren K, et al. Age-dependency of analgesia elicited by intraoral sucrose in acute and persistent pain models. Pain. 2002;97(1–2):93–103.
23. Shah PS, Herbozo C, Aliwalas LL, Shah VS. Breastfeeding or breast milk for procedural pain in neonates. Cochrane Database Syst Rev. 2012;12: Cd004950.
24. Johnston C, Campbell-Yeo M, Fernandes A, Inglis D, Streiner D, Zee R. Skin-to-skin care for procedural pain in neonates. Cochrane Database Syst Rev. 2014;(1):Cd008435.
25. Cignacco E, Denhaerynck K, Nelle M, Buhrer C, Engberg S. Variability in pain response to a non-pharmacological intervention across repeated routine pain exposure in preterm infants: a feasibility study. Acta Paediatr. 2009; 98(5):842–6.
26. Johnsston CC, Filion F, Snider L, Majnemer A, Limperopoulos C, Walker CD, et al. Routine sucrose analgesia during the first week of life in neonates younger than 31 weeks' postconceptional age. Pediatrics. 2002;110(3):523-8.
27. Stevens B, Yamada J, Beyene J, Gibbins S, Petryshen P, Stinson J, et al. Consistent management of repeated procedural pain with sucrose in preterm neonates: is it effective and safe for repeated use over time? Clin J Pain. 2005;21(6):543–8.
28. Gaspardo CM, Miyase CI, Chimello JT, Martinez FE, Martins Linhares MB. Is pain relief equally efficacious and free of side effects with repeated doses of oral sucrose in preterm neonates? Pain. 2008;137(1):16–25.
29. Taddio A, Shah V, Atenafu E, Katz J. Influence of repeated painful procedures and sucrose analgesia on the development of hyperalgesia in newborn infants. Pain. 2009;144(1–2):43–8.
30. Harrison D, Loughnan P, Manias E, Gordon I, Johnston L. Repeated doses of sucrose in infants continue to reduce procedural pain during prolonged hospitalizations. Nurs Res. 2009;58(6):427–34.
31. Johnston CC, Filion F, Snider L, Limperopoulos C, Majnemer A, Pelausa E, et al. How much sucrose is too much sucrose? Pediatrics. 2007;119(1):226.
32. Banga S, Datta V, Rehan HS, Bhakhri BK. Effect of sucrose analgesia, for repeated painful procedures, on short-term neurobehavioral outcome of preterm neonates: a randomized controlled trial. J Trop Pediat. 2016;62(2):101–6.

12

Barriers and enablers to skin-to-skin contact at birth in healthy neonates

Amala James Alenchery[1], Joanne Thoppil[1], Carl Denis Britto[1], Jimena Villar de Onis[4], Lavina Fernandez[2] and P. N. Suman Rao[3*]

Abstract

Background: Skin to skin contact (SSC) at birth is the standard of care for newborns without risk factors. However, implementation of SSC at birth has been far from optimal. A qualitative study was undertaken to determine the barriers, enablers and potential solutions to implementation of SSC at birth in healthy newborn infants in a level III neonatal-care facility in Bangalore, India.

Methods: Consultants and residents/postgraduates (PG) from the departments of Obstetrics ($n = 19$) and Pediatrics ($n = 14$) and nurses ($n = 8$) in the labor room (LR) participated in the study. In depth interviews (IDI) and focus group discussions (FGD) were carried out with an interview guide and a moderators' guide containing inbuilt probes. Subjects of FGD were homogenous. All IDI and FGD were audio-taped, transcribed and analyzed using N VIVO version 9 (using free and tree nodes). Two authors separately coded the transcripts. Major and minor themes were identified. Rigor was ensured by triangulation and theoretical saturation. Informed consent and ethical approval was obtained.

Results: All subjects were aware of SSC at birth, some of its benefits and had practiced SSC. The major barriers identified were lack of personnel (nurses), time constraint, difficulty in deciding on eligibility for SSC, safety concerns, interference with clinical routines, and interdepartmental issues. Recall of an adverse event during SSC was also a major barrier. Furthermore, we found that most participants considered 1 h as impractical; and promoted 5–15 min SSC. Minor themes were gender bias of the newborn and cultural practices.

The participants offered solutions such as assigning a helper exclusively for SSC, allowing a family member into the LR, continuing SSC after initial routines, antenatal counselling, constant reminders in the form of periodic sessions with audiovisual aids or posters in the obstetrics ward, training of new nurses and PG, and inclusion of SSC in medical and nursing curriculum.

Conclusions: The major barriers to SSC at birth are lack of personnel, time constraint and safety concerns. Training, designated health personnel for SSC and teamwork are the key interventions likely to improve SSC at birth.

Keywords: Qualitative study, Barriers, Skin to skin contact at birth

* Correspondence: raosumanv@gmail.com
[3]Department of Neonatology, St. John's Medical College Hospital, Sarjapur Road, Koramangala, Bangalore 560034, India

Background

The transition from intrauterine to extra uterine life represents one of the most dynamic and potentially dangerous events in the human life cycle. This early "sensitive period" after birth during which the newborn adapts to the new world outside the mother's womb requires intimate contact between the infant and mother in order to build a platform for bonding and to improve the physiologic and neurologic development of the child as well as make the mother more confident in her own abilities to nurse her child [1]. Skin to skin contact (SSC) at birth is the placing of the naked newly born baby prone on the mother's bare chest at birth or soon afterward for a minimum duration of at least 1 h. The healthy full-term human infant, placed in SSC after birth, directs himself or herself to the mother's breast and nipple and starts to suckle by about 1 h of age [2].

Health care personnel are uniquely placed to positively influence the mother-infant interaction at birth [3]. It is recommended that healthy infants should be placed and should remain in direct SSC with their mothers immediately after delivery until the first feeding is accomplished [2]. SSC at birth has been shown to have several beneficial effects for the newly born. A meta-analysis of 38 randomized controlled trials including 3472 mother-infant dyads has shown that it improved breastfeeding duration, cardio-respiratory-metabolic stability at birth and temperature. SSC at birth reduces stress associated with birth and facilitates self-regulation. Neurobehavioral benefits and positive parenting impact are evident even after a decade, making SSC at birth the optimal method of care [2].

Despite the reported benefits, direct skin-to-skin contact after birth is not universally practiced. In fact, routines exist today, that separate the mother and her newborn infant as a common practice [4]. There are several barriers to implementation of SSC at birth, even as a component of KMC at the institutional level, health personnel level and maternal or family level [5]; most related to common practice rather than to a medical concern [6].

There is a lack of qualitative studies looking specifically at early SSC, and particularly a dearth of studies exploring the perception of health personnel about SSC at birth from lower-middle income countries (LMICs). Though studies have explored barriers and enablers in the implementation of kangaroo mother care (KMC), this data from KMC implementation may not be applicable to SSC at birth as KMC [7] refers to a standardized method of care of preterm/ low birth weight (LBW) with early, prolonged SSC, frequent breast feeding and early discharge and follow-up [8] whereas SSC is defined as placing the naked newborn prone on the mother's chest and abdomen immediately after birth [2].

A questionnaire based study to understand the barriers for implementation of SSC at birth showed that primary resistance to SSC at birth is at the health care worker level [9]. Furthermore, we hypothesize that most perinatal health care workers are not fully aware of the methodology and guidelines of SSC. This qualitative study is therefore undertaken to explore the barriers, enablers and solutions to promotion of SSC at birth as perceived by the health care personnel.

Methods

Study design

With the aim of understanding the essence of the health workers' experience of the event of "SSC at birth", we undertook the phenomenological life world approach of qualitative research as developed by Husserl and Merleau-Ponty [10], specifically through the use of in-depth interview and focus group discussions. The life world is the world of everyday experience, which is unique for every person, although shared with others. Phenomenological research focuses on experiences in everyday life, as experienced before theorizing, and is a well suited basis to describe and understand human experiences of a specific phenomenon such as health workers' experiences of SSC. It is a meaning oriented approach and includes discovering, analyzing, clarifying and seeking patterns of a certain phenomenon, based on a description of how the life world of humans is experienced, acted out and described. In an interview study this means that the researcher must meet the informants and their experiences in an unprejudiced way and with a reflective, or even a self-reflective attitude.

The study was designed around the work experiences of the pediatric and obstetric staff, as in the Indian context, where SSC falls under the responsibility of the pediatrician and nursing staff with the obstetrician playing some role. Therefore, describing the lived experience of the health workers from nursing, pediatric and obstetric specialties with regard to SSC at birth, we aspired to comprehend the barriers and enablers to the phenomenon of "skin to skin contact at birth".

Setting

The study was conducted in the St. John's Medical College Hospital (Bangalore, India), a tertiary care private medical college hospital, possessing a level III neonatal care facility with an average of 2500 deliveries per year. The hospital provides service to patients from all walks of life, with the motto to help serve the under-privileged societies of the nation. The hospital mainly caters to patients belonging to the lower socio-economic strata and serves as a referral center to smaller rural health-care establishments in surrounding areas, particularly in-utero referrals of high-risk pregnancies. SSC at birth was initiated in the hospital as part of routine care for the healthy newly born in January 2011. Currently, SSC is implemented during daytime only for an average period of about 10 min in the immediate postpartum period.

Participants

The participants included 41 health care workers stationed in the labor room of the hospital, all of whom were contacted in person and agreed to participate in the study. The groups for focus group discussion were homogenous and included personnel belonging to the same category. The health personnel were categorized as: Obstetric consultants ($n = 5$) and Obstetric residents ($n = 14$), Neonatology consultants ($n = 2$), Pediatric residents ($n = 12$) and nurses of the obstetric ward and labor room ($n = 8$). Purposive sampling was conducted from each of these homogenous groups as we had direct access to all health workers in the unit involved in conducting deliveries and administering perinatal care. This was done until no new ideas emerged and we reached data saturation and triangulation. Saturation refers to a state of data redundancy where no new ideas emerge and marks the end point of the interview or discussion and triangulation is a technique in qualitative research which involves convergence of information from different sources in order to obtain different dimensions for the same phenomenon and to validate the consistency of data obtained.

Procedure

An interview guide (Additional file 1: Annexure 1) and a moderators' guide for focus group discussions (FGD) (Additional file 2: Annexure 2), both developed by an iterative process where a questionnaire was administered to several experts (doctors with experience in the field of perinatal research and social scientists) on the particular subject matter, who remained external to the study. Their suggestions were incorporated in the questionnaire. The questionnaire was pilot tested in the first five interviews and redundant items were deleted. This reformulated questionnaire was used to explore the barriers and enablers of SSC at birth as perceived by health personnel. Open ended questions and probes for discussion were inbuilt into the guide for a thorough understanding of the topic. The questionnaires used for the interviews and focus group discussions have been attached as copies.

In depth interviews and focus group discussions were conducted so that the individual and group perspectives could be assessed, after obtaining ethical clearance from the Institutional Ethics Board. Individual interviews were conducted with all senior consultants of the departments, while the more junior faculty - residents, fellows and junior staff nurses - were included in both interviews and focus group discussions in order to encourage emerging ideas, maintain confidentiality and to prevent the hierarchy within departments from skewing the results. Some of the junior faculty were also interviewed individually in order to enhance the quality of data obtained.

In total, 21 face to face in depth interviews (IDI) were conducted by two investigators (AJ and JT) in the NICU and the postnatal wards of the hospital (13 IDI with obstetric personnel, 7 with pediatric personnel and 1 with a labor room nurse in charge. Care was taken to ensure privacy and complete confidentiality. Informed consent was obtained prior to the interview from all subjects. The interviews were audio taped with an average duration of interviews lasting 30 min. Clarifications were sought if any aspect of the transcript was not clear.

The two investigators conducted 4 FGDs with key stakeholders – obstetric residents ($n = 7$), pediatric residents ($n = 7$), neonatal fellows ($n = 4$) and nursing staff ($n = 7$), with the help of the moderator's focus group guide. The subjects for the FGD were homogenous and from the same category. The group discussions were held in a classroom outside the NICU and in the OBG wards classroom. At the time of the FGD, all subjects were given the informed consent form. A co-investigator, a trained social scientist, with experience in conducting FGDs assisted and plotted the sociogram, which gave a visual representation of the dynamics of the group discussion, in order to avoid any dominant or passive members in the same group and to ensure maximal and equal participation from all subjects. Multiple viewpoints and responses were discussed during the FGDs. The FGDs were audio taped. Each discussion lasted approximately 45 min. Clarifications about some aspects of the transcript were done after discussion with the participants.

Of the 41 subjects approached during the study, 17 subjects were included only in IDIs while 20 subjects were included only in the FGDs as part of four separate homogenous groups and there were 4 subjects who were included in both the IDIs and FGDs,

The researchers who interviewed the participants and facilitated the group discussions were independent medical students and did not hold any managerial role or position of authority to reduce any potential bias. The interviews and FGDs were conducted in English, which is the language of communication in this hospital, transcribed verbatim, and anonymized.

Data analysis

The main methodology covered was a deductive analysis based on preliminary analysis and iterative reading of the data. This involved constantly comparing newly emerging themes from the data with a pre-established framework.

A framework analytical approach was used for data analysis. The steps of this analysis were as follows:

1) Familiarization with data and coding
2) Identifying a thematic framework
3) Sorting quotes
4) Placing quotes under the thematic category
5) Mapping and interpreting

Two authors (AJ, JT) initially familiarized themselves with the data by reading and rereading the transcripts which ensured an ease of accessibility to the transcript at a later stage. Then, the focus group discussions and interviews were independently coded to ensure credibility and trustworthiness. Any differences in the coding were resolved by consensual agreement of all authors. This process of familiarization and coding helped to identify new themes and categories that led to an iterative process. Several quotes in the transcripts could be identified with multiple themes and the process was reiterated in order to avoid overlooking any emerging themes [11].

N Vivo version 9 (QSR International, Burlington, Massachusetts) was used to classify the nodes as free and tree nodes. Tree nodes refer to codes which are organised hierarchically into categories and subcategories, while free nodes are emergent themes which are not attached to a pre-existing tree node [12].The nodes developed were used to code the transcripts inductively following a process of constant comparison between the emerging themes/codes and pre-existing codes. Any emergent code was added as free node or attached to a tree node according to its place in the initial thematic framework. Salient quotes were noted. Coding density, which refers to the strength of association between themes was used to identify recurrent themes. The themes with highest coding density were categorized as major themes and the others as minor themes. Based on this, a final thematic model was developed.

Results

Based on the interviews and group discussions, several main barriers emerged, all of which were believed to prevent SSC from being carried out as routine practice for all healthy term neonates. Along with the barriers and enablers, solutions that can help promote SSC were also brought to light. The participants of the study were personnel of the obstetric, pediatric and nursing staff, comprising of males ($n = 8$) and females ($n = 33$), ranging in ages from 24 to 50 years old with the average years of experience being of 15.1 years for the consultants of both departments and 3.2 years for the residents of obstetric department and 3.5 years for the residents of the paediatric and neonatology department.

The importance attributed to SSC among the various departments, the knowledge regarding practice and need for SSC and personal experience of the staff were the foundation for the barriers to SSC at birth, and were similar among the health personnel groups, each focussing on a different subcategory.

The enablers are the existing practices which will help to further establish the practice of SSC, while solutions are merely proposed suggestions which can be utilised by the respective departments in order to promote SSC and furthermore practice it as an established standard of care.

Table 1 shows the main barriers challenging the practice of SSC, enablers that promote the practice and solutions to the perceived barriers.

The figure serves as a graphical summary of the results and serves as a consolidated representation of the barriers to SSC and possible solutions for the same (Fig. 1).

Attempts were made to understand the nature of the perceived difficulties in implementing SSC as a routine practice and the results are as follows.

A. BARRIERS

Table 1 Barriers, Enablers to SSC and Solutions to promote SSC

Barriers	Enablers	Solutions
Skewed health-care staff client ratio in the labor room • Lack of Personnel • Time Constraints	Knowledge of Benefits • Motivation by Pediatricians	Dedicated bystander • Dedicated staff • Relative/family member
Apprehensions related to the procedure • Concern of Safety • Dilemma in decision making		Structured periodic inter-department teaching • Training staff • Reinforcement by Demonstration • Interdepartmental dialogue
Parochialism towards SSC • Lack of Awareness • General lack of belief • Lack of constant motivation	Maternal Acceptance	Antenatal awareness • Creating demand
Interdepartmental Issues Minor barriers • Interference with other clinical procedures • Gender preference for the newborn	Positive Experience	Early SSC – a practical alternative

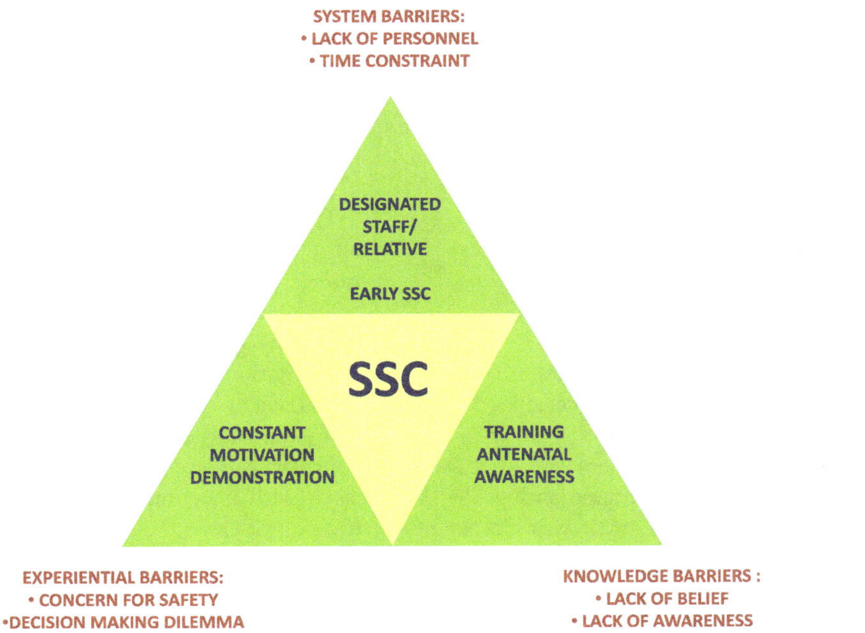
SYSTEM BARRIERS:
• LACK OF PERSONNEL
• TIME CONSTRAINT
DESIGNATED STAFF/ RELATIVE
EARLY SSC
SSC
CONSTANT MOTIVATION DEMONSTRATION
TRAINING ANTENATAL AWARENESS
EXPERIENTIAL BARRIERS:
• CONCERN FOR SAFETY
•DECISION MAKING DILEMMA
KNOWLEDGE BARRIERS :
• LACK OF BELIEF
• LACK OF AWARENESS

Fig. 1 Barriers and solutions to skin to skin contact at birth

Lack of personnel and time constraints owing to the skewed health-care staff to patient ratio were recurring barriers that emerged from all the FGDs and IDIs. Other barriers identified include concerns over the safety of the newborn falling down from the mother's chest, lack of awareness, and doubts in the efficacy of this practice coupled with inadequate motivation to carry out SSC. Interdepartmental disagreements and dilemmas in the eligibility of newborns to undergo SSC were other barriers.

A.1. Skewed health-care staff- client ratio in the labor room

This was a prominent barrier during the night shifts when nurses in the labour room are especially understaffed and overworked by their wide range of duties forcing SSC to be a relatively unimportant priority, particularly when the recommended time for SCC is for an hour. The pediatrician on call has to assess the newborn in addition to a host of other responsibilities in the ward, neonatal care unit and neonatal emergency. This arrangement leads to time constraints making it very unlikely for SSC to be practiced outside regular working hours i.e. 9 am to 4 pm. It is not uncommon for more than one delivery to occur simultaneously in this setting, further stretching resources and making SSC in a situation like this a near impossible task.

N: "Mainly it is the lack of staff. For this one-hour, we can't keep one staff throughout."

Ped: "The pediatricians on duty, being understaffed, have to leave their designated ward duty and attend to the deliveries. Hence, staying with the baby for the entire duration of SSC is not feasible especially when the patient influx is high".

Ped: "Of late, the issues we've had are usually the nurses are in a hurry to finish their work and get done with the delivery, either because they have got more deliveries coming in or they've got admissions coming in or they're short of staff."

A.2. Apprehensions related to the procedure

A major barrier perceived during the course of the study was recall of an adverse event in the labor room wherein a healthy baby became cyanosed during SSC and required resuscitation. The obstetricians felt that as the treating physician, they would be held accountable if there was any untoward event.

Ob-gyn: "We are answerable more than the pediatrician. For 9 months, the patient has seen us, so they'll expect more from us. So it is more of our responsibility. That's why we are a little jittery with care that nothing should happen to the baby and mother."

This was coupled with other concerns like the baby slipping from the mother's chest and falling as well as being uncomfortable making the decision regarding a newborn's eligibility to undergo SSC. Most often, young pediatric residents or fellows are responsible for deciding SSC eligibility, which is not always straightforward.

Ob-gyn: *"Definitely there is fear of the baby falling if we're thinking the baby should be on the mother while doing episiotomy and the mother is tossing and turning in pain."*

Ped: "Deciding on eligibility for SSC is a grey zone"

A.3. Parochialism towards SSC

In a teaching hospital, there is a constant turnover of staff. New staff is not always adequately sensitized to the importance and benefits of SSC, and in this study most of the members of the obstetric department were not aware of the guidelines. In fact, they felt implementing SSC for one whole hour immediately after birth was almost impossible and were unwilling to even consider the possibility. Few even considered it more harmful than beneficial. Several other doctors, especially the new resident doctors felt the same, as they were unaware of the practice and its benefits. Disinterest and general lack of buy-in was a barrier, which seemed to be widespread among all departments. More than logistic issues, the attitude of health care personnel to the process emerged as a barrier.

Ob-gyn: *"Nobody has really told us how it is to be done. We just know that SSC is good for the baby and its being done. But how it is to be done and what is to be done, nobody has really told us. Why it is to be done, how it is beneficial to the mother or baby, no one has taken that extra mile to tell it to us, the gynecologists. Maybe the people doing it will know about it but they have not told us why."*

Ped: "I think the biggest thing is not in lack of personnel, I think it's in the attitude of people; wherein people don't see the need or they don't see the importance of SSC."

Like any other practice that is not a mandated protocol, frequent motivation is essential to ensure that SSC is practiced as a routine procedure. Most of the participants in the study felt that since it was a relatively new practice, it was difficult to remember to promote SSC and it was the responsibility of the pediatricians to be a constant source of motivation.

A nurse on labor room duty expressed that the paediatrician attending the delivery was hastening them to bring the baby away from the mother for routine examination as they had to tend to other sick infants and could not spare one hour of their time solely for SSC. To quote her:

N: "They are busy, so bring the baby, they'll say. They want to collect samples. They say that you can do after we go. Sometimes they do not know we are giving SSC."

A.4. Departmental issues

The nature of SSC as such calls for teamwork and close inter-departmental co-operation. Obstetricians and nurses perceived the onus of SSC to lie on the pediatricians. However, the nurses felt the pediatricians were hastening the shift of the baby from the mother to the resuscitation station, while the pediatricians felt the obstetricians were more inclined to separate the baby from the mother and the obstetricians state their main concern is to ensure progression and completion of labor with no complications and hence, do not concentrate on SSC.

Interestingly, the head nurse in the labor room felt that interdepartmental issues were one of the most addressable barriers to facilitating and promoting SSC by ensuring continuing conversation among the members of the departments.

N: "We cannot identify the staff and say it is your responsibility. If we say that and identify, it is not going to happen smoothly. It is the teamwork; equally the paediatrician, gynaecologist and labour room sister are responsible. Suppose if one of them is not doing it the other person has to remind."

A few minor barriers that were also of concern were the lack of personal experience by the staff, interference with clinical routines, for example, during the period when the shift change of staff occurs, they tend to concentrate on their routine work rather than spending time on establishing and maintaining SSC, and the lack of willingness from the mother. Another minor barrier which emerged was the maternal refusal for SSC due togender preference, which refers to the prevailing preference for the birth a male child by the families in the setting of a hospital in India, a low middle income country (LMIC).

N: *"They [the mothers] are expecting a boy baby and they get a girl. So they push the baby away."*

B. Enablers for SSC

Though there were many constraints that challenged the practice, the factors that motivate the implementation of the practice were:

B.1. Knowledge of benefits of SSC

Knowledge of the benefits of SSC mainly by the nurses and pediatricians was one of the key factors motivating health personnel to implement SSC. They believed that it would actually make a difference. The main source of knowledge regarding SSC was either from the nursing curriculum or from the teachings of a dedicated and motivated paediatrician.

N: "First of all it helps in bonding, then baby's temperature, feeding issues, psychological effects on the mother as well as the baby. It's an opportunity for the mother and baby to bond. It needs to be done."

Motivation by paediatricians

The nurses also stated that the implementation of SSC was to a large extent dependent on the pediatrician attending the labor call. A very motivated pediatric resident would ensure SSC implementation and would even teach the nurses, because they have witnessed the benefits of SSC.

Ped: "We are keen on doing SSC so we are constantly motivating them (nurses)."

N: "The pediatricians are generally around to remind us to do that."

B.2. Positive experiences

A firsthand experience of the benefits was crucial. Obstetricians, pediatricians and nurses who had practiced SSC and had firsthand experience of the benefits were the biggest promoters of SSC.

Ob-gyn: "Yeah, definitely, there is lot of decreased crying, decreased pain for the mother. The mother is not really concerned about her episiotomy and suturing."

N: "The child will be crying and when we put the child on the mother's breast, somehow I've seen how the child stops crying and you know, he feels more comfortable when he's on the mother."

B.3. Maternal acceptance

The level of acceptance of the practice by the mothers and their families were equal and positive despite difference in educational, cultural and religious backgrounds, as perceived by the medical personnel during the interviews and FGDs. Even if some mothers were apprehensive to begin with, their fears were quickly allayed once a nurse held the baby in place.

Hygiene issues of placing a newborn on the mother's bare chest in the labor room were of least concern as most of the doctors and staff believes the exchange of commensal skin flora between the mother and the newborn was beneficial.

C. Solutions

C.1. Dedicated bystander

Even amongst those motivated and aware of the benefits, it was perceived by health personnel across the specialties that a dedicated person for ensuring the safety of the baby would ensure SSC implementation. The dedicated person for ensuring SSC need not be a qualified staff nurse; it could be a relative who holds the baby in SSC.

N: "If one person is given the responsibility of taking care of the SSC, then I think it is possible that we can do (it) for most of the patients. Then in night deliveries, where we are not able to do now, we can do it."

Ob-gyn: "Maybe a responsible attender could be let in like her mother so that they can do the SSC. I mean we are suturing the episiotomy at one end and they can stand in the other end and hold the baby."

C.2. Structured, periodic inter-department teaching

Training staff, subsequent reinforcement by periodic demonstration and consolidation by constant constructive interdepartmental dialogue are imperative to ensure the sustainability of this practice. Considering the high turnover of staff in the institute, ongoing training of nurses is needed. Training of student nurses was perceived as one way of improving the practice. Even the more experienced staff felt that they had to undergo the experience of actually providing SSC in order to subsequently advocate its practice. Revising the guidelines and holding demonstrations in a collaborative manner is necessary to motivate staff and promote adherence to SSC. A team approach where all stakeholders are perceived as equal partners was thought to be a sufficiently inclusive solution.

N: "Whoever has joined newly to OB ward... whoever is assisting in deliveries definitely need to be educated. I think the education can start from all the nursing students who come there."

Ped: "I don't think you can make somebody to believe just by teaching I think they have to see themselves to actually believe in skin to skin contact, so if they see those kind of things with their own eyes I think it will be better rather than teaching them."

N: "If we want to include SSC in our hospital, then I think that the head of neonatology should speak to the head of OBG. We should have a meeting with the unit chiefs, all staff and pgs. This can be easily implemented because there are no costs."

C.3. Antenatal awareness – creating demand

Creating demand by increasing the awareness among the mothers by antenatal education was offered as one solution for improving SSC implementation.

Ob-gyn: "I think posters or written material, any audio-visual aid, definitely will help. And even maybe audio-visual aids for the family in the OB ward, maybe a video where they will be shown what will be done, if they don't have time to go to each of the mothers and counsel them, so that they're more aware and sometimes, at least some patients ask questions and the demand from the patients will also increase."

C.4. Early SSC – A practical alternative for SSC at birth

To overcome their inability to provide 1 h SSC at birth, the health personnel offered the solution of "Early SSC" as opposed to not implementing SSC.

Ob-gyn: "Immediate Skin to Skin is a little difficult to practice but probably after the baby is stabilized and mother is back on the bed, probably EARLY SSC for 1 hour may not be that difficult. Mother is also comfortable in her bed, at that point of time to give the baby SSC for one hour may be a lot easier for the doctors and the staff. Even the sisters, the staff nurse will be happy to do that."

Discussion

SSC at birth though recommended for all newborns who do not need resuscitation at birth, is not routinely practiced in most settings across India. Implementation of SSC at birth in the dynamic delivery room needs a concentrated combined effort from doctors across the different specialties of obstetrics and pediatrics and the labor room nurses who strive towards ensuring labor is safe for the mother and the baby. The ultimate decision as to whether SSC is to be implemented is predominantly made by the pediatricians as the obstetricians are pre-occupied with the welfare of the mother to ensure safe labor process.

The barriers elicited in this study can be grouped under three main factors, namely time constraints (an opportunity barrier), parochialism towards the process (a motivation barrier), and a general lack of buy-in (a motivation barrier),that make it difficult for obstetric staff to improve their clinical behavior as defined by the World Health Organization's Safe Childbirth Checklist Implementation Guide [13].These barriers are described as opportunity barriers, which refers to the "environmental or contextual factors beyond an individual's control (for example: leadership support challenges, human resource, time or supply constraints)", motivation barriers, which refers to a lack of "interest or internal belief" in the procedure, and ability barriers, which refers to a lack of "skill, knowledge, or technical confidence." [14].

This can in turn be expressed in terms of the Behaviour Change Wheel, which is a structured approach for initiating and designing policy changes by using the COM-B (Capability, opportunity, motivation and behaviour) model. This model identifies behaviour to be a part of an ever changing system which is in constant interaction with all the interventions which influence the new policy or intervention and acts as a framework for the same [15].

Though the skewed staff-patient ratio in the labor room is an established fact in LMIC settings, little has been done to bring about a change in the system. The solutions to these seem straightforward in providing additional staff. However, in resource-limited settings, providing more trained personnel can be challenging due to budget constraints, lack of lucrative incentives and a weak retention policy. In some settings, permitting a relative in the labor room is a potential solution which is endorsed in baby friendly hospital initiative (BFHI) manual suggesting that a "family member can stay with the mother and the baby" if no staff is available to stay with mother and baby [6]. The main barrier to allowing a family member into the delivery room is that many hospitals in the region, such as ours, do not permit family members inside the labor room as part of the hospital protocol, due to lack of space and interference with routine procedures during labor and delivery. Also, most of the doctors feel that the mother is in too much pain and under this particular circumstance cannot solely be responsible to hold the baby and participate actively in SSC. However, the benefits of implementing routine SSC to both newborn and mother will greatly outweigh the difficulties in finding a way to accommodate an extra person in the labor room. A hospital staff – a helper /aide (less trained than a nurse) could be another option and could also be used for quality control in addition to ensuring adherence to guidelines. The BFHI manual suggests that "if the delivery room is busy, the mother and baby can be transferred to the ward in skin-to-skin contact, and contact can continue in the ward". This gives rise to a concept of "early SSC" rather than immediate SSC which aims to overcome the barriers of time and personnel constrains as a family member, who is usually present to take care of the mother and baby, can be delegated this responsibility.

Awareness and belief in the practice of SSC at birth came up as both a barrier and an enabler. Within all the limitations and restrictions of the system, the overwhelming belief in the practice is one the key enablers of the practice.

Implementation of potential solutions will only be successful if there is an understanding of the manifold benefits of SSC as well as by actual practice and demonstration of SSC. The awareness needs to be created both in the provider and amongst the patients. From the patient perspective, this should be initiated during antenatal visits when expectant mothers are more receptive to understanding the numerous benefits. These behavioral changes require effective communication aids such as audiovisual aids and antenatal counselling. For the health care worker perspective, "seeing is believing". Learn, Do and Teach would be a good model to adopt as most personnel who have perceived the benefits of SSC such as reduction in pain during episiotomy, consider having had personal experience as one the most important enablers of SSC practice. This model is an extension of the study that looked at two techniques-immersion and education for improving the practice of SSC among health care providers, which concluded that immersion techniques, wherein the participants were educated about the procedure or intervention and being experts in the matter were closely monitored for evolving behavioural changes to accommodate the new technique, had better response towards establishing sustainable practice of SSC when compared to education alone [14].

A collaborative concentrated effort by all concerned personnel is needed for successful implementation since care at birth is a multidisciplinary responsibility. It is important that key stakeholders such as senior obstetricians recognize the importance of SSC at birth. Their concern of safety is reasonable as SSC at birth, like any other medical procedure, is not without a chance of rare adverse events. Safety of the newborn is paramount and reports of apnea and hypoxic brain injury following SSC are known [16]. A single adverse event could convert the personnel to a total non-believer and a threat to the implementation of SSC. There are two issues regarding safety – the first is correct identification of the newborn eligible for SSC at birth and the second, continued monitoring of the baby during SSC. Training all health personnel in the basic steps of neonatal resuscitation would empower them to make the correct decision at birth and would address the first issue; which also came up as a barrier for implementation of SSC. Having a dedicated person to ensure adequate monitoring and safety would overcome the fears expressed by the obstetricians. Further interdepartmental discussions and joint sessions on improving awareness would help in reaching the common goal. In a hierarchical environment such as a medical school, having the senior professors convinced would have a percolating effect on the rest of the department with regard to implementing and adhering to SSC. Consistent motivation by the senior obstetricians, pediatricians and nurses is needed for the execution of this evidence-based practice. Though it is important that the different departments work together, it is perceived that the onus of SSC promotion rests with the pediatrician. Incorporating the practice and benefits of SSC into the medical and nursing curriculum will be an effective way to sensitize the next generation of perinatal professionals to this practice and will act as a long-term solution.

Not surprisingly, the common barriers identified were similar to the barriers identified in a recent systematic review to implementation of Kangaroo mother care in preterm babies [7] which included "Actual increased workload due to KMC", "concerns about medical conditions/care", "Lack of clear guidelines / training", "general lack of buy-in/ belief in efficacy" and "belief that it causes extra work". Another top barrier specific to LMIC was "issues to facility, environment and resources" which referred to the lack of adequate resources as perceived by the mothers. "Support from family, friends, and other mothers" was the top enabler of KMC in the same study and can probably be extrapolated to SSC at birth [7]. Involvement of the grandmother has been postulated as an effective means of promoting KMC at home in African countries [17] and can also be done for SSC. The emotional support offered by families is an important and crucial enabler of practice [18]. "Support from staff or community health workers" was the fourth-highest- ranked enabler for practice in the systematic review but when only LMIC publications were considered, it was only the 7th ranked enabler highlighting that staff support for KMC not only plays a crucial role but also that it needs further strengthening in LMIC. These are readily applicable for SSC at birth.

Limitations of the study

One of the limitations of the study has been that the focus group discussion has been amongst homogenous groups. Labour room being a dynamic setting where the different specialties interact, FGD with participants from the 3 groups could have brought out different issues.

Conclusions

This study provides a set of synthesized factors regarding the system, experiential and knowledge barriers to the implementation of SSC at birth. By providing potential solutions to these barriers and highlighting the enablers of SSC, the results of this study could aid program implementers, policymakers, and researchers to implement and scale up this important tool of SSC at birth that has the potential to improve breastfeeding practices.

Abbreviations

BFHI: baby friendly hospital initiative; FGD: Focus group discussions; IDI: In depth interviews; KMC: Kangaroo mother care; LMIC: Low middle income countries; LR: Labor room; NICU: Neonatal intensive care unit; PG: Post graduates; SSC: Skin-to-skin contact

Acknowledgements

We thank Dr. Ramesh A for his support for the study and acknowledge and thank all the participating health personnel.

Funding

None.

Authors' contributions

AJA, JT and SRPN conceived and designed the study and wrote the manuscript. AJA, JT and CDB conducted the interviews and the focus group discussions. LR conducted the initial focused group discussion and reviewed the design of the study. JVO helped write the manuscript. All authors read and approved the final manuscript.

Competing interests

The authors declare that they have no competing interests.

Author details

[1]Undergraduates, St. John's Medical College Hospital, Bangalore, India. [2]Social Scientist, St. John's Medical College Hospital, Bangalore, India. [3]Department of Neonatology, St. John's Medical College Hospital, Sarjapur Road, Koramangala, Bangalore 560034, India. [4]Maternal Health Research Coordinator, Compañeros En Salud, Chiapas, Mexico.

References

1. Marin GMA, Martin LI, Escobar LA, Villalba FE, Blanco RI, Pol TP. Randomized controlled trial of early skin-to-skin contact: effects on the mother and the newborn. ActaPaediatr 2010; 99(11):1630-1634.
2. Moore ER, Bergman N, Anderson GC, Medley N. Early skin-to-skin contact for mothers and their healthy newborn infants. Cochrane Database Syst Rev. 2016(11). Art. No.: CD003519.
3. DuhnL. The importance of touch in the development of attachment. Adv Neonatal Care 2010; 10(6):294-300.
4. Anderson GC, Chiu SH, Morrison B, Burkhammer M, Ludington S. Skin-to-skin care for breastfeeding difficulties post-birth. In: Field T, editor. Touch and massage therapy in early development. Johnson & Johnson Pediatric Institute. NJ: LLC. New Brunswick; 2004. p. 115–36.
5. Lee HC, Martin-Anderson S, Clinician DRA. Perspectives on barriers to and opportunities for skin to skin contact for premature infants in neonatal intensive care units. Breastfeed Med. 2012;7(2):79–84.
6. Session 5, Birth practices and breastfeeding -STEP 4. Baby-Friendly Hospital Initiative: Revised, Updated and Expanded for Integrated Care. Geneva: World Health Organization; 2009: 85-97.
7. Seidman G, Unnikrishnan S, Kenny E, Myslinski S, Cairns-Smith S, Mulligan B, Barriers EC. Enablers of kangaroo mother care practice: a systematic review. PLoS One. 2015;10(5):e0125643.
8. WHO. Kangaroo Mother Care—A Practical Guide. Department of Reproductive Health and Research, WHO, Geneva; 2003.
9. Kymre IGNICU. Nurses' ambivalent attitudes in skin-to-skin care practice. Int J Qual Stud Health Well-being. 2014;9:e23297.
10. Sadala ML, AdornoRde C. Pheonomenology as a method to investigate the experience lived: a perspective from Husserl and Merleau-Ponty's thought. J AdvNurs. 2002 Feb;37(3):282–93.
11. Gale NK, Heath G, Cameron E, Rashid S, Redwood S. Using the framework method for the analysis of qualitative data in multi-disciplinary health research. BMC Med Res Methodol. 2013;13:117.
12. Data Analysis WL. In qualitative research: a brief guide to using Nvivo. Malays Fam Physician. 2008;3(1):14–20.
13. World Health Organization. "WHO Safe Childbirth Checklist implementation guide: improving the quality of facility-based delivery for mother and newborns." (2015).
14. Brimdyr K, Widström AM, Cadwell K, Svensson K, Turner-Maffei C. A realistic evaluation of two training programs on implementing skin-to-skin as a standard of care. J Perinat Educ. 2012;21(3):149–15.
15. Michie S, van Stralen MM, West R. The behaviour change wheel: a new method for characterising and designing behaviour change interventions. Implement Sci. 2011;6:42.
16. Andres V, Garcia P, Rimet Y, Nicaise C, Apparent SU. Life-threatening events in presumably healthy newborns during early skin-to-skin contact. Pediatrics. 2011;127(4):e1073–6.
17. Blencowe H, Molyneux E. Setting up kangaroo mother Care at Queen Elizabeth Central Hospital, Blantyre—a practical approach. Malawi med. Journal. 2005;17:39–42.
18. Leonard A, Mayers P. Parents' lived experience of providing kangaroo care to their preterm infants. Health SA Gesondheid. 2008;13(4):16–28.

13

Early-onset neonatal hyperkalemia associated with maternal hypermagnesemia

Kenichi Tanaka[1], Hiroko Mori[1], Rieko Sakamoto[2], Shirou Matsumoto[2], Hiroshi Mitsubuchi[1], Kimitoshi Nakamura[2] and Masanori Iwai[1*]

Abstract

Background: Neonatal nonoliguric hyperkalemia (NOHK) is a metabolic abnormality that occurs in extremely premature neonates at approximately 24 h after birth and is mainly due to the immature functioning of the sodium (Na^+)/potassium (K^+) pump. Magnesium sulfate is frequently used in obstetrical practice to prevent preterm labor and to treat preeclampsia; this medication can also cause hypermagnesemia and hyperkalemia by a mechanism that is different from that of NOHK. Herein, we report the first case of very early-onset neonatal hyperkalemia induced by maternal hypermagnesemia.

Case presentation: A neonate born at 32 weeks of gestation developed hyperkalemia (K^+ 6.4 mmol/L) 2 h after birth. The neonate's blood potassium concentration reached 7.0 mmol/L 4 h after birth, despite good urine output. The neonate and his mother had severe hypermagnesemia caused by intravenous infusion of magnesium sulfate given for tocolysis due to pre-term labor.

Conclusion: The early-onset hyperkalemia may have been caused by the accumulation of potassium ions transported through the placenta, the shift of potassium ions from the intracellular to the extracellular space in the infant due to the malfunctioning of the Na^+/K^+ pump and the inhibition of renal distal tube potassium ion secretion, there is a possibility that these mechanisms were induced by maternal and fetal hypermagnesemia after maternal magnesium sulfate administration. Because neonatal hyperkalemia poses a significant risk for the development of life-threatening cardiac arrhythmia, this case highlights the necessity of maternal blood magnesium monitoring during magnesium sulfate administration and neonatal blood potassium monitoring when there is severe maternal hypermagnesemia at delivery.

Keywords: Neonatal nonoliguric hyperkalemia, Progressive early-onset hyperkalemia, Maternal hypermagnesemia, Na^+/K^+-ATPase, Renal outer medullary potassium channel

Background

Neonatal nonoliguric hyperkalemia (NOHK) is a frequently observed electrolyte imbalance that occurs in nonoliguric premature infants during the first days after birth [1]. NOHK results secondary to potassium shift from the intracellular space to the extracellular space partly because of the malfunctioning of the Na^+/K^+ pump due to the immature activity of Na^+/K^+-ATPase [2]. It can cause life-threatening cardiac arrhythmia as a severe complication [3].

Magnesium is a modulator of the Na^+ and K^+ ion transport systems in numerous tissues, and hypermagnesemia inhibits K^+ ion transport from the extracellular to the intracellular space through the Na^+/K^+ pump [4]. Additionally, hypermagnesemia inhibits renal distal tube K^+ ion secretion by the renal outer medullary K^+ (ROMK) channel, which is an inward-rectifying K^+ ion channel responsible for basal K^+ ion secretion [5, 6]. An overdose of magnesium sulfate, frequently used in obstetrical practice for the prevention of preterm labor and to treat preeclampsia, can cause maternal hypermagnesemia [7]. Because the magnesium ion administered to the mother readily crosses the placenta, infants born to mothers with hypermagnesemia often develop transient

* Correspondence: miwai@kuh.kumamoto-u.ac.jp
[1]Division of Neonatology, Kumamoto University Hospital, 1-1-1 Honjo, Chuo-ku, Kumamoto 860-8556, Japan

hypermagnesemia during the first days after birth [8]. Moreover, it has been reported maternal and neonatal magnesium concentrations were highly correlated [9].

Although transient hyperkalemia during magnesium sulfate therapy in two pregnant drug abusers has been reported [7], there has been no report on neonatal transient hyperkalemia caused by maternal magnesium sulfate therapy. Here, we present the case of a male infant at 32 weeks gestation (weight 1268 g) that developed hyperkalemia immediately after birth due to neonatal and maternal transient hypermagnesemia after administration of magnesium sulfate.

Case presentation

A 29-year-old Japanese woman in her second pregnancy was being treated for pregnancy-induced hypertension and preeclampsia with a drip infusion of magnesium sulfate at 30 weeks 2 days gestation. The dose of continuously infused magnesium sulfate was 0.1 g/h on day 1, 0.5 g/h on day 2–5, and 1.0 g/h on day 6–12. The dose was increased to 2.0 g/h to control an imminent preterm delivery on day 12, just before an emergency transfer to our hospital. During this treatment, maternal serum magnesium levels were not monitored. The mother had no medical conditions or any intake of other medications within these 12 days, which could have influenced blood potassium concentration.

On admission to our hospital, the patient could not mobilize independently because of hypotonia caused by severe hypermagnesemia and hypocalcemia (Table 1). On the same day, she delivered a male infant through vaginal birth. Her laboratory analysis at 7 h before and 7 h after delivery showed that the serum concentration of potassium, sodium, and creatinine ranged from 4.3 to 6.0 mmol/L, 133 to 128 mmol/L, and 0.85 to 0.95 mg/dL, respectively. These levels returned to within normal ranges at 5 days after delivery.

The male infant was born at 32 weeks gestation weighing 1268 g and with Apgar scores of 8 at 1 min and 9 at 5 min. He was immediately admitted to the neonatal intensive care unit in our hospital. There was no evidence of respiratory distress syndrome on chest radiograph, and he had a stable microbubble test. His heart rate was 130 beats per minute, and the arterial blood pressure was 42/22 mmHg, with normal contraction of the left ventricle confirmed by echocardiographic examination. His muscle tone was determined to be within the normal range by two expert neonatologists. The size and shape of both kidneys on ultrasonography were within the normal range, and his first urine was observed at 2 h after birth.

Laboratory data showed that his venous blood potassium concentration was 6.4 mmol/L at 2 h after birth and reached 7.0 mmol/L at 4 h after birth even though he had sufficient urine output (Table 1, Fig. 1). Glucose-insulin combined therapy was administered for 54 h with an insulin infusion rate between 0.9 units/kg/day and 1.9 units/kg/day to maintain his serum potassium concentration below 6.0 mmol/L. All blood samples were obtained from a catheter inserted directly into the right radial artery. During the therapy, he was not given potassium. His urine output was 4.1 mL/kg/h during the first 8 h, 6.2 mL/kg/h during the next day, and 3.3 mL/kg/h during the third day after birth with insufficient urinary potassium excretion (Table 1).

Laboratory analysis of his umbilical blood also showed hypermagnesemia at birth, which gradually subsided (Table 1, Fig. 1). The serum calcium concentration remained over 7.3 mg/dL with intravenous drip administration of calcium sulfate. Although transient

Table 1 The progression of blood and urine laboratory data of the mother and the infant

	Mother			Infant			
Sampling time	Day of delivery (7 h before delivery)	1 day after delivery (7 h after delivery)	5 days after delivery (at discharge)	Day of birth	1 day after birth	2 days after birth	30 days after birth
Mg (mg/dL)	9.9	5.9	–	8.7	7.7	5.9	2.0
Ca (mg/dL)	6.3	6.2	8.0	8.5	8.0	8.8	9.7
P (mg/dL)	–	–	–	10.4	8.7	6.2	6.9
K (mmol/L)	4.3	6.0	4.8	6.4	6.0	5.2	3.4
Na (mmol/L)	133	128	138	131	136	139	140
Cre (mg/dL)	0.85	0.95	0.56	0.82	1.07	1.10	0.32
BUN (mg/dL)	20.3	25.7	14.1	22.2	25.0	19.8	3.5
Urine K (mmol/L)	–	–	–	13	16	3	–
FeK (%)	–	–	–	36.5	24.9	4.4	–

Mg serum magnesium concentration, *Ca* serum calcium concentration, *K* serum potassium concentration, *Na* serum sodium concentration, *Cre* serum creatinine concentration, *BUN* Blood urea nitrogen, serum, *FeK* Fractional excretion of potassium, *Urine K* Urine potassium concentration (a spot urine specimen)

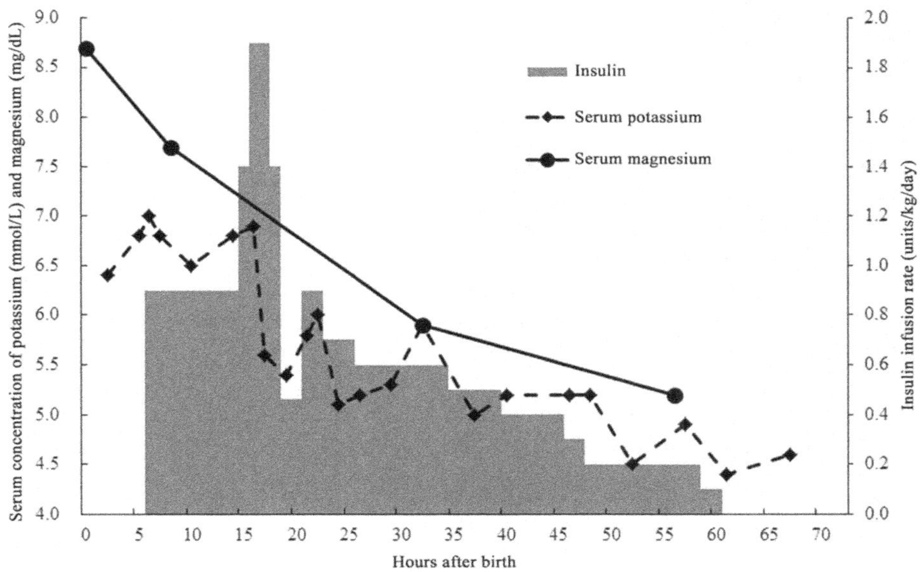

Fig. 1 The neonate's clinical course until 72 h after birth. The clinical course of the patient is shown. The main indicators include the serum potassium and magnesium concentrations and infusion rate of insulin until 72 h after birth

hyponatremia was observed at 6 h after birth, it recovered in 24 h without sodium administration.

After resolution of NOHK, the neonate's serum concentrations of potassium and magnesium were within the normal range. He was discharged from our hospital at 72 days after birth with no clinical complications and had normal growth and development at 3 years of age.

Discussion

NOHK is a metabolic disorder that usually occurs in extremely premature neonates; therefore, the onset at 32 weeks old in the neonate presented in this case is less expected. Furthermore, the clinical course in this case was very unique in terms of the early onset at 2 h after birth and prolonged for 54 h under glucose-insulin combined therapy.

One possible explanation as to the cause of the early onset hyperkalemia is maternal hyperkalemia caused by hypermagnesemia [7]. Usually, the fetal plasma K^+ ion concentration is higher than the maternal plasma concentrations [10] because of active K^+ ion transport across the placenta [11]. In this case, the maternal potassium concentration increased from 4.3 mmol/L at 7 h before delivery to 6.0 mmol/L at 7 h after delivery. It is therefore possible that the excess K^+ ions might have crossed from the mother to the fetus through the placenta and might have partially contributed to early onset neonatal hyperkalemia.

Alternatively, the prolonged hyperkalemia may have been secondary to a shift in K^+ ions from the intracellular to the extracellular space. In premature infants with NOHK, erythrocyte Na^+/K^+-ATPase activity is significantly lower and the malfunctioning of the Na^+/K^+ pump induces a K^+ ion shift from the intracellular to the extracellular space [1, 2]. This case may illustrate that even in an infant at 32 weeks gestation, Na^+/K^+-ATPase activity may be immature and result in malfunctioning of the Na^+/K^+ pump. In addition to prematurity, neonatal hypermagnesemia may produce a K^+ ion shift from the intracellular to the extracellular space because of the high concentration of magnesium ions, which modulates the Na^+/K^+ ion transport systems in numerous tissues and inhibits the Na^+/K^+ pump exchange [4].

An additional mechanism whereby neonatal hypermagnesemia results in hyperkalemia is through the inhibition of renal distal tubule K^+ ion secretion. Magnesium is thought to inhibit renal distal tube K^+ ion secretion by suppressing the ROMK channel, which is an inward-rectifying K^+ ion channel responsible for basal K^+ ion secretion [5, 6]. In the neonate described in this case, post-delivery urine output was sufficient; however, the fractional excretion of potassium (FeK) at 0, 1, and 2 days after birth was 36.5, 24.9, and 4.4%, respectively, and these levels of excretion are lower than the average FeK ($40 \pm 5\%$) in NOHK during the first few days after birth [12]. The amount of urinary excretion of potassium is larger in an infant with NOHK than an infant with normokalemia [13]. However, in this case, it is interesting that urinary excretion of potassium was suppressed despite hyperkalemia, because of hypermagnesemia.

Thus, this progressive early-onset hyperkalemia may be caused by maternal and fetal hypermagnesemia. The underlying mechanism of this hyperkalemia is mainly assumed to be secondary to hypermagnesemia and subsequent malfunctioning of the Na^{+}/K^{+}-ATPase and inhibition of secretion in the ROMK channel.

Conclusion

Maternal and fetal hypermagnesemia can induce rapidly progressive hyperkalemia in neonates. Because hyperkalemic infants are at high risk of developing life-threatening cardiac arrhythmias, we highlight the necessity of maternal blood magnesium monitoring during intravenous infusion of magnesium sulfate for tocolysis, as well as neonatal blood potassium monitoring when there is maternal severe hypermagnesemia at delivery.

Abbreviations

NOHK: Neonatal nonoliguric hyperkalemia; ROMK: Renal outer medullary K^{+}

Acknowledgements

The authors would like to thank Dr. Endo for thoughtful comments during the writing of this manuscript.

Funding

This work was not funded by institutional, financial or material support from external sources.

Authors' contributions

KT reviewed the literature and prepared the manuscript. HMo and SM helped to draft the manuscript. RS was involved in collection of the clinical details. HMi and NK assisted with manuscript revision. MI reviewed the literature, prepared the manuscript, and is the corresponding author. All authors read and approved the final version of the manuscript.

Competing interests

The authors declare that they have no competing interests.

Author details

[1]Division of Neonatology, Kumamoto University Hospital, 1-1-1 Honjo, Chuo-ku, Kumamoto 860-8556, Japan. [2]Department of Pediatrics, Graduate School of Life Science, Kumamoto University, 1-1-1 Honjo, Chuo-ku, Kumamoto 860-8556, Japan.

References

1. Sato K, Kondo T, Iwao H, Honda S, Ueda K. Internal potassium shift in premature infants: cause of nonoliguric hyperkalemia. J Pediatr. 1995;126:109–13.
2. Baumgart S. Acute problems of prematurity: balancing fluid volume and electrolyte replacements in very low birth weight (VLBW) and extremely low birth weight (ELBW) neonates. In: Oh W, Guignard JP, Baumgart S, editors. Nephrology and fluid/electrolyte physiology. Philadelphia: Saunders; 2008. p. 161–83.
3. Hu PS, Su BH, Peng CT, Tsai CH. Glucose and insulin infusion versus kayexalate for the early treatment of non-oliguric hyperkalemia in very-low-birth-weight infants. Acta Paediatr Taiwan. 1999;40:314–8.
4. Bara M, Guiet-Bara A, Durlach J. Regulation of sodium and potassium pathways by magnesium in cell membranes. Magnes Res. 1993;6:167–77.
5. Heller BI, Hammarsten JF, Stutzman FL. Concerning the effects of magnesium sulfate on renal function, electrolyte excretion, and clearance of magnesium. J Clin Invest. 1953;32:858–61.
6. Huang CL, Kuo E. Mechanism of hypokalemia in magnesium deficiency. J Am Soc Nephrol. 2007;18:2649–52.
7. Spital A, Greenwell R. Severe hyperkalemia during magnesium sulfate therapy in two pregnant drug abusers. South Med J. 1991;84:919–21.
8. Rantonen T, Kääpä P, Jalonen J, Ekblad U, Peltola O, Välimäki I, et al. Antenatal magnesium sulphate exposure is associated with prolonged parathyroid hormone suppression in preterm neonates. Acta Paediatr. 2001;90:278–81.
9. Sherwin CM, Balch A, Campbell SC, Fredrickson J, Clark EA, Varner M, et al. Maternal magnesium sulphate exposure predicts neonatal magnesium blood concentrations. Basic Clin Pharmacol Toxicol. 2014;114:318–22.
10. Shennan DB, Boyd CA. Ion transport by the placenta: a review of membrane transport systems. Biochim Biophys Acta. 1987;906:437–57.
11. Ashoor IF, de Jesús-González N, Somers MJ. Fluid and electrolyte physiology in the fetus and neonate. In: Chishti AS, Alam S, Kiessling SG, editors. Kidney and urinary tract diseases in the newborn. Berlin Heidelberg: Springer; 2014. p. 77–98.
12. Omar SA, DeCristofaro JD, Agarwal BI, LaGamma EF. Effect of prenatal steroids on potassium balance in extremely low birth weight neonates. Pediatrics. 2000;106:561–7.
13. Stefano JL, Norman ME, Morales MC, Goplerud JM, Mishra OP, Delivoria-Papadopoulos M. Decreased erythrocyte Na+, K+ -ATPase activity associated with cellular potassium loss in extremely low birth weight infants with nonoliguric hyperkalemia. J Pediatr. 1993;122:276–84.

Clinical and genetic characteristics of patients with fatty acid oxidation disorders identified by newborn screening

Eungu Kang[1], Yoon-Myung Kim[2], Minji Kang[3], Sun-Hee Heo[3], Gu-Hwan Kim[4], In-Hee Choi[4], Jin-Ho Choi[2], Han-Wook Yoo[2,4] and Beom Hee Lee[2,4*]

Abstract

Background: Fatty acid oxidation disorders (FAODs) include more than 15 distinct disorders with variable clinical manifestations. After the introduction of newborn screening using tandem mass spectrometry, early identification of FAODs became feasible. This study describes the clinical, biochemical and molecular characteristics of FAODs patients detected by newborn screening (NBS) compared with those of 9 patients with symptomatic presentations.

Methods: Clinical and genetic features of FAODs patients diagnosed by NBS and by symptomatic presentations were reviewed.

Results: Fourteen patients were diagnosed with FAODs by NBS at the age of 54.8 ± 4.8 days: 5 with very-long-chain acyl-CoA dehydrogenase (VLCAD) deficiency, 5 with medium chain acyl-CoA dehydrogenase (MCAD) deficiency, 1 with primary carnitine deficiency, 1 with carnitine palmitoyltransferase 1A (CPT1A) deficiency, 1 with long-chain 3-hydroxyacyl-CoA dehydrogenase or mitochondrial trifunctional protein (LCAHD/MTP) deficiency, and 1 with short chain acyl-CoA dehydrogenase (SCAD) deficiency. Three patients with VLCAD or LCHAD/MTP deficiency developed recurrent rhabdomyolysis or cardiomyopathy, and one patient died of cardiomyopathy. The other 10 patients remained neurodevelopmentally normal and asymptomatic during the follow-up. In 8 patients with symptomatic presentation, FAODs manifested as LCHAD/MTP deficiencies by recurrent rhabdomyolysis or cadiomyopathy (6 patients), and VLCAD deficiency by cardiomyopathy (1 patient), and CPT1A deficiency by hepatic failure (1 patient). Two patients with LCHAD/MTP deficiencies died due to severe cardiomyopathy in the neonatal period, and developmental disability was noted in CPT1A deficiency (1 patient).

Conclusions: NBS helped to identify the broad spectrum of FAODs and introduce early intervention to improve the clinical outcome of each patient. However, severe clinical manifestations developed in some patients, indicating that careful, life-long observation is warranted in all FAODs patients.

Keywords: Fatty acid oxidation disorders, Newborn screening, Genotype-phenotype correlation, Treatment outcome

* Correspondence: bhlee@amc.seoul.kr
[2]Department of Pediatrics, Asan Medical Center Children's Hospital, University of Ulsan College of Medicine, 88, Olympic-ro 43-Gil, Songpa-Gu, Seoul 05505, Korea
[4]Medical Genetics Center, Asan Medical Center Children's Hospital, University of Ulsan College of Medicine, 88, Olympic-ro 43-Gil, Songpa-Gu, Seoul 05505, Korea

Background

Fatty acid oxidation (FAO) is a key metabolic pathway for maintaining energetic substrates used to maintain metabolic homeostasis. FAO is important for some high-energy-requiring organs and provides the main energy supply during prolonged fasting, febrile illness, cold exposure, or muscular exertion. The prime pathway for the degradation of fatty acids is mitochondrial fatty acid oxidation, which is composed of the uptake and activation of fatty acids, carnitine cycles, beta-oxidation cycle, and electron transfer [1].

More than 15 distinct disorders have been described as affecting FAO; These include glutaric aciduria type 2, primary carnitine deficiency and deficiencies of carnitine palmitoyltransferase 1A (CPT1A), carnitine acylcarnitine translocase (CACT), very long chain acyl-CoA dehydrogenase (VLCAD), long chain hydroxyacyl-CoA dehydrogenase or mitochondrial trifunctional protein (LCHAD/MTP), medium chain acyl-CoA dehydrogenase (MCAD), medium/short chain hydroxyacyl-CoA dehydrogenase (M/SCHAD), and short chain acyl-CoA dehydrogenase (SCAD) [2–4].

After the introduction of newborn screening by tandem mass spectrometry analysis of acylcarnitines, the detection of FAO disorders (FAODs) has increased. The estimated combined incidence of all FAODs is 1 in 9000, which is calculated from reports out of Australia, Germany, and the USA, but it seems to be much lower in Asian countries [5]. The estimated prevalence of long chain fatty acid oxidation disorders in Korea is 1 in 15,800, which is more frequently diagnosed following the introduction of tandem mass spectrometry newborn screening [6].

FAODs present with a heterogeneous clinical phenotype at various ages of onset, from neonate to adulthood. The most severe form manifests with hypertrophic cardiomyopathy, hepatic encephalopathy, or severe hypoketotic hypoglycemia in the neonatal period or infancy. The less-severe, later-onset myopathic form is characterized by exercise-induced myopathy and rhabdomyolysis [7, 8].

The diagnosis of FAODs are based on the measurement of abnormal acylcarnitines and confirmed by enzyme assay or molecular analysis. Early identification of FAODs became possible using expanded newborn screening using tandem mass spectrometry, which measures acylcarnitine levels in dried blood spots. Identification of FAODs in newborn screening is very important because intervention in the presymptomatic period helps improve patient prognosis [9].

In this respect, here we describe fourteen patients with diverse FAODs identified by newborn screening, and compare their clinical outcome and genetic characteristics with those of 8 patients diagnosed by symptomatic presentation. Our experience indicates the effectiveness of newborn screening for the early diagnosis of FAOD, especially in the presymptomatic period. However, careful observation and appropriate management is warranted to improve the clinical outcome of the affected patients.

Methods

Patients

A total of fourteen patients were diagnosed with FAODs by newborn screening between May 2002 and February 2016 at the department of Medical Genetics, Asan Medical Center Children's Hospital, Seoul, Korea. Clinical features of these patients were compared with nine FAOD patients identified by symptomatic presentation, including rhabdomyolysis, cardiomyopathy, or developmental delay.

The Institutional Review Board at Asan Medical Center approved this study. Appropriate written informed consent was obtained from the parents of all participants.

Methods

Presenting manifestations, biochemical findings including plasma acylcarnitines, molecular analysis, and clinical course of each patient were reviewed retrospectively.

All patients diagnosed by newborn screening tests were referred to our department due to abnormal newborn screening results. Dried blood spot samples were obtained at the hospital where the patients were born and tandem mass spectrometry analysis was performed at commercial biochemical laboratories. Newborns with abnormal initial screening result were requested for repeated tandem mass spectrometry. If a second screening results were still exceeding the cut off value, molecular genetic analyses was performed and the diagnosis of FAOD was confirmed after receiving a positive confirmation test.

Acylcarnitine was measured by Liquid Chromatography-Tandem Mass Spectrometry, as previously described [6]. Genomic DNA was isolated from peripheral blood leukocytes. PCR was performed for all coding exons and exon–intron boundaries of *SLC22A5* for primary carnitine deficiency, *CPT1A* for CPT1A deficiency, *ACADVL* for VLCAD deficiency, *HADHA* and *HADHB* for LCHAD/MTP deficiencies, *ACADM* for MCAD deficiency, and *ACADS* for SCAD deficiency. Direct sequencing was performed on a ABI 3130 genetic analyzer (Applied Biosystems, Foster City, CA, USA) using a BigDye Terminator cycle sequencing kit (Applied Biosystems). In silico prediction analyses were performed for novel missense and splicing variants, using PolyPhen-2 (http://genetics.bwh.harvard.edu/pph2) and SIFT (http://sift.jcvi.org).

Results

Clinical characteristics of patients with FAODs identified by newborn screening

FAODs were identified in 14 patients by newborn screening: VLCAD deficiency (5 patients), MCAD deficiency (5 patients), primary carnitine deficiency (1 patient), CPT1A deficiency (1 patient), LCHAD/MTP deficiencies (1 patient), and SCAD deficiency (1 patient). Newborn screening using tandem mass spectrometry was performed at 3.2 ± 0.2 days after birth and the diagnosis of FAOD was confirmed by molecular genetic analyses at the mean age of 54.7 ± 40.8 days (range: 16–153 days). Plasma C14:1 and C14:2 were elevated in VLCAD deficiency, C14OH, C16OH and C18:1OH levels in LCHAD/MTP deficiencies, C6 and C8 in MCAD deficiency, C2 and C4 in SCAD deficiency, and C0/(C16 + C18) in CPT1A deficiency. C0 level was markedly decreased in primary carnitine deficiency.

Molecular characteristics of patients with FAODs identified by newborn screening

Germline mutations of the gene responsible for each FAOD were identified in 90% of alleles (9 out of 10 alleles) in VLCAD deficiency, 90% (9 out of 10 alleles) in MCAD deficiency, 100% (2 out of 2 alleles) in LCHAD/MTP, primary carnitine, CPT1A, and SCAD deficiencies (Table 1). In VLCAD deficiency, 5 out of 7 mutations were novel mutations, c.[104_105ins10] (p.[Pro35fs*27]), c.[104_105ins5] (p.[Pro35fs*25]), c.[103_112dup] (p.[Arg38-Profs*26]), c.[996_997ins(T)] (p.[Ala333Cysfs*26]), and c.[552C > G] (p.[Ile184Met])). Two novel mutations, c.[748G > T] (p.[Val250Leu]) and c.[1015C > T] (p.[Arg339-Ter]), were detected in CPT1A deficiency. All other mutations were previously reported (Table 1) [10–20].

Clinical outcomes of patients with FAODs identified by newborn screening

The mean age at last follow-up for the 14 patients was 2.5 ± 2.0 years (range: 49 days–6.5 years). All patients had been educated to avoid prolonged fasting. Medium chain triglyceride diets with long chain fat restriction were recommended in the 5 patients with VLCAD deficiency and 1 patient with LCHAD/MTP deficiency. L-carnitine was given to 5 patients with MCAD deficiency even though the carnitine levels were within normal range, 1 patient with primary carnitine deficiency, and 1 patient with CPT1A deficiency.

Significant clinical manifestations that required emergency management were noted in 4 patients with VLCAD deficiency or LCHAD/MTP deficiency: recurrent rhabdomyolysis (2 patients), hypertrophic cardiomyopathy (2 patients), or sudden infantile death (1 patient). The remaining 2 patients with VLCAD deficiency and all patients with MCAD deficiency, SCAD deficiency, primary carnitine deficiency, or CPT1A deficiency were free of a metabolic crisis during the follow-up period. Additionally, the 13 surviving patients showed normal development without any neurologic deficit during the follow-up period (Table 1).

Molecular and clinical characteristics of patients with FAODs identified by symptomatic presentation

During the same study period, a total of 8 patients were diagnosed with FAODs by symptomatic presentation (Table 2).

One patient was diagnosed with VLCAD deficiency due to hypertrophic cardiomyopathy and rhabdomyolysis at the age of 2 months. This patient had two novel frameshift mutations in the *ACADVL* gene (p.A333fs and p.S590 fs). During the follow-up period of 3.5 years, this patient suffered from recurrent rhabdomyolysis and cardiomyopathy. LCHAD/MTP deficiencies were detected by cardiomyopathy with severe lactic acidosis at 1–5 days after birth (2 patients) and recurrent rhabdomyolysis at the median age of 9–48 months (4 patients). *HAHDA* or *HAHDB* mutations were identified in all six patients, including one novel mutation, c.[1211dup] (p.[G404 fs*2]). During the median follow-up period of 5.3 years (range: 4 days–12.7 years), the two patients with cardiomyopathy died at ages of 4 days and 9 days. The remaining four patients experienced recurrent rhabdomyolysis and sensorimotor polyneuropathy. No patient developed pigmentary retinopathy during follow-up. No patient was identified with MCAD or primary carnitine deficiency by symptomatic presentation during the study period.

One patient with CPT1A deficiency was identified by recurrent hepatopathy, nephromegaly, rhabdomyolysis, and hemolytic anemia [21]. Plasma acylcarnitine analysis revealed elevated free carnitine and ratio of free carnitine to C16 + C18. Compound heterozygous pathogenic mutations were identified in the *CPT1A* gene. Recurrent hepatic failure and intellectual disability was shown during 6.6 years of follow-up. At the age of 7, the patient's intelligence quotient (IQ) was less than 35 and Korean Childhood Autism Rating Scale (K-CARS) score was 44, suggesting severe intellectual disability and severe autism.

Discussion

The current study described the clinical and genetic features of 14 patients with FAODs identified by newborn screening, compared to those of 8 patients diagnosed with FAODs based on their symptomatic presentations.

The results of our current study indicate some important findings. Newborn screening helped to identify the broad spectrum of FAODs compared to FAODs with symptomatic presentation. These findings

Table 1 Clinical, biochemical, and genetic characteristics of patients with fatty acid oxidation disorders diagnosed by newborn screening

No	Age at diagnosis	Age at last follow-up	Phenotype	Acylcarnitine		Gene	Allele 1	Allele 2
				Sample	Elevated acylcarnitine (value)			
Very long chain acyl-CoA dehydrogenase deficiency								
1	39 days	3.7 years	recurrent rhabdomyolysis and hypertrophic cardiomyopathy after 7 months old	DBS	C14 (2.504 μM; ref., 0.006–0.166), C14:1 (1.097 μM; ref., 0.006–0.166)	*ACADVL*	c.[104_105ins10] (p.[P35fs*27]) [a]	c.[104_105ins5] (p.[P35fs*25]) [a]
2	33 days	5.8 years	recurrent rhabdomyolysis after 11 months	DBS	C14:1 (n.a.), C14 (n.a.), C14:2 (n.a.)	*ACADVL*	c.[1349G > A] (p.[R450H])	c.[1349G > A] (p.[R450H])
3	25 days	10 months	hypertrophic cardiomyopathy	DBS	C14:2 (0.581 μM; ref., 0.006–0.166), C14:1 (1.391 μM; ref., 0.034–0.599)	*ACADVL*	c.[103_112dup] (p.[R38P*26]) [a]	c.[1532G > A] (p.[R511Q])
4	49 days	3.3 years	1 episode of rhabdomyolysis	DBS	C14:1 (6.62 μM; ref., < 0.85)	*ACADVL*	c.[996_997ins(T)] (p.[A333C*26]) [a]	c.[552C > G] (p.[I184M]) [a]
5	48 days	2.0 years	asymptomatic	Plasma	C14 (0.184 μmol/L; ref., < 0.15), C14:2 (0.215 μmol/L; ref., < 0.13)	*ACADVL*	c.[1349G > A] (p.[R450H])	?
Medium chain acyl-CoA dehydrogenase deficiency								
6	16 days	4.5 years	asymptomatic	DBS	C8 (0.68 μM; ref., < 0.31)	*ACADM*	c.[617G > A] (p.[R206H])	c.[1189 T > A] (p.[Y397N])
7	36 days	3.5 years	asymptomatic	DBS	C6 (n.a.), C8 (n.a.), C10:1 (n.a.), C10 (n.a.)	*ACADM*	c.[1085G > A] (p.[G362E])	c.[1189 T > A] (p.[Y397N])
8	51 days	6.9 years	asymptomatic	DBS	C6 (0.46 μM; ref., < 0.22), C8 (1.66 μM; ref., < 0.35)	*ACADM*	c.[449_452del] (p.[Y150Rfs*4])	c.[1189 T > A] (p.[Y397N])
9	56 days	1.4 years	asymptomatic	DBS	C8 (2.98 μM; ref., < 0.37), C10:1 (0.58 μM; ref., < 0.40)	*ACADM*	c.[449_452del] (p.[Y150Rfs*4])	c.[1085G > A] (p.[G362E])
10	153 days	1.4 years	asymptomatic	Plasma	C6 (0.868 μmol/L; ref., < 0.18), C8 (5.067 μmol/L; ref., < 0.27), C10:1 (1.387 μmol/L; ref., < 0.46)	*ACADM*	c.[1189 T > A] (p.[Y397N])	?
Primary carnitine deficiency								
11	53 days	3.2 years	mild CK elevation, normal development	Plasma	C0 (4.1 μmol/L; ref., 12–46), Total carnitine (6.1 μmol/L; ref., 19–59)	*SLC22A5*	c.[396G > A] (p.[W132*])	c.[1400C > G] (p.[S467C])
Carnitine palmitoyltransferase 1A deficiency								
12	41 days	5 months	normal development	Plasma	C0 (80.839 μmol/L; ref., < 62.10), C0/(C16 + C18) (123.5)	*CPT1A*	c.[748G > T] (p.V250 L) [a]	c.[1015C > T] (p.[R399*]) [a]
Long chain hydroxyacyl-CoA dehydrogenase/mitochondrial trifunctional protein deficiencies								
13	26 days		Family history of sibling who died of lactic acidemia during the neonatal period. Died at age 49	DBS	C16OH (n.a.), C16OH/C16 (n.a.), C18:1OH (n.a.), C14 (n.a.), C14OH (n.a.)	*HADHA*	c.[1689 + 2 T > G] (deletion of exon 16)	c.[1689 + 2 T > G] (deletion of exon 16)
Short chain acyl-CoA dehydrogenase deficiency								
14	141 days	5 months	asymptomatic	Plasma	C4 (4.51 μmol/L; ref., < 1.06)	*ACADS*	c.[164C > T] (p.[P55L])	c.[1041A > G] (p.[E344G])

[a]indicates novel mutations. *DBS* dried blood spot samples, *n.a.* not available

were comparable to previous reports regarding the newborn screening program [8, 22]. In addition, the relative frequency of each FAOD was reflected; VLCAD, LCHAD/MTP, and MCAD deficiencies were common FAODs identified by newborn screening. Alternatively, other FAODs, including primary carnitine deficiency, CPT1A or SCAD deficiencies, were identified in a small number of patients. Of note, VLCAD or LCHAD/MTP deficiencies were the most common among the FAODs identified either by newborn screening or by symptomatic presentation, whereas all patients with another common FAOD, MCAD deficiency, were identified by newborn screening, as symptomatic presentation of MCAD deficiency is expected to be very rare.

Table 2 Clinical, biochemical, and genetic characteristics of patients with fatty acid oxidation disorders diagnosed by clinical signs and symptoms

No	Age at diagnosis	Age at last follow-up	Phenotype	Acylcarnitine		Gene	Allele 1	Allele 2
				Sample	Elevated acylcarnitine (value)			
Long chain hydroxyacyl-CoA dehydrogenase/mitochondrial trifunctional protein deficiencies								
1	2.7 years	11.3 years	Recurrent rhabdomyolysis, sensorimotor polyneuropathy, difficulty running and climbing stairs	DBS	C10OH (n.a.), C18OH (n.a.)	*HADHB*	c.[340A > G] (p. [N114D])	c.[739C > T] (p.[R247C])
2	2.1 years	11.9 years	Recurrent rhabdomyolysis, sensorimotor polyneuropathy, difficulty running, positive Gowers' sign	DBS	C10 (n.a.), C12 (n.a.), C14:1 (n.a.), C14OH (n.a.), C16OH (n.a.), C18:1OH (n.a.)	*HADHB*	c.[340A > G] (p. [N114D])	c.[919A > G] (p.[N307D])
3	4.8 years	6.8 years	Recurrent rhabdomyolysis, sensorimotor polyneuropathy, difficulty running	DBS	C14OH (n.a.), C16OH (n.a.), C18OH (n.a.), C18:1OH (n.a.)	*HADHB*	c.[340A > G] (p. [N114D])	c.[1148C > T] (p.[S383 L])
4	10.6 years	23.3 years	Recurrent rhabdomyolysis, sensorimotor polyneuropathy, walk with assistance	DBS	C14OH (0.156 μM; ref., 0.003–0.87), C16OH (0.228 μM; ref., 0.003–0.083), C18OH (0.072 μM; ref., 0.003–0.055)	*HADHB*	c.[919A > G] (p.[N307D])	c.[1165A > G] (p.[N389D])
5	1 day	–	Severe cardiomyopathy at first day of life. Died of lactic acidosis at 4 days old	DBS	C16OH, (0.86 μM; ref., < 0.15), C18OH (0.33 μM; ref., < 0.1), C18:1OH (0.48 μM; ref., < 0.08), C14:1 (0.66 μM; ref., < 0.35), C14 (1.35 μM; ref., < 0.86), C16:1 (0.54 μM; ref., < 0.25)	*HADHA*	c.[1793_1974del] (p.[H598Rfs*33])	c.[1793_1974del] (p.[H598Rfs*33])
6	5 days	–	Presented with tachypnea and metabolic acidosis at 5 days old. Died at 9 days old due to cardiomyopathy	DBS	C14 (n.a.), C14OH (n.a.), C16OH (n.a.), C18OH (n.a.), C18:1OH (n.a.)	*HADHB*	c.[1136A > G] (p.[H379R])	c.[1211dup] (p.[G404 fs*2]) [a]
Very long chain acyl-CoA dehydrogenase deficiency								
7	2 months	3.9 years	Hypertrophic cardiomyopathy, recurrent rhabdomyolysis	DBS	C14:1 (n.a.), C14 (n.a.)	*ACADVL*	c.[997_998ins(T)] (p.[A333*]) [a]	c.[1770_1773del] (p.[S590*]) [a]
Carnitine palmitoyltransferase 1A deficiency								
8	33 months	6.8 years	Recurrent hepatic failure, nephromegaly, hemolytic anemia, rhabomyolysis, developmental delay	Plasma	C0 (68.86 μmol/L; ref., < 62.10), C0/(C16 + C18) (1639)	*CPT1A*	c.[837_838insT] (p.[I279*])	c.[947G > A] (p.[R316Q])

[a]indicates novel mutations. *DBS* dried blood spot samples, *n.a.* not available

The purpose of newborn screening is to identify patients with inborn metabolic disorders in their presymptomatic period and intervene to prevent a metabolic crisis and improve their clinical outcome. In our current study, a fair outcome was observed in the patients with MCAD, CPT1A or primary carnitine deficiency identified by newborn screening. However, clinical outcomes were not significantly different among patients with long-chain FAODs, including VLCAD deficiency and LCHAD/MTP deficiencies identified either by newborn screening or by symptomatic presentation; most long-chain FAOD patients developed recurrent rhabdomyolysis and hypertrophic cardiomyopathy regardless of presymptomatic management.

The difference in outcomes among patients with FAODs appears to be related to disease characteristics and pathogenic effect of the mutations in addition to the mode of identification. In VLCAD or LCHAD/MTP deficiencies, patients identified by newborn screening experience a broad spectrum of severity even though the majority of patients were asymptomatic at diagnosis; symptoms develop in some patients even before newborn screening results were available, or some patients may remain asymptomatic through the long-term follow-up period [23–25]. Most of our patients with VLCAD or LCHAD/MTP deficiencies (4 out of 6) experienced recurrent rhabdomyolysis or severe cardiomyopathy. These severe phenotypes are related to complete inactivating or null alleles [25–28]. This correlation became more meaningful when the phenotype-genotype correlation was evaluated in all patients with VLCAD or LCHAD/MTP deficiencies, irrespective of the mode of identification. Seven patients with severe types of mutations, such as frameshift, nonsense, or splicing mutations, experienced severe phenotypes. Particularly, early death from severe cardiomyopathy was noted in 3 patients with severe mutations in LCHAD/MTP deficiencies. On the other hand, patients with missense mutations only either remained asymptomatic or experienced milder phenotypes (Tables 1 and 2).

As a long-term complication, peripheral polyneuropathy developed in four patients with LCHAD/MTP deficiencies, which has been reported in up to 80% of cases. In addition, pigmentary retinopathy develops in up 15–30% of patients [29, 30]. The mechanism responsible for these complications is not fully understood, although accumulation of 3-hydroxy fatty acid intermediate may be responsible [8]. Because the follow-up period was short for the patients in our current report, observation for these long-term complications is necessary.

The benign clinical course of MCAD deficiency can also be explained in part by the mutation type; most of the mutations were missense and only a small proportion of severe mutations such as frame-shift were noted. However, a life-long follow-up evaluation is required for patients with MCAD deficiency, considering the development of late-onset metabolic episodes. Between 3 and 24 months of age, patients may experience hypoketotic hypoglycemia, vomiting, lethargy, encephalopathy during febrile illness, or prolonged fasting. Sudden unexplained death may be the first presentation of MCAD deficiency [31, 32]. Even some adult patients may suffer from rhabdomyolysis, hepatic failure, encephalopathy or cardiac arrest triggered by alcohol consumption, pregnancy, or prolonged fasting [9, 33].

SCAD deficiency has also been classified as a benign condition because most of the newborns with SCAD deficiency as identified by newborn screening do not develop a clinical phenotype without any medical intervention. There exist controversies whether SCAD deficiency is benign biochemical phenotype, a clinical disorder with incomplete penetrance, or a clinically relevant part of multi-factorial or a multi-genetic disorder [34, 35]. Previously, some patients reported as having severe developmental delay, dysmorphic features and epilepsy, which would have been attributed to unknown genetic defects rather than to SCAD deficiency.

The CPT1A deficiency patient identified by newborn screening harbor heterozygous of two novel mutations. The patient remained asymptomatic during follow-up period, which was relatively short considering that CPT1A deficiency patients usually present by the age of 2 years [36]. The major manifestation of CPT1A deficiency is hepatic encephalopathy followed by febrile illness or prolonged fasting [21]. Even for a patient with neonatal presymptomatic presentation, late-onset hepatic failure develops, requiring lifelong evaluation. There exists a possibility that the novel missense mutation may not be deleterious, yet longer follow-up is needed in our patient in case of developing the symptomatic manifestations.

Conclusions

Newborn screening for FAODs revealed the relative frequency of each disease subtype and their general clinical characteristics. This screening helped to reduce the mortality and morbidity of each patient with FAODs, but their broad spectrum of disease severity was also encountered regardless the mode of diagnosis, which was explained in part by their respective genotype. Careful, life-long observation of patients with FAODs is required to improve clinical outcome.

Abbreviations

CPT1A: Carnitine palmitoyltransferase 1A; FAO: Fatty acid oxidation; FAODs: Fatty acid oxidation disorders; LCAHD/MTP: Long-chain 3-hydroxyacyl-CoA dehydrogenase or mitochondrial trifunctional protein; M/SCHAD: Medium/short chain hydroxyacyl-CoA dehydrogenase; MCAD: Medium chain acyl-CoA dehydrogenase; NBS: Newborn screenings; SCAD: Short chain acyl-CoA dehydrogenase; VLCAD: Very long chain acyl-CoA dehydrogenase

Acknowledgments

Not applicable.

Funding

This study was supported by a grant from the National Research Foundation of Korea, funded by the Ministry of Education, Science, and Technology (NRF-2015R1D1A1A01058192).

Authors' contributions

EK, HWY and BHL designed the study. EK and BHL drafted the manuscript. All authors (EK, YMK, MK, SHH, GHK, IHC, JHC, HWY, and BHL) were involved in analyzing and interpreting data. All authors read and approved the final manuscript.

Competing interests

No potential conflict of interest relevant to this article was reported.

Author details

[1]Department of Pediatrics, Hanyang University Guri Hospital, Hanyang University College of Medicine, Guri, Korea. [2]Department of Pediatrics, Asan Medical Center Children's Hospital, University of Ulsan College of Medicine, 88, Olympic-ro 43-Gil, Songpa-Gu, Seoul 05505, Korea. [3]Asan Insitute for Life Sciences, Asan Medical Center Children's Hospital, 88, Olympic-ro 43-Gil, Songpa-Gu, Seoul 05505, Korea. [4]Medical Genetics Center, Asan Medical Center Children's Hospital, University of Ulsan College of Medicine, 88, Olympic-ro 43-Gil, Songpa-Gu, Seoul 05505, Korea.

References

1. Houten SM, Wanders RJ. A general introduction to the biochemistry of mitochondrial fatty acid beta-oxidation. J Inherit Metab Dis. 2010;33(5):469–77.
2. Wanders RJ, Vreken P, den Boer ME, Wijburg FA, van Gennip AH, IJlst L. Disorders of mitochondrial fatty acyl-CoA beta-oxidation. J Inherit Metab Dis. 1999;22(4):442–87.
3. Rinaldo P, Matern D, Bennett MJ. Fatty acid oxidation disorders. Annu Rev Physiol. 2002;64:477–502.
4. Gregersen N, Andresen BS, Pedersen CB, Olsen RK, Corydon TJ, Bross P. Mitochondrial fatty acid oxidation defects–remaining challenges. J Inherit Metab Dis. 2008;31(5):643–57.
5. Lindner M, Hoffmann GF, Matern D. Newborn screening for disorders of fatty-acid oxidation: experience and recommendations from an expert meeting. J Inherit Metab Dis. 2010;33(5):521–6.
6. Yoon HR, Lee KR, Kang S, Lee DH, Yoo HW, Min WK, Cho DH, Shin SM, Kim J, Song J, et al. Screening of newborns and high-risk group of children for inborn metabolic disorders using tandem mass spectrometry in South Korea: a three-year report. Clin Chim Acta. 2005;354(1–2):167–80.
7. Gregersen N, Andresen BS, Corydon MJ, Corydon TJ, Olsen RK, Bolund L, Bross P. Mutation analysis in mitochondrial fatty acid oxidation defects: exemplified by acyl-CoA dehydrogenase deficiencies, with special focus on genotype-phenotype relationship. Hum Mutat. 2001;18(3):169–89.
8. Spiekerkoetter U. Mitochondrial fatty acid oxidation disorders: clinical presentation of long-chain fatty acid oxidation defects before and after newborn screening. J Inherit Metab Dis. 2010;33(5):527–32.
9. Schatz UA, Ensenauer R. The clinical manifestation of MCAD deficiency: challenges towards adulthood in the screened population. J Inherit Metab Dis. 2010;33(5):513–20.
10. Choi JH, Yoon HR, Kim GH, Park SJ, Shin YL, Yoo HW. Identification of novel mutations of the HADHA and HADHB genes in patients with mitochondrial trifunctional protein deficiency. Int J Mol Med. 2007;19(1):81–7.
11. Waddell L, Wiley V, Carpenter K, Bennetts B, Angel L, Andresen BS, Wilcken B. Medium-chain acyl-CoA dehydrogenase deficiency: genotype-biochemical phenotype correlations. Mol Genet Metab. 2006;87(1):32–9.
12. Purevsuren J, Kobayashi H, Hasegawa Y, Mushimoto Y, Li H, Fukuda S, Shigematsu Y, Fukao T, Yamaguchi S. A novel molecular aspect of Japanese patients with medium-chain acyl-CoA dehydrogenase deficiency (MCADD): c.449-452delCTGA is a common mutation in Japanese patients with MCADD. Mol Genet Metab. 2009;96(2):77–9.
13. Yokoi K, Ito T, Maeda Y, Nakajima Y, Ueta A, Nomura T, Koyama N, Kato I, Suzuki S, Kurono Y, et al. Acylcarnitine profiles during carnitine loading and fasting tests in a Japanese patient with medium-chain acyl-CoA dehydrogenase deficiency. Tohoku J Exp Med. 2007;213(4):351–9.
14. Ensenauer R, Winters JL, Parton PA, Kronn DF, Kim JW, Matern D, Rinaldo P, Hahn SH. Genotypic differences of MCAD deficiency in the Asian population: novel genotype and clinical symptoms preceding newborn screening notification. Genet Med. 2005;7(5):339–43.
15. Jethva R, Ficicioglu C. Clinical outcomes of infants with short-chain acyl-coenzyme a dehydrogenase deficiency (SCADD) detected by newborn screening. Mol Genet Metab. 2008;95(4):241–2.
16. Pedersen CB, Kolvraa S, Kolvraa A, Stenbroen V, Kjeldsen M, Ensenauer R, Tein I, Matern D, Rinaldo P, Vianey-Saban C, et al. The ACADS gene variation spectrum in 114 patients with short-chain acyl-CoA dehydrogenase (SCAD) deficiency is dominated by missense variations leading to protein misfolding at the cellular level. Hum Genet. 2008;124(1):43–56.
17. Smelt AH, Poorthuis BJ, Onkenhout W, Scholte HR, Andresen BS, van Duinen SG, Gregersen N, Wintzen AR. Very long chain acyl-coenzyme a dehydrogenase deficiency with adult onset. Ann Neurol. 1998;43(4):540–4.
18. Hoffmann L, Haussmann U, Mueller M, Spiekerkoetter U. VLCAD enzyme activity determinations in newborns identified by screening: a valuable tool for risk assessment. J Inherit Metab Dis. 2012;35(2):269–77.
19. Nezu J, Tamai I, Oku A, Ohashi R, Yabuuchi H, Hashimoto N, Nikaido H, Sai Y, Koizumi A, Shoji Y, et al. Primary systemic carnitine deficiency is caused by mutations in a gene encoding sodium ion-dependent carnitine transporter. Nat Genet. 1999;21(1):91–4.
20. Koizumi A, Nozaki J, Ohura T, Kayo T, Wada Y, Nezu J, Ohashi R, Tamai I, Shoji Y, Takada G, et al. Genetic epidemiology of the carnitine transporter OCTN2 gene in a Japanese population and phenotypic characterization in Japanese pedigrees with primary systemic carnitine deficiency. Hum Mol Genet. 1999;8(12):2247–54.
21. Lee BH, Kim YM, Kim JH, Kim GH, Kim JM, Kim JH, Woo KH, Yang SH, Kim CJ, Choi IH, et al. Atypical manifestation of carnitine palmitoyltransferase 1A deficiency: hepatosplenomegaly and nephromegaly. J Pediatr Gastroenterol Nutr. 2015;60(3):e19–22.
22. Landau YE, Waisbren SE, Chan LM, Levy HL. Long-term outcome of expanded newborn screening at Boston children's hospital: benefits and challenges in defining true disease. J Inherit Metab Dis. 2017;40(2):209–18.
23. Karall D, Brunner-Krainz M, Kogelnig K, Konstantopoulou V, Maier EM, Moslinger D, Plecko B, Sperl W, Volkmar B, Scholl-Burgi S. Clinical outcome, biochemical and therapeutic follow-up in 14 Austrian patients with long-chain 3-Hydroxy acyl CoA dehydrogenase deficiency (LCHADD). Orphanet J Rare Dis. 2015;10:21.
24. Sykut-Cegielska J, Gradowska W, Piekutowska-Abramczuk D, Andresen BS, Olsen RK, Oltarzewski M, Pronicki M, Pajdowska M, Bogdanska A, Jablonska E, et al. Urgent metabolic service improves survival in long-chain 3-hydroxyacyl-CoA dehydrogenase (LCHAD) deficiency detected by symptomatic identification and pilot newborn screening. J Inherit Metab Dis. 2011;34(1):185–95.
25. Pena LD, van Calcar SC, Hansen J, Edick MJ, Walsh Vockley C, Leslie N, Cameron C, Mohsen AW, Berry SA, Arnold GL, et al. Outcomes and genotype-phenotype correlations in 52 individuals with VLCAD deficiency diagnosed by NBS and enrolled in the IBEM-IS database. Mol Genet Metab. 2016;118(4):272–81.
26. Spiekerkoetter U, Lindner M, Santer R, Grotzke M, Baumgartner MR, Boehles H, Das A, Haase C, Hennermann JB, Karall D, et al. Management and outcome in 75 individuals with long-chain fatty acid oxidation defects: results from a workshop. J Inherit Metab Dis. 2009;32(4):488–97.
27. Spiekerkoetter U, Sun B, Khuchua Z, Bennett MJ, Strauss AW. Molecular and phenotypic heterogeneity in mitochondrial trifunctional protein deficiency due to beta-subunit mutations. Hum Mutat. 2003;21(6):598–607.
28. Boutron A, Acquaviva C, Vianey-Saban C, de Lonlay P, de Baulny HO, Guffon N, Dobbelaere D, Feillet F, Labarthe F, Lamireau D, et al. Comprehensive cDNA study and quantitative analysis of mutant HADHA and HADHB transcripts in a French cohort of 52 patients with mitochondrial trifunctional protein deficiency. Mol Genet Metab. 2011;103(4):341–8.
29. den Boer ME, Dionisi-Vici C, Chakrapani A, van Thuijl AO, Wanders RJ, Wijburg FA. Mitochondrial trifunctional protein deficiency: a severe fatty acid oxidation disorder with cardiac and neurologic involvement. J Pediatr. 2003;142(6):684–9.
30. Spiekerkoetter U, Bennett MJ, Ben-Zeev B, Strauss AW, Tein I. Peripheral neuropathy, episodic myoglobinuria, and respiratory failure in deficiency of the mitochondrial trifunctional protein. Muscle Nerve. 2004;29(1):66–72.
31. Iafolla AK, Thompson RJ Jr, Roe CR. Medium-chain acyl-coenzyme a dehydrogenase deficiency: clinical course in 120 affected children. J Pediatr. 1994;124(3):409–15.
32. Chace DH, DiPerna JC, Mitchell BL, Sgroi B, Hofman LF, Naylor EW. Electrospray tandem mass spectrometry for analysis of acylcarnitines in dried postmortem blood specimens collected at autopsy from infants with unexplained cause of death. Clin Chem. 2001;47(7):1166–82.
33. Lang TF. Adult presentations of medium-chain acyl-CoA dehydrogenase deficiency (MCADD). J Inherit Metab Dis. 2009;32(6):675–83.
34. Jethva R, Bennett MJ, Vockley J. Short-chain acyl-coenzyme a dehydrogenase deficiency. Mol Genet Metab. 2008;95(4):195–200.
35. Nochi Z, Olsen RKJ, Gregersen N. Short-chain acyl-CoA dehydrogenase deficiency: from gene to cell pathology and possible disease mechanisms. J Inherit Metab Dis. 2017;40(5):641–55.
36. Baruteau J, Sachs P, Broue P, Brivet M, Abdoul H, Vianey-Saban C, Ogier de Baulny H. Clinical and biological features at diagnosis in mitochondrial fatty acid beta-oxidation defects: a French pediatric study of 187 patients. J Inherit Metab Dis. 2013;36(5):795–803.

Diagnosis and therapeutic monitoring of inborn errors of metabolism in 100,077 newborns from Jining city in China

Chi-Ju Yang[1], Na Wei[2], Ming Li[1], Kun Xie[3], Jian-Qiu Li[3], Cheng-Gang Huang[3], Yong-Sheng Xiao[3], Wen-Hua Liu[3] and Xi-Gui Chen[1*]

Abstract

Background: Mandatory newborn screening for metabolic disorders has not been implemented in most parts of China. Newborn mortality and morbidity could be markedly reduced by early diagnosis and treatment of inborn errors of metabolism (IEM). Methods of screening for IEM by tandem mass spectrometry (MS/MS) have been developed, and their advantages include rapid testing, high sensitivity, high specificity, high throughput, and low sample volume (a single dried blood spot).

Methods: Dried blood spots of 100,077 newborns obtained from Jining city in 2014-2015 were screened by MS/MS. The screening results were further confirmed by clinical symptoms and biochemical analysis in combination with the detection of neonatal deficiency in organic acid, amino acid, or fatty acid metabolism and DNA analysis.

Results: The percentages of males and females among the 100,077 infants were 54.1% and 45.9%, respectively. Cut-off values were established by utilizing the percentile method. The screening results showed that 98,764 newborns were healthy, and 56 out of the 1313 newborns with suspected IEM were ultimately diagnosed with IEM. Among these 56 newborns, 19 (1:5267) had amino acid metabolism disorders, 26 (1:3849) had organic acid metabolism disorders, and 11 (1:9098) had fatty acid oxidation disorders. In addition, 54 patients with IEM were found to carry mutations, and the other 2 patients had argininemia.

Conclusions: Fifty-six cases of metabolic disorders in Jining were confirmed via newborn screening (NBS) by MS/MS. Early diagnosis and treatment are crucial for the survival and well-being of affected children. A nationwide NBS program using MS/MS is recommended, especially in poor areas of China.

Keywords: Tandem mass spectrometry, Inborn errors of metabolism (IEM), Aminoacidemia, Organic acidemia, Fatty acid oxidation disorders

Background

Newborn screening (NBS) is a public health program for the screening of infants shortly after birth for a list of conditions that are treatable but not clinically evident in the newborn period that could cause severe illness or death without early detection and treatment [1]. The NBS program aims to diagnose infants born with certain genetic, metabolic and functional disorders [2]. By early diagnosis and treatment, severe neurologic damage can be avoided in advance. NBS is designed to provide early diagnosis and treatment before significant and irreversible damage occurs [3, 4].

With the increasing number of disorders for which screening methods are available, there is a greater need for clinical diagnosis and differential diagnosis of genetic metabolic disorders. Traditional screening methods have not met this need because their speeds of testing were slow and their false positive rates were relatively high, greatly limiting their suitability for large-scale neonatal screening [5]. In the 1980s, tandem mass spectrometry (MS/MS) was introduced into newborn screening. The

* Correspondence: chenxigui1122@163.com
[1]Center of Neonatal Disease Screening, Maternal and Child Health Care Hospital, Number 12, Gongxiao Road, Jining, Shandong Province, People's Republic of China

use of MS/MS in newborn screening makes it possible to screen for a wide range of previously unscreened inborn errors of metabolism (IEM) using a single test [6]. The disorder profile of IEM includes aminoacidemias, fatty acid oxidation (FAO) disorders and organic acidemias. Early screening and diagnosis may help to decrease mortality and morbidity rates in children with IEM. Tandem mass spectrometry (MS/MS) techniques are now routinely used to screen more than 30 types of IEM, including aminoacidopathies, organic acid disorders and fatty acid oxidation disorders, given their advantages such as rapid testing, high sensitivity, high specificity, high throughput and a low sample volume (a single blood spot). By simply analyzing a dry blood spot (DBS), MS/MS was able to provide significant technical support to the diagnosis of IEM by detecting the characteristics of amino acids and acylcarnitines, thereby facilitating the screening, diagnosis and treatment of IEM [7, 8].

China is the world's most populous country. There are approximately 20 million newborns in China every year, among whom 400 to 500 thousand have inherited metabolic disorders, and the incidence of these disorders is very high [9]. From 2000 to 2009, 1, 495,132 neonates were screened in Taiwan, among whom 170 patients were diagnosed with an inherited metabolic disorder. The total incidence rate was 1:6219, including 107 cases of amino acid metabolism disorder, 51 cases of organic acid metabolism disorder and 12 cases of fatty acid metabolism disorder [10]. In the mainland, Xinhua Hospital in Shanghai introduced MS/MS technology into diagnosis of IEM in 2003. Since then, a total of 269,341 newborns have been screened, in whom 14 types of inherited metabolism disorders were detected, totaling 74 cases with an incidence rate of 1:3640. Subsequently, the neonatal screening center of Guangzhou City began to use tandem mass spectrometry to provide screening services for 30 types of inherited metabolic disorders in 2007. The neonatal screening center of Zhejiang Province provided screening for 26 kinds of genetic metabolic diseases with tandem mass spectrometry in 2008 and expanded this program to newborn screening in 2009. From 2009 to September 2010, approximately 129,415 newborns were screened. In total, 13 types of disorders of amino acids, organic acids and fatty acid metabolism were detected, for a total of 23 cases with an incidence rate of 1:5626. More than 50 screening centers for neonatal diseases have carried out the program in China [11].

However, because of economic and technological limitations, the expansion of the NBS program in China has been slow. Jining, one of the most populated cities in Shandong Province in China, carried out a program to screen for inherited metabolic disorders in newborns with MS/MS, aiming at improving the health of the population and the potential of clinical medicine. In 2014, the Jining municipal government added newborn screening for inherited metabolic disorders by tandem mass spectrometry to the city's birth defects tertiary prevention engineering and provided funding for the screening costs to promote the application of this technology.

With MS/MS newborn screening, a variety of common genetic metabolic disorders can be detected simply. The occurrence of disability or death and other serious consequences of IEM in children can be avoided by early detection and timely treatment, thus improving the health of the newborns and reducing the incidence of birth defects in local areas, as well as decreasing the economic burden on patients, families and society.

In this study, 100,077 newborns attended the screening, and we report the estimated incidences of inborn errors of amino acid, organic acid and fatty acid metabolism in suspected children referred for screening in Jining city.

Methods

DBS samples were collected from 100,077 (54,141 male and 45,936 female) infants in Jining city between 2014 and 2015. Each DBS was collected by sticking the inside or outside heel edge and then drawing a few drops of blood on filter paper (United States S&S903). The blood was allowed to thoroughly saturate the paper, and the sample was air dried for several hours. The filter paper was then sent to the neonatal center by cold chain transportation within 5 working days. The Ethics Committee of Jining Maternal and Child Health Care Hospital & Ethics Committee of Shandong province approved the study protocol (authorization number: JNCH-0128).

Reagents

The analysis was performed using a commercially available LC-MS/MS kit permitted for sale in the Chinese market (NeoBase™ Non-derivatized MS/MS Kit, Perkin Elmer, MA, USA).

Pretreatment of DBS

A 3.2-mm-diameter disc of saturated paper was separated from the filter paper and dropped into a 96-well U-bottomed plate. For extraction, 100 μL of extraction solution (containing a mixture of the respective stable-isotope-labeled internal standard) was added to each well. The plate was sealed by viscous film and incubated for 45 min at 45 °C on a horizontal orbital microplate shaker set at 650 rpm. The extracted solutions were transferred to a V-bottomed plate and covered with aluminum foil. Then, the samples were incubated at room temperature for 2 h. Finally, the plate was placed in the autosampler for testing.

Eleven amino acids, specifically, alanine (ALA), citrulline (CIT), arginine (ARG), glycine (Gly), leucine/isoleucine

(Leu/Ile/Pro-OH), methionine (MET), ornithine (ORN), phenylalanine (PHE), proline (PRO), tyrosine (Tyr), and valine (VAL); 31 acylcarnitines, namely, C0, C2, C3, C3DC/C4OH, C4, C4DC/C5OH, C5, C5:1, C5DC/C6OH, C6, C6DC, C8, C8:1, C10, C10:1, C10:2, C12, C12:1, C14, C14:1, C14:2, C14OH, C16, C16:1, C16OH, C16:1OH, C18, C18:1, C18:2, C18OH, and C18:1OH; and one ketone, succinylacetone (SA), were analyzed.

Apparatus settings

Acylcarnitines and amino acids extracted from each DBS were analyzed on a triple quadrupole tandem mass spectrometer equipped with an ACQUITY TQ Detector (Waters, MA, USA) and coupled to a Waters 1525 binary HPLC pump. Mass spectrometry was performed in multiple reaction monitoring (MRM) mode. The abundance of each compound was quantified by calculating the signal intensity ratio of the compound to its internal standard.

Confirmation of diseases

The diagnostic procedure was as follows:

1. The MS/MS test was repeated, and the results were compared to the data from the first test. 2. The levels of urinary organic acids were determined by GC-MS, or high-precision DNA mass spectrometry analysis was performed for the 39 genetic mutations related to the clinical disorders of neonatal organic acid, amino acid, and fatty acid metabolism.

Results

Basic characteristics

Among the 100,077 newborns from whom screening samples were collected, the 54,141 males accounted for 54.1% of the cohort, and the 45,936 females accounted for 45.9%. The age of blood collection from the newborns ranged from 3 to 37 days, with an average age of (5.2 ± 3.8) days.

Analysis of the screening results

According to the neonatal screening results, 98,764 infants were healthy, and 1313 were suspected to have IEM (shown in Table 1), for a positive rate of 1.31%. Among these 1313 suspected cases, 1152 were recalled for retesting (87.74%), with the final results being negative, and the remaining 161 (12.26%) cases were recalled for further diagnostic assessment. Ultimately, 56 cases of IEM were confirmed.

Analysis of diagnosed diseases

From the results of further confirmatory tests, 56 out of the 1313 suspected cases were finally diagnosed with IEM. Among these 56 infants, 19 (1:5267) had amino acid disorders, 26 (1:3849) had organic acid disorders, and 11 (1:9098) had fatty acid oxidation disorders. Moreover, 54 of these individuals carried mutations, while the other 2 patients had argininemia.

Aminoacidemias

Three types of aminoacidemias were detected in this study (16 cases with PKU, 2 cases with argininemia and 1 case with cystathionine γ-lyase deficiency), and the total prevalence rate was 1:5267. The data also indicated that PKU was the most common amino acid disorder in Jining city, as it is in other provinces in China. Other aminoacidemias were rare, such as the remaining two types, argininemia (2 patients, 10.5%) and cystathionine γ-lyase deficiency (1 patient, 5.3%) (Table 2). In the patients with PKU, the Phe level in blood was highly elevated, accompanied by an increase in the Phe/Tyr ratio. According to the confirmatory test, the gene mutation of phenylalanine hydroxylase (PAH) was the main cause of PKU. For the 2 cases of argininemia, no mutated genes were found. For the 1 case of cystathionine γ-lyase deficiency, a gene mutation of MAT1A led to this disease.

FAO disorders

There were 11 infants diagnosed with FAO disorders, for a total prevalence rate of 1:9098 (eight cases of primary carnitine deficiency [PCD], two cases of medium-chain acyl-CoA dehydrogenase [MCAD] deficiency, and one case of short-chain acyl-CoA dehydrogenase [SCAD] deficiency) (Table 3). PCD was caused by mutation of the *SLC22A5* gene, with a low blood C0 level as a hallmark. Patients with MCAD deficiency can be identified based on high blood C8 levels, which is due to mutation of the *ACADM* gene. SCAD deficiency is caused by mutation of the *ACADS* gene. This disease can be confirmed by an elevated blood C4 level and by high ethylmalonic acid levels in urine.

Organic acidemias

The most common organic acidemias in this group of patients was methylmalonic acidemia (MMA, 16, 59.3%), followed by 3-methylcrotonyl CoA carboxylase (3-MCC) deficiency (5, 18.5%), ethylmalonic encephalopathy (EE, 4, 14.8%) and β-ketothiolase deficiency (BKD, 1, 3.7%) (Table 4). Two types of gene mutations were confirmed from the blood samples of patients with MMA: MMACHC and MUT. Almost all patients with MMA (14/16, 88%) were in the group with MMACHC gene mutations. The confirmatory tests showed that methylmalonic acidemia and homocysteinemia resulted from a defect in the steps leading to adenosylcobalamin (AdoCbl) synthesis. In the remainder of the patients with MMA, the disorder was confirmed to result from a defect in the apoenzyme L-methylmalonyl-CoA mutase

Table 1 MS/MS screening profiles

MS/MS analytes	Cut-off value (μmol/L)	Possible disorder(s)	Number of cases	Ratio
Amino acids				
↑PHE	> 100	Phenylketonuria	29	2.21%
↑PHE/TYR	> 1.5			
↑MET	> 55	Hypermethioninemia	53	4.04%
↑MET/PHE	> 0.95	Cystathionine-γ-lyase deficiency	36	2.74%
↑LEU	> 300	Maple syrup urine disease	14	1.07%
↑LEU/PHE	> 5.46			
↑VAL	> 300			
↑TYR	> 290	Tyrosinemia	101	7.69%
↑TYR/PHE	> 7			
↑SA	> 1	Tyrosinemia type I	22	1.68%
↑CIT	> 40	Citrullinemia	22	1.68%
↑CIT/PHE	> 0.7			
↑ARG	> 60	Argininemia	37	2.82%
↓CIT	< 7	Carbamoyl-phosphate synthase deficiency	139	10.59%
↑ORN	> 350	Hyperornithinemia	27	2.06%
↑PRO	> 420	Hyperprolinemia	30	2.28%
Organic Acids				
↑C3	> 4	Methylmalonic acidemia	121	9.22%
↑C3/C2	> 0.17	Propionic acidemia	34	2.59%
↑C3DC + C4OH	> 0.35	Malonic acidemia	15	1.14%
↑C4	> 0.45	Glutaric acidemia type II	2	0.15%
↑C5	> 0.43	Isovaleric acidemia	138	10.51%
↑C5/C2	> 0.04			
↑C5DC + C6OH	> 0.2	Glutaric acidemia type I	1	0.08%
↑C4DC + C5OH	> 0.4	3-methylcrotonyl-CoA carboxylase deficiency	14	1.07%
		Multiple carboxylase deficiency	90	6.85%
↑(C4DC + C5OH)/C8	> 11	3-OH-3-methylglutaryl-CoA lyase deficiency	12	0.91%
↑C5:1	> 0.02	Beta-ketothiolase deficiency	9	0.69%
↑C8	> 0.15			
Fatty acid oxidation disorders				
↓C0	< 10	Carnitine uptake defect	216	16.45%
↑C0	> 50	Carnitine palmitoyltransferase I deficiency	10	0.76%
↑C0/(C16 + C18)	> 45			
↓C16	< 0.45			
↑C4	> 0.45	Short-chain acyl-CoA dehydrogenase deficiency	24	1.83%
↑C4/C2	> 0.03	Ethylmalonic encephalopathy	65	4.95%
↑C8	> 0.15	Medium-chain acyl-CoA dehydrogenase deficiency	22	1.68%
↑C8/C10	> 1.5			
↑C6	> 0.1			
↑C10:1	> 0.15			
↑C14:1	> 0.25	Very long-chain acyl-CoA dehydrogenase deficiency	9	0.69%
↑C14:1/C16	> 0.09			

Table 1 MS/MS screening profiles *(Continued)*

MS/MS analytes	Cut-off value (μmol/L)	Possible disorder(s)	Number of cases	Ratio
↑C14	> 0.4			
↑C16	> 6.5	Carnitine palmitoyltransferaseII deficiency	3	0.23%
↑C18	> 1.9	Carnitine-acylcarnitine translocase deficiency	5	0.38%
↑C18:1	> 3.5			
↑C16OH	> 0.04	Long-chain hydroxyacyl-CoA dehydrogenase deficiency	4	0.30%
↑C18OH	> 0.03	Trifunctional protein deficiency	9	0.69%
↑C18:1OH	> 0.05			

(MCM) due to a mutation of the MUT gene. Aside from MMA, other organic acidemias were rare. The number of patients with EE was 4. The diagnostic marker of EE was similar to that of SCAD deficiency, which can be distinguished by analyzing the organic acid content in urine. In patients with EE, the ethylmalonic acid level was elevated. Infants with 3-MCC, the 3-hydroxyisovaleric acid and 3-methylcrotonyl glycine levels in urine were specifically elevated. Regarding BKD, which was caused by gene mutation of ACAT1, 2-methyl-3-hydroxyl butyric acid and methylcrotonyl glycine levels in urine showed specific increases.

Discussion

Early detection and treatment for IEM can effectively prevent or reduce serious developmental and neurological damage. MS/MS is a useful tool for diagnosing different types of IEM, such as organic acidemias or aminoacidopathies [12–14]. With its feature of high throughput, MS/MS is suitable both for diagnosis of patients in the clinic and for newborn screening [7, 15]. Although the MS/MS method has been used for diagnosis for many years in China, its use has mainly been concentrated in high-end laboratories of developed areas [16]. NBS by MS/MS is not currently a national project, and corresponding supporting policy is lacking. For some poor areas that cannot afford the cost of diagnostic screening, there is also a lack of data regarding NBS. Therefore, it is difficult to establish an effective cut-off value of the screening index for guidance of the screening of IEM. In this study, 100,077 infants in Jining city underwent screening for IEM, and laboratory screening cut-off values were established based on the results. The percentage of infants with IEM was approximately 0.56‰ (56 cases were confirmed), which was lower than the positive detection rate in the other regions of Asia [17, 18], probably because of different screening criteria, screening areas or sample collection methods [18, 19].

Amino acid disorders accounted for 33.9% of all cases of IEM, and PKU was the most common type. Except for one HPA case, which was caused by mutation of the *PTS* gene, the HPA cases were related to mutation of the *PAH* gene. The rate of PKU was 50% below that of the entire country, which may be because PKU patients in some areas were not detected at an early age. According to our data, the median age of PKU patients was 16 days (range: 10-40 days). Once PKU diagnosis was confirmed, therapy was initiated, a strict diet with measures such as drinking a special formula was implemented, and regular checks were conducted to confirm that the phenylalanine concentration in blood remained in the range of 120~ 600 μmol/L. With effective treatment, the physical and mental development of the PKU patients in our study were equivalent to those of healthy children of the same age.

By analyzing the concentration of Arg in blood and urine, two cases of argininemia were confirmed, although the associated gene mutation was still unknown. The MS/MS screening results showed that patients with cystathionine-γ-lyase deficiency had higher Met levels and Met/Phe ratios. By detecting the amino acids in plasma, we observed that the concentrations of methionine and cystathionine were high, while the cysteine concentration was lower than in normal samples. The c.791G > A mutation in the *MAT1A* gene was found to be responsible for this disorder.

Table 2 Abnormal MS/MS results of aminoacidemias

Aminoacidemias (*n* = 19)	n (%)	Age at Diagnosis (day)	Abnormal parameter	Concentration mean (range)(μmol/l)	Reference range (μmol/l)	Mutated gene
Phenylketonuria (PKU)	16(84.2)	10-40	Phe	987.39 (139.92-2607.82)	21-100	PAH, PTS
			Phe/Tyr	15.66 (1.75-37.76)	0.12~ 1.1	
Argininemia (ARG)	2(10.5)	41-48	Arg	92.24 (73.97-110.50)	1.5-65	–
Cystathionine-γ-lyase deficiency	1(5.3)	35	MET	87.97	11-45	MAT1A
			MET/PHE	2.81	0.2-0.8	

Table 3 Abnormal MS/MS results of fatty acid oxidation disorders

Fatty acid oxidation disorders (*n* = 11)	n (%)	Age at Diagnosis (day)	Abnormal parameter	Concentration mean (range)(μmol/l)	Reference range (μmol/l)	Mutated gene
Primary carnitine deficiency(PCD)	8(72.7)	25-76	C0	4.32(2.40-6.43)	10-55	SLC22A5
Medium-chain acyl-CoA dehydrogenase (MCAD)	2(18.2)	45-49	C8	2.07(0.63-3.51)	0.01-0.15	ACADM
			C10	0.18(0.15-0.21)	0.02-0.22	
Short-chain acyl-CoA dehydrogenase (SCAD)	1(9.1)	102	C4	1.94	0.07-0.45	ACADS

According to other studies, FAO disorders were not common in the Asian population [20, 21], and our data showed that FAO disorders accounted for 17.9% of all IEM cases. PCD was the most common type of FAO disorder in this study, and patients were identified between 1 month and 3.5 months of age. With oral supplementation of carnitine and avoidance of hunger, patients with PCD were not different from normal babies. Only two MCAD cases were found in this study and were caused by the c.449-452delCTGA mutation in the *ACADM* gene. The remaining case was SCAD deficiency with the c.1031A > G mutation in the *ACADS* gene. Other types of FAO disorders are also rare in the Chinese population. However, blood sampling was not performed under strictly fasting conditions for most infants, and patients with some types of FAO disorders may have been missed, thus underestimating the incidence of FAO disorders.

Organic acidemias accounted for 48.2% of IEM cases in this study, and MMA, 3-MMC and EE were the three most common types. The patients with MMA accounted for 61.6% (16 patients) of the patients with organic acidemias, consistent with the findings in other countries [22–24] that also indicated MMA as the most common organic acidemia. In the patients with MMA, there were two types of therapy, depending on whether vitamin B_{12} ($VitB_{12}$) treatment was effective. Fortunately, $VitB_{12}$ was useful for most of the patients, except for one with a mutation in the *MUT* gene. For the one patient, the successful method was diet therapy with a special formula removing several natural amino acids, such as Leu and Val. With the therapy, most were normal, except that one had motor disorders because of the parents stopping $VitB_{12}$ treatment of their own accord. It was a pity for the family, as they knew little about the damage of inherited metabolic disorders. This experience serves as an alarm for us to consider not only the technology but also the need for people to understand the damage of IEM. Additionally, the program could provide genetic counseling for families with babies suffering from IEM.

Other organic acidemias are relatively rare but also lead to physical or nerve damage. The patients with EE had persistent lactic acidosis. The biochemical characteristics are typical of ethylmalonic aciduria, with a high concentration of methylsuccinic acid in urine and a high C4 concentration and C4/C3 ratio in blood. The patients with 3-MMC presented hypoglycemia with low ketone levels, sleepiness and vomiting. The BKD patient suffered from intermittent ketoacidosis accompanied by sleepiness and even coma. With early diagnosis and treatment, infants with IEM grew in a healthy state. Our study indicated that if patients with organic acidemias were not diagnosed and treated at an early stage of the disorder, irreversible sequelae of the nervous system usually occurred. In addition, except for 2 cases with argininemia, the remaining 54 patients had gene mutations that were detected. Among the 54 patients with gene mutations, 6 patients carried homozygous mutations (5 patients with primary carnitine deficiency, 1 with methylmalonic acidemia), and the remaining 48 carried heterozygous mutations. Except for one mutation in the *PTS* gene, the gene mutations of PKU patients were centered on the *PAH* gene. In total, 13 types of mutations in the *PAH* gene and 2 in the *PTS* gene were

Table 4 Abnormal MS/MS results of organic acidemias

Organic acidemias (*n* = 26)	n (%)	Age at Diagnosis (day)	Abnormal parameter	Concentration mean (range)(μmol/l)	Reference range (μmol/l)	Mutated gene
Methylmalonic academia (MMA)	16 (61.6)	13-121	C3	7.50 (4.27-18.94)	0.28-4.3	MMACHC, MUT
			C3/C2	0.90 (0.24-1.85)	0.02-0.17	
Ethylmalonic encephalopathy (EE)	4 (15.4)	30-47	C4	1.47 (1.22-1.64)	0.07-0.45	ACADS
			C4/C3	1.59 (1.47-1.77)	0.04-0.4	
3-methylcrotonyl CoA carboxylase deficiency (3-MCC)	5 (19.2)	21-57	C4DC + C5OH	6.36 (0.94-14.94)	0.06-0.4	MCCC1
β-ketothiolase deficiency (BKD)	1 (3.8)	37	C5:1	0.47	0-0.02	ACAT1

detected. Almost every patient with PKU carried unique gene mutations, which indicated that the gene mutations causing PKU were diverse, as in patients with MMA. In total, 11 types of mutations in the *MMACHC* gene and 2 in the *MUT* gene were detected, with c.609G > A being the most frequent mutation. PCD was the third most common disorder related to IEM. By DNA analysis, the gene mutation of all patients was c.1400C > G in the *SLC22A5* gene.

Conclusions

Extensive newborn screening by the MS/MS method is important for early diagnosis and effective treatment of IEM. Because people in different areas may have different blood indices for many factors, establishing a specific cut-off value for quickly and accurately diagnosing IEM is necessary. In this study, IEM could be accurately diagnosed by the combination of the MS/MS method and DNA analysis. Based on the established methods of newborn screening in Jining city, other areas of China, especially some poor areas, can obtain effective clinical guidance for the diagnosis of IEM. This guidance is helpful for saving the lives of newborns and reducing the governmental economic burden.

Abbreviations

AdoCbl: Adenosylcobalamin; ALA: Alanine; ARG: Arginine; BKD: β-ketothiolase deficiency; CIT: Citrulline; DBS: Dry blood spot; EE: Ethylmalonic encephalopathy; FAO: Fatty acid oxidation; GLY: Glycine; HPA: Hyperphenylalaninemia; HPLC: High-performance liquid chromatography; IEM: Inborn errors of metabolism; MCAD: Medium-chain acyl-CoA dehydrogenase; MCM: L-methylmalonyl-CoA mutase; MET: Methionine; MMA: Methylmalonic acidemia; MRM: Multiple reaction monitoring; MS/MS: Tandem mass spectrometry; NBS: Newborn screening; ORN: Ornithine; PCD: Primary carnitine deficiency; PHE: Phenylalanine; PKU: Phenylketonuria; PRO: Proline; SA: Succinylacetone; SCAD: Short-chain acyl-CoA dehydrogenase; TYR: Tyrosine; VAL: Valine; VitB12: Vitamin B12

Acknowledgements

We are grateful to Zhejiang Biosan Biochemical Technologies Co., Ltd., for facilitating this study with the tandem mass spectrometry (MS/MS) analysis.

Funding

There was no funding support. The corresponding author had full access to all the data in the study and was fully responsible for the decision to submit for publication.

Authors' contributions

CJY, NW, and ML designed and performed the experiments and analyzed the data. KX, JQL, and CGH analyzed the data and wrote the paper. YSX and WHL performed the experiment. XGC designed the experiments, analyzed the data, and wrote the paper. All authors read and approved the final manuscript.

Competing interests

The authors declare that they have no competing interests.

Author details

[1]Center of Neonatal Disease Screening, Maternal and Child Health Care Hospital, Number 12, Gongxiao Road, Jining, Shandong Province, People's Republic of China. [2]Clinical Laboratory of Linyi People's Hospital, Linyi, Shandong Province, People's Republic of China. [3]Zhejiang Biosan Biochemical Technologies Co., Ltd., Hangzhou, Zhejiang Province, People's Republic of China.

References

1. Maternal and Child Health Bureau. Newborn screening: Towards a uniform screening panel and system. 2005. http://mchb.hrsa.gov/programs/newbornscreening/screeningreport.pdf. Accessed 26 May, 2012.
2. March of Dimes. Newborn screening tests for your baby. 2012. https://www.marchofdimes.org/baby/newborn-screening-tests-for-your-baby.aspx. Accessed 26 May 2016.
3. Dietzen DJ, Rinaldo P, Whitley RJ, Rhead WJ, Hannon WH, Garg UC, et al. National academy of clinical biochemistry laboratory medicine practice guidelines: follow-up testing for metabolic disease identified by expanded newborn screening using tandem mass spectrometry; executive summary. Clin Chem. 2009;55:1615–26. https://doi.org/10.1373/clinchem.2009.131300.
4. Watson MS, Mann MY, Lloyd-Puryear MA, Rinaldo P, Howell RR. Newborn screening: toward a uniform screening panel and system—executive summary. Pediatrics. 2006;117:S296–307. https://doi.org/10.1542/peds.2005-2633I.
5. Liu W. Tandem mass spectrometry – developmental trend of newborn screening. Chin J Women Child Health. 2011;2:42–4.
6. Wilcken B, Wiley V, Hammond J, Carpenter K. Screening newborns for inborn errors of metabolism by tandem mass spectrometry. N Engl J Med. 2003;348:2304–12. https://doi.org/10.1056/NEJMoa025225.
7. Chace DH, Kalas TA. A biochemical perspective on the use of tandemmass spectrometry for newborn screening and clinical testing. Clin Biochem. 2005;38:296–309. https://doi.org/10.1016/j.clinbiochem.2005.01.017.
8. Copeland S. A reviewof newborn screening in the era of tandemmass spectrometry: what's new for the pediatric neurologist? Semin Pediatr Neuro. 2008;15:110–6.
9. Gao L, Gq S, Zhang SH. Clinical study of screening and diagnosis of metabolic defect by gas chromatography-mass spectrometry of urine. Mod J Integr Trad Chin West Med. 2008;17:20–1.
10. Niu D, Chien Y, Chiang C, Ho H, Hwu W, Kao S, et al. Nationwide survey of extended newborn screening by tandem mass spectrometry in Taiwan. J Inherit Metab Dis. 2010;33:295–305. https://doi.org/10.1007/s10545-010-9129-z.
11. Huang XW, Yang JB, Tong F, Yang RL, Mao HQ, Zhou XL, et al. Screening for neonatal inborn errors of metabolism by electrospray ionization-tandemmass spectrometry and follow-up. Chin J Pediatr. 2011;49:765–70.
12. Rashed MS, Ozand PT, Harrison ME, Watkins PJF, Evans S, Baillie TA. Electrospray tandem mass spectrometry in the diagnosis of organic acidemias. Rapid Commun Mass Spectrom. 1994;8:129–33. https://doi.org/10.1002/rcm.1290080124.
13. Rashed MS, Ozand PT, Bucknall MP, Little D. Diagnosis of inborn errors of metabolism from blood spots by acylcarnitines and amino acids profiling using automated electrospray tandem mass spectrometry. Pediatr Res. 1995; 38:324–31. https://doi.org/10.1203/00006450-199509000-00009.
14. Attia N, Sakati N, Al Ashwal A, al Saif R, Rashed M, Ozand PT. Isovaleric acidemia appearing as diabetic ketoacidosis. J Inherit Metab Dis. 1996;19: 85–6. https://doi.org/10.1007/BF01799353.
15. Pasquali M, Monsen G, Richardson L, Alston M, Longo N. Biochemical findings in common inborn errors of metabolism. Am J Med Genet C. 2006; 142C:64–76. https://doi.org/10.1002/ajmg.c.30086.
16. Huang XW, Yang LL, Tong F, Yang RL, Zhao ZY. Screening for inborn errors of metabolism in high-risk children: a 3-year pilot study in Zhejiang Province, China. BMC Pediatr. 2012;12:18. https://doi.org/10.1186/1471-2431-12-18.
17. Yoon HR, Lee KR, Kang S, Lee DH, Yoo HW, Min WK, et al. Screening of newborn and symptomatic group of children for inborn metabolic disorders using tandem mass spectrometry in South Korea: a three-year report. Clin Chim Acta. 2005;354:167–80.

18. Han LS, Ye J, Qiu WJ, Gao XL, Wang Y, Gu XF. Selective screening for inborn errors of metabolism on clinical patients using tandem mass spectrometry in China: a four-year report. J Inherit Metab Dis. 2007;30:507–14. https://doi.org/10.1007/s10545-007-0543-9.
19. Gu XF, Han LS, Gao XL, Yan YL, Ye J, Qiu WJ. A pilot study of selective screening for high risk children with inborn errors of metabolism using tandem mass spectrometry in China. Chin J Pediatr. 2004;42:401–4.
20. Vilarinho L, Rocha H, Sousa C, Marcão A, Fonseca H, Bogas M, et al. Four years of expanded newborn screening in Portugal with tandem mass spectrometry. J Inherit Metab Dis. 2010;33(Suppl 3):S133–8. https://doi.org/10.1007/s10545-010-9048-z.
21. Nagaraja D, Mamatha SN, De T, Christopher R. Screening for inborn errors of metabolism using automated electrospray tandem mass spectrometry: study in high-risk Indian population. Clin Biochem. 2010;43:581–8. https://doi.org/10.1016/j.clinbiochem.2009.12.009.
22. Shigematsu Y, Hirano S, Hata I, Tanaka Y, Sudo M, Sakura N, et al. Newborn mass screening and selective screening using electrospray tandem mass spectrometry in Japan. J Chrmatogr B. 2002;776:39–48.
23. Dionisi-Vici C, Rizzo C, Burlina AB, Caruso U, Sabetta G, Uziel G, et al. Inborn errors of metabolism in the Italian pediatric population: a national retrospective survey. J Pediatr. 2002;140:321–9. https://doi.org/10.1067/mpd.2002.122394.
24. Lim JS, Tan ES, John CM, Poh S, Yeo SJ, Ang JS, et al. Inborn error of metabolism (IEM) screening in Singapore by electrospray ionization-tandem mass spectrometry (ESI/MS/MS): an 8 year journey from pilot to current program. Mol Genet Metab. 2014;113:53–61. https://doi.org/10.1016/j.ymgme.2014.07.018.

16

Efficacy of levetiracetam for neonatal seizures in preterm infants

Ji Yoon Han, Chung Joon Moon, Young Ah Youn, In Kyung Sung and In Goo Lee*

Abstract

Background: Neonatal seizures remain a significant clinical problem, and therapeutic options are still not diverse with limited efficacy. Levetiracetam (LEV) is a relatively new and wide spectrum anti-seizure medication with favorable pharmacokinetics and safety profile. In the recent decades, LEV has been increasingly used for the treatment of neonatal seizures. The aim of this study was to describe the experience of using LEV as the first line anti-seizure medication for preterm infants.

Methods: A retrospective analysis of 37 preterm infants who were treated with LEV as the first-line anti-seizure medication was performed.

Results: Mean gestational age of the 37 preterm infants was 31.5 ± 1.9 weeks (range, 26 to 36^{+6} weeks). Twenty-one infants (57%) were seizure-free while given LEV at the end of the first week, and no additional anti-seizure medication was required. Loading doses of LEV ranged from 40 to 60 mg/kg (mean 56 mg/kg) and the maintenance dose ranged from 20 to 30 mg/kg (mean 23 mg/kg). No adverse effect was observed.

Conclusions: Levetiracetam can be a good and safe choice for treatment of neonatal seizures in preterm infants. Prospective double blind controlled studies are needed in the future.

Keywords: Levetiracetam, Neonatal seizures, Preterm infants

Background

Neonatal seizures are clinically defined as abnormal, stereotyped and paroxysmal dysfunctions in the central nervous system (CNS), occurring within the first 28 days after birth in full-tem infants or before 44 weeks of gestational age in preterm infants. It is the most common neurological event in neonates, indicating a variety of different pre-, peri-, or postnatal diseases of the CNS. Seizures occur more often during the neonatal period compare to other periods in the life span. They affect up to 1.5–3.5/1000 in full-term infants and 10–130/1000 in preterm infants [1], with a consistently identified trend a greater risk for seizures in preterms than full-term infants.

Various reports have suggested that prolonged seizures may lead to poor neurodevelopmental outcome [2–4]; thus appropriate treatment of neonatal seizures is important in reducing long-term neurologic disabilities. Conventionally, the first-line anti-seizure medication for the treatment of neonatal seizures is phenobarbital (PB), despite suboptimal efficacy (only around 50%) and altered pharmacodynamics effects in neonates. Furthermore, currently, a consensus has not been reached regarding the second-line anti-seizure medication such as fosphenytoin, benzodiazepine, levetiracetam (LEV), or lidocaine [5, 6].

LEV is a relatively new and wide spectrum anti-seizure medication which is designed to act through synaptic vesicle glycoprotein 2A (SV2A), which is a protein believed to be involved in the release of neurotransmitters [7]. LEV has a unique mechanism of action, novel structure, and very favorable pharmacokinetic and safety profile in neonates [8, 9]. However, insufficient data are available on the efficacy or safety of LEV in preterm infants with seizures. The purpose of this study was to examine the safety and efficacy of LEV for controlling seizures in preterm infants.

* Correspondence: hanji024@naver.com
Department of Pediatrics, College of Medicine, Seoul St. Mary's Hospital, The Catholic University of Korea, 222 Banpodaero, Seochogu, Seoul 137-701, South Korea

Methods

We performed a retrospective chart review of neonates treated in the neonatal intensive care unit at Seoul St. Mary's Hospital from January 2013 to January 2015. Infants were eligible for inclusion if they met the following criteria: 1) preterm birth (< 37 weeks); and 2) received LEV during the neonatal period (0 to 28 days after the birth). Exclusion criteria were: 1) infants whose seizures were caused by electrolyte disturbances (i.e., hypoglycemia, hyponatremia, or hypocalcemia): or 2) infants whose seizures were responsive to pyridoxine. We retrospectively analyzed 37 preterm neonates (18 males and 19 females) who received LEV monotherapy or combination therapy including LEV. Neonatal seizures were diagnosed based on clinical manifestations, neurological and physical examinations, laboratory findings, and continuous video-electroencephalography (EEG) findings during the ictal period for at least 48 h. All patients had electroencephalographic confirmation of seizures and continuous monitoring until seizure control (ranging from 48 h to 8 days).

The onset of seizures was classified as occurring within 24 h, between 24 to 48 h, between 2 and 7 days, and over 7 days to 4 weeks after birth. Types of seizures were defined according to Volpe's classification, including subtle, tonic, clonic, myoclonic, and mixed types [10].

Anti-seizure medications were considered effective if the seizure terminated within one hour after administration without recurring at least 48 h. Anti-seizure medications were considered safe and tolerable if patients had no neurological/physical abnormalities during treatment period and showed no changes in vital signs, electrocardiography, or clinical laboratory parameters. Laboratory parameters included whole blood cell counts, electrolytes, liver enzyme, gas analysis, and ammonia. LEV was mixed with normal saline and initially loaded intravenously (IV) over one hour. After the initial loading, LEV was administered twice daily. Additional application of PB (IV) was used as the second anti-seizure medication, and phenytoin (IV), midazolam (IV), topiramate (orally), or valproic acid (orally) was used as the third anti-seizure medication.

All patients underwent Bayley scales of infant developments (3rd edition) at 1 year after birth and developmental delay was defined as significant delay (> 2 standard deviation below age-matched peers) in the following areas: gross and fine motor; speech and language; cognition; personal and social development. This study was approved by the institutional review board (KC12RAS10602) of The Catholic University of Korea, Seoul St. Mary's Hospital, Korea.

Results

Gestational ages and body weights

The gestational age of 37 preterm infants ranged from 26 to 36^{+6} weeks. Their birth weights ranged from 590 g to 3300 g (Table 1). Three infants (8%) had extremely low birth weights (less than 1000 g), 10 (27%) had very low birth weights (less than 1500 g), 14 (38%) had low birth weights (2499 g or less), and 10 (27%) had normal birth weights (2500–4200 g).

Onset of neonatal seizures

Neonatal seizures occurred within 30 min to 45 days after birth (according to gestational ages: from 27 to 44 weeks). Three infants (8%) had seizures within 24 h, 7 infants (19%) had seizures within 48 h, 14 infants (38%) had seizures within 7 days, and 13 infants (35%) had seizures after 7 days. Twenty-four infants (65%) among all the patients showed seizures within one week after birth.

Types of neonatal seizures

Subtle seizures occurred in more than half of the participants (19 infants, 51.4%). Other types of seizures included clonic (5 infants, 17%), tonic (7 infants, 19%), myoclonic (1 infant, 2%), and mixed seizures (5 infants, 13%).

Nine infants (47%) showed pedaling motions or swimming movements of upper extremities, 6 infants (31%) showed apnea and blood pressure elevation, 2 infants (11%) showed ocular movements or nystagmus, and 2 infants (11%) showed chewing motions.

Brain MRI findings

Brain sonogram or magnetic resonance imaging (MRI) was performed on all preterm infants and 35 infants (94%) showed abnormal findings. The most common finding was hypoxic ischemic encephalopathy (HIE) (15 infants, 41%). Six infants (16%) had germinal matrix hemorrhage, 14 infants (38%) had intraventricular/subdural/subarachnoid hemorrhage, 1 infant had cortical dysplasia (3%), and 1 infant (3%) had bacterial meningitis.

Response to anti-seizure medication

LEV was administrated intravenously (IV) as the first-line anti-seizure medication and PB was used as the second

Table 1 Demographic features of patients

		Number of patients ($n = 37$, %)
Sex	Male	18 (49)
	Female	19 (51)
Gestational age	Mean	31.5 ± 1.9 weeks
	< 28^{+0} weeks	5 (14)
	28 > to 36^{-6} weeks	32 (86)
Birth weight	Mean	1840 ± 102 g
	< 1000 g	3 (8)
	1000~ 1500 g	10 (27)
	1500~ 2500 g	14 (38)
	> 2500 g	10 (27)

anti-seizure medication (Fig. 1). LEV (40–60 mg/kg, mean dose 56 mg/kg) was mixed with normal saline and initially loaded over one hour; after initial loading, LEV (20-30 mg/kg, mean dose 23 mg/kg) was administered twice per day. For infants who continued to have seizures after LEV administration, additional infusion of PB (IV, 20 mg/kg) was used as the second anti-seizure medication, and phenytoin (IV, 20 mg/kg), midazolam (IV continuous infusion, 0.1–0.3 mg/kg/h), topiramate (orally, 5–8 mg/kg), or valproic acid (IV, 10–15 mg/kg) was used as the third anti-seizure medications. Overall, seizures terminated in 21 of 37 of the neonates (57%) after receiving LEV, and no additional anti-seizure medications were required (Fig. 1). Sixteen infants (43%) required additional anti-seizure medications during LEV treatment. Seizure cessation was achieved 9 infants (24%) after administration of both LEV and PB. The remaining 7 infants (9%) continued with seizures until a third line anti-seizure medication (phenytoin, topiramate, midazolam, or valproic acid) were administered.

Twenty-one infants (57%) were seizure free under LEV by the end of the first week. Of the remaining, 13 (35%) were seizure free by the 5th week, and 3 (8%) were seizure free by the 11th week after initiating the treatment. In 19 infants (51%), LEV was discontinued after 2–4 weeks of being seizure free.

The mean duration of anti-seizure medication therapy was 42 ± 21 days (range, 15 to 189 days); 36 ± 17 days under LEV monotherapy and 54 ± 21 days under polytherapy. Twenty-three patients (62%) were discharged with LEV, 11 patients (30%) were discharged with additional anti-seizure medications, and 3 patients (8%) were discharged without anti-seizure medication.

Adverse reactions of LEV

There were no documented adverse drug reactions during or after LEV administration. No serious or consistent emergent laboratory abnormalities were observed. All patients were monitored for increased irritability or somnolence; however no clear adverse reactions including rash and tremor were observed during the study.

Follow-up and neurological outcomes

Physical, neurological, and developmental examinations were performed for all patients at 1 year after birth. There are no mortality in 37 infants. Twenty-eight patients (75%) were free of seizures and had been completely weaned off all anti-seizure medications. Fourteen infants (38%) showed developmental delay, and 9 infants (25%) had post-neonatal epilepsy with receiving anti-seizure medications.

Discussion

Neonatal seizures are neurological emergencies and must be treated promptly since seizures can aggravate neuronal injury in the immature brain and contribute to the pathogenesis of later neurodevelopmental disabilities or post-neonatal epilepsy [2]. There are only a few treatment options in neonates with seizures because anti-seizure medications such as PB, phenytoin, and benzodiazepines are rarely effective in controlling epileptogenesis in neonates, and the known risk of adverse effect on cognition effect of PB in infants [11].

Levetiracetam is an anti-seizure medication originally approved for the use in children 4 years old and above in 2005. It received approval for the administration to infants 1 month old (for oral application) and above in 2011. Favorable features of LEV include linear pharmacokinetics, rapid absorption (within 30 min), nonhepatic elimination, lack of protein binding (< 10%), no drug-drug interaction with other medications, and relatively short half-life compared to PB [7]. The availability of its oral and intravenous formulations has made it very useful as an off-label anti-seizure medication in the treatment of neonatal seizures. It has been found that LEV does not increase apoptosis in a developing rodent brain or interfere with neuroprotective

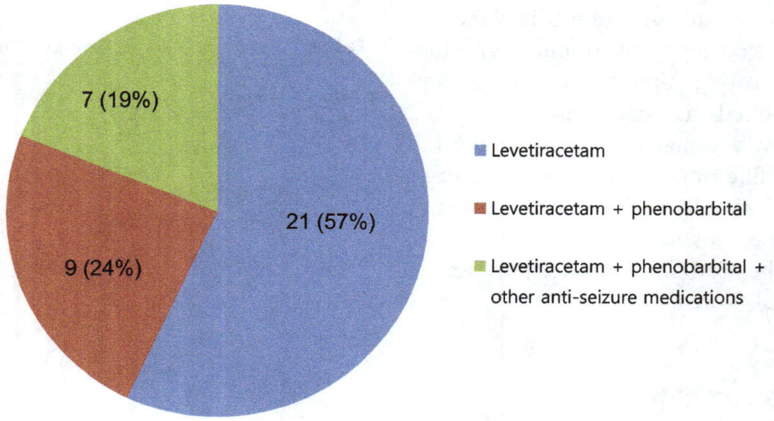

Fig. 1 Response of neonatal seizures to anti-seizure medications ($N = 37$)

up-regulation of hypoxia inducible transcription factor 1 (HIF-1a) [12]. It can also decrease neurodegeneration in rodent models of hypoxic-ischemia [13] or epilepsy [14]. Due to maturational differences and adverse complications of the brain, preterm infants of less than 30 weeks of gestation have a higher incidence of seizures compared to neonates older than 30 weeks [15]. Seizures are a sign of neuronal injury and approximately 40%–60% of all neonatal seizures are attributable to HIE [2]. In our study, the most common brain MRI finding was also HIE (41%). Repeated seizures may be deleterious to the developing brain without disturbing ventilation or perfusion by increasing central nervous system metabolic demand, leading to the release of excitatory amino acid such as glutamate [16]. Neonatal seizures have not been directly shown to lead to neuronal cell death and they are clearly associated with alterations in neurogenesis or synaptic organization [17]. Therefore, continued seizures have a poor prognosis and may lead to serious sequelae such as intellectual disability and motor deficit.

Studies using animal models have shown that LEV does not lead to neuronal apoptosis in immature brain or disrupt synaptic development and may even have neuroprotective properties [18]. Kilicdag et al. [19] demonstrated that administration of LEV after hypoxia significantly reduced the number of apoptotic cells in the cerebral cortex and hippocampus compared to the control in an animal model ($p < 0.006$). When given prophylactically to HIE-induced neonatal rodents, LEV can significantly reduce seizure activity and duration of ictal EEG activity [20]. These findings suggest that LEV may be a viable choice for treating neonatal seizures in HIE. Decreased efficacy and adverse neurodevelopmental prognosis of conventional anti-seizure medications have generated an interest in the use of LEV for the treatment of neonatal seizures.

Despite published data on children and adolescents, only a few have evaluated the efficacy and safety of LEV in neonatal seizures. Several studies have shown the efficacy and safety of LEV in neonatal seizures with diverse etiologies over the past decade [21–32] (Table 2). These studies have demonstrated that LEV may be effective in neonatal seizures when conventional anti-seizure medications have failed. Overall results have shown that LEV may have an overall effect of 50%–80% seizure reduction. These data suggest that LEV can be effective for the treatment of neonatal seizures [25, 26], with a favorable tolerability and side-effect profile comparable to PB. In our study, the use of LEV as the first anti-seizure medication demonstrated seizure cessation within 24 h in 57% (21/37) of patients. Ramantani et al. [24] have also reported the efficacy of LEV in a prospective study using LEV as the first anti-seizure medication. Thirty neonates (79%) including preterm infants were seizure-free under LEV by the end of the 1st week. Such variations in LEV efficacy may be due to the difference in etiology, types of seizures, methods of diagnosis, definitions of efficacy, use of concomitant anti-seizure medications, and dose of LEV.

Anti-seizure medications such as NMDA receptor antagonists (i.e., ketamine or felbamate), GABA agonists (i.e., PB or benzodiazepine), and sodium channel blockers (i.e., phenytoin or carbamazepine) have been considered to potentiate neurodegeneration in the developing brain of animal models [33]. Dissimilar to other conventional anti-seizure medications, LEV has shown favorable neurodevelopment outcomes and lack of neurodegenerative effects in early animal studies, making LEV a fair treatment option in neonatal seizures. Because SV2a is found in the whole brain, LEV can be used to treat multiple types of seizures that arise from various regions of the brain, as seen in neonatal seizures.

Our study also monitored safety parameters including vital signs and laboratory findings. None of these parameters revealed any adverse effects following LEV administration. These findings have motivated us to institute a protocol for neonatal seizures including preterm infants. Furthermore no serious adverse reactions were seen in our patients. These results were consistent with the most of the data previously reports. A 2007 survey showed that 47% of pediatric neurologists recommended LEV's off-label use for treating neonatal seizures [34]. Although LEV seems to be safe and effective in neonatal seizures, whether its use will be approved as the first-line anti-seizure medication or as monotherapy remains unclear. Moreover, the pharmacokinetics and safety of LEV appears to be more reasonable than those of conventional anti-seizure medications (i.e., PB, phenytoin or benzodiazepine) in neonatal seizures. Larger prospective studies in newborn patients are needed to investigate LEV as an effective and safe treatment choice for neonatal seizures.

Our results suggest that LEV is a potentially good option to as the first-line anti-seizure medication for treating neonatal seizures including preterm infants. However, our study had some limitations, including a small sample size and its retrospective nature. Our data showed a favorable profile of LEV in neonatal seizures, but additional future researches are needed to clarify its efficacy and safety. Also, long-term observation of neurodevelopmental outcome is necessary in order to establish a proper alternative to traditional anti-seizure medications in neonates with seizures.

Conclusion

Although this study does not provide conclusive evidence for using LEV in neonatal seizures, treatment with LEV did not result in any adverse reactions and was generally well tolerated. Our data will aid in the decision for using LEV as a treatment option in preterm infants with neonatal seizures, which can improve neurological outcome. Further research studies with larger datasets of prospective randomized control study on LEV use are needed to clarify the efficacy and safety of LEV.

Table 2 Levetiracetam studies in neonatal seizures

Study	Year of publication	No. of patients	Gestational age	Anti-seizure medications used before LEV	LEV dose	Results	Remarks
Shoemaker et al. [21]	2007	3	25^{+6}–41^{+6} weeks	PB, MDZ, fPHT	LD: 60 mg/kg (oral) MD: 30 mg/kg	All 3 patients showed seizure-free with LEV monotherapy.	
Furwentsches et al. [22]	2010	6	37^{+1}–41^{+3} weeks	PB	ID: 10 mg/kg MD: 50 mg/kg	All 6 patients showed seizure-free within 6 days.	Prospective
Ledet et al. [23]	2010	1	40^{+5} weeks	PB	LD: 40 mg/kg, MD: 40 mg/kg	Seizure-free	Acute lymphoblastic leukemia
Ramantani et al. [24]	2011	38	28–36^{+6} weeks	none	ID: 10–20 mg/kg MD:45–60 mg/kg	Thirty infants (79%) seizure-free under LEV at the end of 1st week.	Prospective
Khan et al. [26]	2011	22	37^{+5}–41^{+2} weeks	PB, fPHT	LD: 10–50 mg/kg MD: 50 mg/kg	Nineteen of 22 patients (86%) demonstrated immediate seizure cessation at 1 h.	LEV as 1st AED in 3 patient
Abend et al. [27]	2011	23	35–41 weeks	PB, PHT	ID: 5–22 mg/kg MD: 10–80 mg/kg	50% seizure reduction in 35% (8/23), including seizure termination in 7 (30%)	LEV as 1st AED in 4 patient
Sharpe et al.	2012	18	37–41 weeks	PB	LD: 20–40 mg/kg MD: 5–10 mg/kg	Six (33%) of the 18 required no additional AEDs after LEV administration.	
Rakshasbhuvankar et al. [28]	2013	8	22^{+6}-ferm weeks	PB, PTH, MDZ, CZP	ID: 10 mg/kg MD: 10–35 mg/kg	Six (75%) of the eight neonates had an excellent response with either cessation of reduction in seizures by at least 80%.	
Khan et al. [25]	2013	12	23^{+3}–36 weeks	PB	LD: 25–50 mg/kg MD: 50 mg/kg	Nine of 11 patients (82%) reached seizure cessation within 24 h of receiving LEV.	LEV as 1st AED in 3 patient
Kirmani et al. [29]	2014	22	NA	NA	LD: 10–50 mg/kg MD: NA	Seizure cessation was achieved in 86% (19/22) of patients one hour after the loading dose.	
Neininger et al. [32]	2015	72	23^{+2}–41^{+7} weeks	PB, PTH, MZD, DIZ	ID: 4.9–106.2 mg/kg (mean 20.3 mg/kg) MD: 41.7 mg/kg		LEV as 1st AED in 15 patient,
Shin et al. [30]	2017	18	24^{+3}–40^{+2} weeks	PB, PHT	ID: 4.9–59.5 mg/kg (mean 20 mg/kg) MD: 4.5–99.5 mg/kg (mean 29 mg/kg)	Seventeen patients (94%) had seizure cessation within 1 week and 16 (84%) remained seizure-free at 30 days under LEV therapy.	LEV as 1st AED in 1 patient
Venkatesan et al. [31]	2017	32	35–42^{+4} weeks	PB	LD: 20–150 mg/kg (mean 63 mg/kg) MD: 30–100 mg/kg (mean 65 mg/kg)	Thirty two neonates received LEV after PB, the seizures stopped in 27 (84%) patients.	LEV as 1st AED in 2 patient
Our study		37	26–36^{+6} weeks	None	LD: 40–60 mg/kg MD: 40–60 mg/kg	Seizures were stopped in 21 (57%) of 37 of neonates after receiving LEV, and no additional AEDs were required	

PB phenobarbital, *MDZ* midazolam, *PHT* phenytoin, *fPHT* fosphenytoin, *CZP* clonazepam, *DIZ* diazepam, *LD* loading dose, *MD* maintenance dose, *ID* Initial dose, *NA* not available

Abbreviations
EEG: Electroencephalography; HIE: Hypoxic ischemic encephalopathy; LEV: Levetiracetam; MRI: Magnetic resonance image; PB: Phenobarbital

Funding
None.

Acknowledgements
The authors have no acknowledgements to make.

Authors' contributions
Ji Yoon Han carried out statistical analyses and drafted the manuscript. In Goo Lee participated in the design of this study, data collection, and interpretation of the data. Chung Joon Moon carried out the data collection and interpretation of data. Young Ah Youn and In Kyung Sung participated in data collection and statistical analysis. Ji Yoon Han and In Goo Lee participated in study design and coordination. All authors read and approved the final manuscript.

Competing interests
The authors declare that they have no competing interests.

References

1. Bassan H, Bental Y, Shany E, Berger I, Froom P, Levi L, Shiff Y. Neonatal seizures: dilemmas in workup and management. Pediatr Neurol. 2008;38(6): 415–21.
2. Silverstein FS, Jensen FE. Neonatal seizures. Ann Neurol. 2007;62(2):112–20.
3. Kharoshankaya L, Stevenson NJ, Livingstone V, Murray DM, Murphy BP, Ahearne CE, Boylan GB. Seizure burden and neurodevelopmental outcome in neonates with hypoxic–ischemic encephalopathy. Developmental Medicine & Child Neurology. 2016;58(12):1242–8.
4. Pisani F, Facini C, Pelosi A, Mazzotta S, Spagnoli C, Pavlidis E. Neonatal seizures in preterm newborns: a predictive model for outcome. Eur J Paediatr Neurol. 2016;20(2):243–51.
5. van Rooij LG, Hellström-Westas L, de Vries LS. Treatment of neonatal seizures. Semin Fetal Neonatal Med. 2013;18(4):209–15.
6. Donovan M, Griffin B, Kharoshankaya L, Cryan J, Boylan G. Pharmacotherapy for neonatal seizures: current knowledge and future perspectives. Drugs. 2016;76(6):647–61.
7. Merhar SL, Schibler KR, Sherwin CM, Meinzen-Derr J, Shi J, Balmakund T, Vinks AA. Pharmacokinetics of levetiracetam in neonates with seizures. The Journal of pediatrics. 2011;159(1):152–4. e153
8. Briggs DE, French JA. Levetiracetam safety profiles and tolerability in epilepsy patients. Expert Opin Drug Saf. 2004;3(5):415–24.
9. Sharpe CM, Capparelli EV, Mower A, Farrell MJ, Soldin SJ, Haas RH. A seven-day study of the pharmacokinetics of intravenous levetiracetam in neonates: marked changes in pharmacokinetics occur during the first week of life. Pediatr Res. 2012;72(1):43–9.
10. Volpe JJ. Neurology of the newborn. Elsevier Health Sciences. 2008;
11. Booth D, Evans DJ. Anticonvulsants for neonates with seizures. Cochrane Database Syst Rev. 2004;(4):CD004218.
12. Trollmann R, Schneider J, Keller S, Strasser K, Wenzel D, Rascher W, Ogunshola OO, Gassmann M. HIF-1-regulated vasoactive systems are differentially involved in acute hypoxic stress responses of the developing brain of newborn mice and are not affected by levetiracetam. Brain Res. 2008;1199:27–36.
13. Hanon E, Klitgaard H. Neuroprotective properties of the novel antiepileptic drug levetiracetam in the rat middle cerebral artery occlusion model of focal cerebral ischemia. Seizure. 2001;10(4):287–93.
14. Marini H, Costa C, Passaniti M, Esposito M, Campo GM, Ientile R, Adamo EB, Marini R, Calabresi P, Altavilla D. Levetiracetam protects against kainic acid-induced toxicity. Life Sci. 2004;74(10):1253–64.
15. Scher MS, Aso K, Beggarly ME, Hamid MY, Steppe DA, Painter MJ. Electrographic seizures in preterm and full-term neonates: clinical correlates, associated brain lesions, and risk for neurologic sequelae. Pediatrics. 1993;91(1):128 34.
16. Thibeault-Eybalin M-P, Lortie A, Carmant L. Neonatal seizures: do they damage the brain? Pediatr Neurol. 2009;40(3):175–80.
17. Holmes GL. Effects of seizures on brain development: lessons from the laboratory. Pediatr Neurol. 2005;33(1):1–11.
18. Forcelli PA, Janssen MJ, Vicini S, Gale K. Neonatal exposure to antiepileptic drugs disrupts striatal synaptic development. Ann Neurol. 2012;72(3):363–72.
19. Kilicdag H, Daglıoglu K, Erdogan S, Guzel A, Sencar L, Polat S, Zorludemir S. The effect of levetiracetam on neuronal apoptosis in neonatal rat model of hypoxic ischemic brain injury. Early Hum Dev. 2013;89(5):355–60.
20. Talos DM, Chang M, Kosaras B, Fitzgerald E, Murphy A, Folkerth RD, Jensen FE. Antiepileptic effects of levetiracetam in a rodent neonatal seizure model. Pediatr Res. 2013;73(1):24–30.
21. Shoemaker M, Rotenberg J. Levetiracetam for the treatment of neonatal seizures. J Child Neurol. 2007;22(1):95–8.
22. Fürwentsches A, Bussmann C, Ramantani G, Ebinger F, Philippi H, Pöschl J, Schubert S, Rating D, Bast T. Levetiracetam in the treatment of neonatal seizures: a pilot study. Seizure. 2010;19(3):185–9.
23. Ledet DS, Wheless JW, Rubnitz JE, Morris EB. Levetiracetam as monotherapy for seizures in a neonate with acute lymphoblastic leukemia. Eur J Paediatr Neurol. 2010;14(1):78–9.
24. Ramantani G, Ikonomidou C, Walter B, Rating D, Dinger J. Levetiracetam: safety and efficacy in neonatal seizures. Eur J Paediatr Neurol. 2011;15(1):1–7.
25. Khan O, Cipriani C, Wright C, Crisp E, Kirmani B. Role of intravenous levetiracetam for acute seizure management in preterm neonates. Pediatr Neurol. 2013;49(5):340–3.
26. Khan O, Chang E, Cipriani C, Wright C, Crisp E, Kirmani B. Use of intravenous levetiracetam for management of acute seizures in neonates. Pediatr Neurol. 2011;44(4):265–9.
27. Abend NS, Gutierrez-Colina AM, Monk HM, Dlugos DJ, Clancy RR. Levetiracetam for treatment of neonatal seizures. J Child Neurol. 2011: 0883073810384263.
28. Rakshasbhuvankar A, Rao S, Kohan R, Simmer K, Nagarajan L. Intravenous levetiracetam for treatment of neonatal seizures. J Clin Neurosci. 2013;20(8): 1165–7.
29. Kirmani BF. Levetiracetam–An Alternative Option in Preterm Neonates for Acute Seizure Management. Mol Cell Epilepsy. 2014;1:e19.
30. Shin JW, Jung YS, Park K, Lee SM, Eun HS, Park MS, Park KI, Namgung R. Experience and pharmacokinetics of Levetiracetam in Korean neonates with neonatal seizures. Korean journal of pediatrics. 2017;60(2):50–4.
31. Venkatesan C, Young S, Schapiro M, Thomas C. Levetiracetam for the treatment of seizures in neonatal hypoxic ischemic encephalopathy. J Child Neurol. 2017;32(2):210–4.
32. Neininger MP, Ullmann M, Dahse AJ, Syrbe S, Bernhard MK, Frontini R, Kiess W, Merkenschlager A, Thome U, Bertsche T, et al. Use of Levetiracetam in neonates in clinical practice: a retrospective study at a German university hospital. Neuropediatrics. 2015;46(5):329–34.
33. Ikonomidou C. Triggers of apoptosis in the immature brain. Brain Dev. 2009; 31(7):488–92.
34. Silverstein FS, Ferriero DM. Off-label use of antiepileptic drugs for the treatment of neonatal seizures. Pediatr Neurol. 2008;39(2):77–9.

Clostridium difficile stool shedding in infants hospitalized in two neonatal intensive care units is lower than previous point prevalence estimates using molecular diagnostic methods

Andrea Green Hines[1,2], Alison Freifeld[1], Xing Zhao[2], Ann Anderson Berry[3], Lynne Willett[3], Peter C. Iwen[4] and Kari A. Simonsen[2*]

Abstract

Background: The point prevalence of *Clostridium difficile* stool shedding in hospitalized infants from two neonatal intensive care units (NICUs) was examined utilizing standard clinical testing compared with duplex PCR to identify toxigenic and non-toxigenic *C. difficile* strains.

Methods: All infants from the two NICUs affiliated with a single academic medical center were eligible for inclusion. Stool collection was blinded to patient characteristics and occurred during a one week period at each NICU and repeated with a second weeklong collection 6 months later to increase sample size. Stools were tested for *C. difficile* using EIA (GDH/toxin A/B) with samples testing +/+ or +/− subsequently evaluated by Loop-Mediated Isothermal Amplification (LAMP) and by duplex PCR amplification of *tcdB* and *tpi* (housekeeping) genes. Cytotoxicity assays were performed on all samples positive for *C. difficile* by any modality.

Results: Eighty-four stools were collected from unique infants for evaluation. EIA results showed 6+/+ [7.1%], 7 +/− [8.3%], and 71 −/− [84.5%] samples. All 6 EIA +/+ were confirmed as toxigenic *C. difficile* by LAMP; 6/7 EIA +/− were negative by LAMP with one identified as invalid. Duplex PCR concurred with LAMP in all 6 stools positive for toxigenic *C. difficile*. PCR identified 2 EIA −/− stools positive for *tpi*, indicating shedding of non-toxigenic *C. difficile*. Cytotoxicity assay was positive in 4/6 duplex PCR positive samples and negative for all stools that were EIA +/− but negative by molecular testing.

Conclusions: *C. difficile* blinded point prevalence in infants from two NICUs was 7.1% by molecular methods; and lower than expected based on historical incidence estimates. In house duplex PCR had excellent concordance with clinically available LAMP and EIA tests, and added detection of non-toxigenic *C. difficile* strain shedding. Evolving NICU care practices may be influencing the composition of infant gut microbiota and reducing the point prevalence of *C. difficile* shedding in NICU patient stools.

Keywords: Clostridium difficile, Infant, Epidemiology, Molecular epidemiology

* Correspondence: kasimonsen@unmc.edu
[2]Pediatric Infectious Diseases, University of Nebraska Medical Center, Omaha, NE, USA

Background

The epidemiology of *Clostridium difficile* infection (CDI) has shifted in the last decade and is now affecting populations previously at low risk to include healthy adults, peripartum women and young children [1]. Based on several recent studies, traditional risk factors for CDI, including antimicrobial exposure and recent hospitalization are absent in a major proportion of cases [2–4]. These epidemiological shifts in CDI have prompted renewed investigation into potential reservoirs and vectors for transmission. Asymptomatic shedders of *C. difficile*, including infants, have been suggested as playing a role [5–11]. A single-center study demonstrated that based on multilocus variable number of tandem repeats analysis (MLVA), 29% of hospital acquired CDI (HA-CDI) cases were highly related to *C. difficile* isolates from asymptomatic patients that were collected before the HA-CDI isolate [7]. A more recent investigation noted that asymptomatic *C. difficile* carriers increased the risk of nosocomial CDI in other hospitalized patients [12]. A wide range of asymptomatic colonization rates with toxigenic and non-toxigenic *C. difficile* have been reported in both hospitalized and community-dwelling infants from 11 to 71% [8, 10, 13–29]. NICU infants have been reported to have a prevalence of *C. difficile* colonization of between 15 and 78% based on several previously published studies performed in the U.S. and elsewhere [13, 18–20, 25, 30–42] (see Table 1). These studies also showed that confirmation testing using the cytotoxicity assay or PCR showed prevalence of toxigenic *C. difficile* to range from 0 to 67%.

During the last three decades substantial advances in NICU care have occurred. These include earlier feeding, emphasis on human milk feedings, use of more broad-spectrum antibiotics as well as additional efforts to control antimicrobial exposure through stewardship, and the survival of very low birth weight infants with prolonged, complicated hospital stays. Despite these important medical practice changes and the evolution of more precise molecular laboratory tests for toxigenic *C. difficile*, the prevalence of *C. difficile* has not been re-evaluated in U.S. NICU settings with molecular technology.

Table 1 Prior NICU studies examining *C. difficile* prevalence

Author, Year of Study	Location	Test Methods	Prevalence of *C. difficile*
Kim, 1981 [37]	U.S.	Culture + cytotoxicity assay	21% culture +, 14% toxin +
Blakey, 1982 [31]	Australia	Culture	0–35% culture +[a]
Donta, 1982 [18]	U.S.	Cytotoxicity assay	54.9% toxin +
Sherertz, 1982 [25]	U.S.	Culture	59% culture +
Malamou-Ladas, 1983 [39]	England	Culture	54% culture +
Al-Jumaili, 1984 [13]	England	Culture + cytotoxicity assay	71% culture +, 45% toxin +
Lishman, 1984 [38]	England	Culture + cytotoxicity assay	78% culture +, 67% toxin +
Phua, 1984 [40]	England	Culture + cytotoxicity assay	21% culture +, 0% toxin +
Zedd, 1984 [42]	U.S.	Culture	41% culture +
Cardines, 1988 [32]	Italy	Culture + cytotoxicity assay + PAGE[b]	63% culture +, 0% toxin + (per cytotoxicity assay), 16% toxigenic strain + (per PAGE)
el-Mohandes, 1993 [34]	U.S.	Culture + cytotoxicity assay	15–33% culture +, 71–100% toxin +[c]
Kato, 1994 [36]	Japan	Culture + PCR for toxins A and B	61% culture +, 6% toxin +[d]
Tina, 1994 [41]	Italy	Culture + EIA for toxins A and B	43.6% culture +, 31.2% toxin +
Enad, 1997 [19]	U.S.	EIA for toxin A	52% EIA +
Alfa, 2002 [30]	Canada	PCR for *C. difficile* 16S gene	21% *C. difficile* 16S gene +
Chang, 2012 [33]	Korea	PCR for *C. difficile* 16S gene + PCR for toxins A and B	34.7–53.1% *C. difficile* 16S gene+[e] 23.5–30.8% toxin +
Ferraris, 2012 [35]	France	PCR for *C. difficile* 16S gene	42.1% *C. difficile* 16S gene+
Faden, 2015 [20]	U.S.	EIA GDH Ag/toxins A/B *C. difficile* culture	25.7% +[f]

[a]Study measured prevalence at days 0–4, 5–8, 9–12, 13–16, 17–20 and > 20 days, thus providing a prevalence range
[b]SDS-polyacrylamide gel electrophoresis (PAGE) of EDTA-extracted proteins used to identify toxigenic strains
[c]Study measured prevalence after 1 week of enteral feeding, at 15 +/− 1 days of life; 2 more specimens were collected at 2 week intervals, 24 +/− 1 and 32 +/− 2 days of life, thus providing a prevalence range
[d]PCR for toxins A and B were performed on only 32 of 41 *C. difficile* culture+ infants
[e]Study measured prevalence within 72 h of birth, 1, 2, and 4–6 weeks of age thus providing a prevalence range
[f]Test modality of positivity unspecified

We examined the current point prevalence of *C. difficile* stool shedding in hospitalized infants from two affiliated NICUs utilizing a rapid and novel duplex PCR which was developed and validated in our laboratory [43]. This duplex PCR detected the presence of two genes, (*tpi* and *tcdB*) and we proposed the NICU as a high prevalence unit for validation of the PCR method.

All *C. difficile* strains, toxigenic and non-toxigenic, possess the housekeeping gene *tpi* (triose phosphatase isomerase). The *tcdB* gene encodes for the *C. difficile* toxin B. A non-toxigenic strain was defined as the detection of the *tpi* gene alone while a toxigenic strain was defined as the detection of both *tpi* and *tcdB* genes. We hypothesized that with both the epidemiologic changes in CDI as well as the advances in NICU care, the prevalence of *C. difficile* stool shedding may be rising, and heighten concerns for risk to hospital patients and the hospital environment.

Methods

All infants hospitalized in two NICUs (NICU A and B) producing stool during the study period were included in the point prevalence survey. The institutional IRB reviewed and approved the protocol and waived informed consent as no patient identifiers were maintained for the study.

Collection of the stool samples occurred over two separate weeks in each NICU. At NICU A, stool samples were collected in March and in September; at NICU B, stool samples were collected in April and in September. NICU A is a Level III, 36-bed NICU and NICU B is a Level IV, 42-bed NICU. At the beginning of each study week and at the time of any new NICU admission during the study week, five sticker labels containing unique study numbers were placed at the bedside of each NICU patient. Each NICU bedside nurse collected patient's stool soiled diapers, placed the diaper in a sealed container labeled with the study number and date and subsequently deposited the specimen container into a specially labeled bin located in the NICU. Nurses were instructed to collect up to five stool soiled diapers per patient. This collection methodology ensured patient non-duplication at the clinical level with blinding of the study team. Each NICU had a neonatologist on the study team who was also able to ensure non-duplication and who did not have access to the stool results on a per patient level. A study researcher collected the stool samples from the bin periodically each day and transported them to the research laboratory.

Stool from each NICU patient's soiled diapers was divided into five 1 mL aliquots and frozen at -20^0 C until DNA extraction and PCR testing. The procedure is briefly described: DNA extraction was performed with liquid stool combined with lysis reagents and processed in a 1 ml-capacity lysis microreactor (LMR) which employed intense mixing with heating resulting in bacterial cell lysis. A surface-treated polystyrene strip bound DNA released by lysis from the mixture and permitted transfer of the DNA on the strip to the PCR cuvette. A rapid thermocycler (Philisa Thermal Cycler, Streck, Inc., Omaha, NE) was used to specifically amplify a conserved region of both toxigenic and non-toxigenic *C. difficile tpi* gene and a non-repeat region of the toxigenic *C. difficile tcdB* gene using primers designed using online multiplex PCR primer design software called "Primo Multiplex 3.4". (http://www.changbioscience.com/primo/primoml.html). The forward *tpi* gene primer was TATATGTGCACCATTTACTTTATT and the *tpi* reverse primer was AACTTTACAAACATCTTTAGTTTTT, generating a 320 bp PCR product. The forward *tcdB* gene primer was TTAGCAGGAATTTCAGCAGGT and the reverse *tcdB* gene primer was ATGACCTGAAC CACCTTCCA, generating a 249 bp product. Each 25 μl reaction contained a final concentration of 0.2 mM dNTPs, 5.5 mM $MgSO_4$, 0.5 U KOD Hot Start DNA polymerase, 1X PCR buffer (PCR kit, EMD Chemicals, Inc), 0.4 mg/ml BSA (Ambion, Inc), 0.2 μM forward and 0.2 μM reverse primers (Sigma-Aldrich, St. Louis, MO). Amplification was completed in 19 min as more fully described in a previous study [43]. The thermal protocol included an enzyme activation step at 95 °C for 30 s followed by 45 cycles of 95 °C for 6 s and 56 °C for 6 s, and 72 °C for 6 s. Gel electrophoresis was utilized for identifying bands corresponding to the molecular weights for *tpi* and *tcdB* amplified fragments (Fig. 1).

All stool samples were additionally tested for *C. difficile* antigen glutamate dehydrogenase (GDH and *C. difficile* toxins A and/or B by enzyme immunoassay (EIA) (*C. diff* Quik Chek Complete, Alere Inc., Waltham, MA). Samples that were discordant (+/−) or positive/positive (+/+) for GDH and toxins A/B had reflex testing using LAMP technology (illumigene®, Meridian Bioscience, Inc., Cincinnati, OH). These commercially available tests were performed by the hospital clinical laboratory for comparison of the research method to current standard of care clinical tests. Cytotoxicity assays were performed on all samples positive by any modality. The *Clostridium difficile* Toxin/Antitoxin kit (TechLab, Blacksburg, VA) was used for the detection of *C. difficile* toxin in stool specimens by following manufacturer's instructions. Specimens that showed characteristic cytotoxin activity after inoculation of MRC-5 tissue culture cells (rounding of the cells) which were neutralized by *C. difficile* antitoxin were considered positive for *C. difficile* toxin.

Results

Eighty-four stool samples from unique infants were collected during the study (Fig. 2). The number of samples collected from each NICU was unknown as no patient

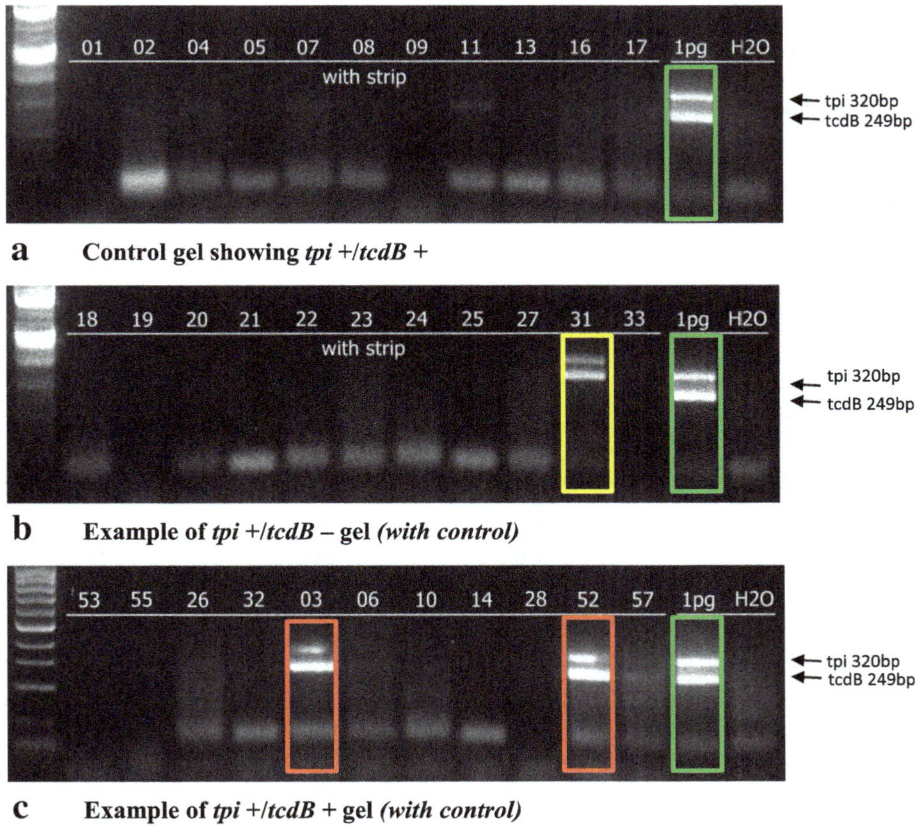

Fig. 1 Gel electrophoresis examples for *C. difficile tpi* and *tcdB* results reporting. **a**. Control gel showing *tpi* +/*tcdB* +. **b**. Example of *tpi* +/*tcdB* – gel *(with control)*. **c**. Example of *tpi* +/*tcdB* + gel *(with control)*

identifiers were maintained with the specimens. Seventy-one samples were EIA –/–, 7 samples were EIA +/– and 6 were EIA +/+. All 6 EIA +/+ samples were confirmed as toxigenic *C. difficile* by LAMP technology and also concurred with the results of the in house duplex PCR. Therefore, the point prevalence of toxigenic *C. difficile* in our NICU population was 7.1% (6/84). Cytotoxicity assay was performed on positive samples (by any test) for additional confirmation and was positive for 4/6 duplex PCR samples that were positive for toxigenic *C. difficile*; 2 samples could not be confirmed. Six of the 7 EIA +/– samples were negative for toxigenic *C. difficile* by LAMP technology and one sample was invalid. Our duplex PCR and the cytotoxicity assay were negative for all 7 of these samples. Our duplex PCR was negative for 69 of the 71 EIA –/– samples. The other 2 EIA –/– samples were positive for the *tpi* gene but negative for *tcdB*, indicating non-toxigenic *C. difficile*. Thus, the overall point prevalence of toxigenic ($n = 6$) and non-toxigenic ($n = 2$) *C. difficile* shedding in our NICU population was 9.5% (8/84) (Table 2).

Discussion

The point prevalence of *C. difficile* stool shedding in hospitalized infants from two affiliated NICUs was examined utilizing standard clinical testing (EIA with reflexive molecular identification via LAMP) and an in house duplex PCR that identified toxigenic and non-toxigenic *C. difficile* strains. We hypothesized that the prevalence of NICU *C. difficile* shedding would be higher than previous reports in part due to increased sensitivity of molecular testing compared to the testing modalities used in most previous studies (culture, cytotoxicity assay and EIA). The increased sensitivity of molecular testing contributing to the increase in *C. difficile* prevalence has been observed in previous studies [44–47]. Additionally, we surmised that the epidemiologic changes in CDI as well as the advances in NICU care would contribute to a higher prevalence of *C. difficile* shedding in NICUs over time. However, on the contrary, we demonstrated a prevalence of 7.1% for toxigenic *C. difficile* and 9.5% for both toxigenic and non-toxigenic *C. difficile* strains, which is substantially less than previously published reports suggesting a mean

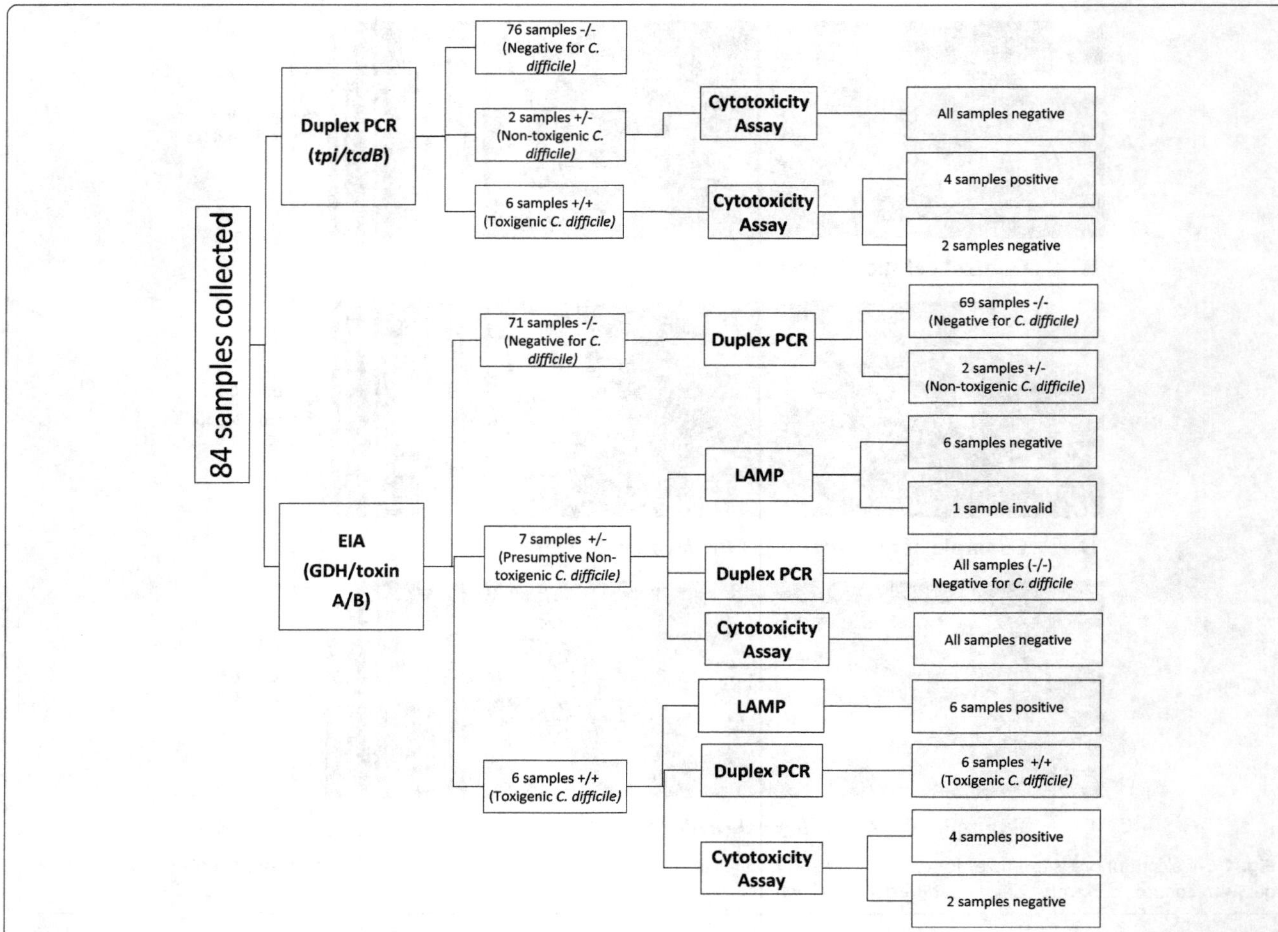

Fig. 2 Pathway for testing of stool samples collected from NICU babies using duplex PCR and standard clinical lab methods for the detection of *Clostridium difficile*

prevalence of at least 21% in the NICU population [13, 18–20, 25, 30–42]. Our secondary aim was achieved in that our stool lysis technique and rapid duplex PCR had excellent concordance with commercial EIA and LAMP testing, and moderately good concordance with cytotoxicity tests. This suggests that the duplex PCR could be used more broadly for rapid, accurate clinical diagnosis and for further epidemiologic studies of *C. difficile* stool shedding with and without toxin production. Stool isolates testing +/− on EIA but negative by both LAMP and duplex PCR may have been from GDH cross-reactivity with other organisms [48, 49].

Table 2 NICU stool samples positive for *C. difficile* by one or more modalities

Number of samples (n)	EIA GDH/toxin A/B	LAMP technology	Duplex PCR (*tpi/tcdB*)	Cytotoxicity assay
2	−/− Negative	Not done	+/− Nontoxigenic *C. difficile*	Negative
4	+/+ Toxigenic *C. difficile*	Positive	+/+ Toxigenic *C. difficile*	Positive
2	+/+ Toxigenic *C. difficile*	Positive	+/+ Toxigenic *C. difficile*	Negative
7	+/− Presumptive Nontoxigenic *C. difficile*	Negative[a]	−/− Negative	Negative

[a]one sample specimen was invalid

The identified difference between the prevalence of NICU *C. difficile* shedding in our study and previous studies may still be a reflection of advances in NICU practices. One important practice change is the emphasis of using human milk for feedings, perhaps decreasing the colonization of *C. difficile* in the infant gut [17, 22, 50, 51]. Another hypothesis for this change is the evolution of infection control measures with greater emphasis on caregiver hand hygiene and a transition from open ward NICUs to private patient rooms. These improvements in infection control within a NICU could decrease the transmission and thus prevalence of *C. difficile* shedding in the NICU environment.

Our study had several limitations. As no patient identifiers were maintained with the stool specimens, we were unable to obtain any clinical data on the infants. We were therefore unable to investigate possible clinical correlates with *C. difficile* shedding in these NICU infants. We did not test for the B1/NAP1/027 strain, which may contribute to increased incidence and severity of CDI, since we found a low prevalence of NICU *C. difficile*. Additionally, the use of previously frozen stool specimens may have impacted the sensitivities of the tests.

Additional NICU-based studies examining the clinical correlations of infant *C. difficile* colonization and shedding are needed to further answer questions regarding the epidemiologic changes in CDI. A lower point prevalence of NICU *C. difficile* as defined by our study is meaningful in that it informs sample size calculation for future work of clinical correlates of asymptomatic *C. difficile* colonization in the NICU. Potential future directions in NICU *C. difficile* colonization and shedding research include a follow-up survey of NICU infants with specific attention to mode of delivery, use of antibiotics, timing of initial feeding and number of hospitalization days. Additionally, as the epidemiology of CDI evolves, studies are needed to evaluate the potential for colonized NICU infants to serve as a reservoir or vector for transmission of toxigenic *C. difficile* strains to healthcare workers, the hospital environment, and vulnerable populations within and outside the hospital.

Abbreviations

CDI: *Clostridium difficile* infection; EIA: Enzyme immunoassay; GDH: Glutamate dehydrogenase; HA-CDI: Hospital acquired *Clostridium difficile* infection; LAMP: Loop-mediated isothermal amplification; LMR: Lysis microreactor; MLVA: Multilocus variable number of tandem repeats analysis; NICU: Neonatal Intensive Care Unit

Acknowledgements

The authors would like to acknowledge Dr. Henrik Viljoen, PhD for contributions to the development of the duplex PCR methodology utilized in the study, Alyssa Hornay for technical support in performing the cytotoxicity assay, and the Cheryl Lozier Pediatric Research Foundation for providing financial support to the study.

Funding

1. Cheryl Lozier Research Foundation- funding for PCR reagents and supplies.
2. University of Nebraska Medical Center, Clinical Research Center-funding for comparative clinically-available tests (EIA and LAMP).

Authors' contributions

AGH contributed to study design, data collection, analysis, and interpretation, and manuscript writing. AF contributed to study conception and design, data analysis and interpretation and manuscript writing. XZ contributed to study conception and design, data collection, analysis, and interpretation. Performed study-related PCR and gel electrophoresis. AAB contributed to study design, data collection, analysis, and interpretation and manuscript writing. LW contributed to study design, data collection, analysis, and interpretation and manuscript critical revisions. PCI contributed to study design, data analysis and interpretation, cytotoxicity assay performance, and critical manuscript revisions. KAS contributed to study design, data collection, analysis and interpretation and manuscript writing. All authors have given final approval for the submitted version of the manuscript.

Competing interests

The authors declare that they have no competing interests.

Author details

[1]Adult Infectious Diseases, University of Nebraska Medical Center, Omaha, NE, USA. [2]Pediatric Infectious Diseases, University of Nebraska Medical Center, Omaha, NE, USA. [3]Neonatology, University of Nebraska Medical Center, Omaha, NE, USA. [4]Pathology and Microbiology, University of Nebraska Medical Center, Omaha, NE, USA.

References

1. Lessa FC, Gould CV, McDonald LC. Current status of Clostridium difficile infection epidemiology. Clin Infect Dis. 2012;55(Suppl 2):S65–70.
2. Centers for Disease Control and Prevention (CDC). Severe Clostridium difficile-associated disease in populations previously at low risk–four states, 2005. MMWR Morb Mortal Wkly Rep. 2005;54(47):1201–5.
3. Chitnis AS, Holzbauer SM, Belflower RM, Winston LG, Bamberg WM, Lyons C, Farley MM, Dumyati GK, Wilson LE, Beldavs ZG, Dunn JR, Gould LH, Maccannell DR, Gerding DN, McDonald LC, Lessa FC. Epidemiology of community-associated Clostridium difficile infection, 2009 through 2011. JAMA Intern Med. 2013;173(14):1359–67.
4. Kuntz JL, Chrischilles EA, Pendergast JF, Herwaldt LA, Polgreen PM. Incidence of and risk factors for community-associated Clostridium difficile infection: a nested case-control study. BMC Infect Dis. 2011;11:194.
5. Riggs MM, Sethi AK, Zabarsky TF, Eckstein EC, Jump RL, Donskey CJ. Asymptomatic carriers are a potential source for transmission of epidemic and nonepidemic Clostridium difficile strains among long-term care facility residents. Clin Infect Dis. 2007;45(8):992–8.
6. Clabots CR, Johnson S, Olson MM, Peterson LR, Gerding DN. Acquisition of Clostridium difficile by hospitalized patients: evidence for colonized new admissions as a source of infection. J Infect Dis. 1992;166(3):561–7.
7. Curry SR, Muto CA, Schlackman JL, Pasculle AW, Shutt KA, Marsh JW, Harrison LH. Use of multilocus variable number of tandem repeats analysis genotyping to determine the role of asymptomatic carriers in Clostridium difficile transmission. Clin Infect Dis. 2013;57(8):1094–102.
8. Hecker MT, Riggs MM, Hoyen CK, Lancioni C, Donskey CJ. Recurrent infection with epidemic Clostridium difficile in a peripartum woman whose infant was asymptomatically colonized with the same strain. Clin Infect Dis. 2008;46(6):956–7.
9. McFarland LV, Surawicz CM, Greenberg RN, Bowen KE, Melcher SA, Mulligan ME. Possible role of cross-transmission between neonates and mothers with recurrent Clostridium difficile infections. Am J Infect Control. 1999;27(3):301–3.
10. Rousseau C, Poilane I, De Pontual L, Maherault AC, Le Monnier A, Collignon A. Clostridium difficile carriage in healthy infants in the community: a potential reservoir for pathogenic strains. Clin Infect Dis. 2012;55(9):1209–15.

11. Stoesser N, Crook DW, Fung R, Griffiths D, Harding RM, Kachrimanidou M, Keshav S, Peto TE, Vaughan A, Walker AS, Dingle KE. Molecular epidemiology of Clostridium difficile strains in children compared with that of strains circulating in adults with Clostridium difficile-associated infection. J Clin Microbiol. 2011;49(11):3994–6.
12. Blixt T, Gradel KO, Homann C, Seidelin JB, Schønning K, Lester A, Houlind J, Stangerup M, Gottlieb M, Knudsen JD. Asymptomatic carriers contribute to nosocomial Clostridium difficile infection: a cohort study of 4508 patients. Gastroenterology. 2017;152(5):1031–41. e2
13. Al-Jumaili IJ, Shibley M, Lishman AH, Record CO. Incidence and origin of Clostridium difficile in neonates. J Clin Microbiol. 1984;19(1):77–8.
14. Bacon AE, Fekety R, Schaberg DR, Faix RG. Epidemiology of Clostridium difficile colonization in newborns: results using a bacteriophage and bacteriocin typing system. J Infect Dis. 1988;158(2):349–54.
15. Bolton RP, Tait SK, Dear PR, Losowsky MS. Asymptomatic neonatal colonisation by Clostridium difficile. Arch Dis Child. 1984;59(5):466–72.
16. Collignon A, Ticchi L, Depitre C, Gaudelus J, Delmee M, Corthier G. Heterogeneity of Clostridium difficile isolates from infants. Eur J Pediatr. 1993;152(4):319–22.
17. Cooperstock M, Riegle L, Woodruff CW, Onderdonk A. Influence of age, sex, and diet on asymptomatic colonization of infants with Clostridium difficile. J Clin Microbiol. 1983;17(5):830–3.
18. Donta ST, Myers MG. Clostridium difficile toxin in asymptomatic neonates. J Pediatr. 1982;100(3):431–4.
19. Enad D, Meislich D, Brodsky NL, Hurt H. Is Clostridium difficile a pathogen in the newborn intensive care unit? A prospective evaluation. J Perinatol. 1997; 17(5):355–9.
20. Faden HS, Dryja D. Importance of asymptomatic shedding of Clostridium difficile in environmental contamination of a neonatal intensive care unit. Am J Infect Control. 2015;43(8):887–8.
21. Holst E, Helin I, Mardh PA. Recovery of Clostridium difficile from children. Scand J Infect Dis. 1981;13(1):41–5.
22. Jangi S, Lamont JT. Asymptomatic colonization by clostridium difficile in infants: implications for disease in later life. J Pediatr Gastroenterol Nutr. 2010;51(1):2–7.
23. Larson HE, Barclay FE, Honour P, Hill ID. Epidemiology of Clostridium difficile in infants. J Infect Dis. 1982;146(6):727–33.
24. Penders J, Stobberingh EE, van den Brandt PA, van Ree R, Thijs C. Toxigenic and non-toxigenic Clostridium difficile: determinants of intestinal colonisation and role in childhood atopic manifestations. Gut. 2008;57(7):1025–6.
25. Sherertz RJ, Sarubbi FA. The prevalence of Clostridium difficile and toxin in a nursery population: a comparison between patients with necrotizing enterocolitis and an asymptomatic group. J Pediatr. 1982;100(3):435–9.
26. Stark PL, Lee A, Parsonage BD. Colonization of the large bowel by Clostridium difficile in healthy infants: quantitative study. Infect Immun. 1982;35(3):895–9.
27. Svedhem A, Kaijser B, MacDowall I. Intestinal occurrence of campylobacter fetus subspecies jejuni and Clostridium difficile in children in Sweden. Eur J Clin Microbiol. 1982;1(1):29–32.
28. Viscidi R, Willey S, Bartlett JG. Isolation rates and toxigenic potential of Clostridium difficile isolates from various patient populations. Gastroenterology. 1981;81(1):5–9.
29. Wongwanich S, Pongpech P, Dhiraputra C, Huttayananont S, Sawanpanyalert P. Characteristics of Clostridium difficile strains isolated from asymptomatic individuals and from diarrheal patients. Clin Microbiol Infect. 2001;7(8):438–41.
30. Alfa MJ, Robson D, Davi M, Bernard K, Van Caeseele P, Harding GK. An outbreak of necrotizing enterocolitis associated with a novel clostridium species in a neonatal intensive care unit. Clin Infect Dis. 2002;35(Suppl 1):S101–5.
31. Blakey JL, Lubitz L, Barnes GL, Bishop RF, Campbell NT, Gillam GL. Development of gut colonisation in pre-term neonates. J Med Microbiol. 1982;15(4):519–29.
32. Cardines R, Luzzi I, Menichella G, Virgili Q, Mastrantonio P. Clostridium difficile in preterm neonates. Microbiologica. 1988;11(3):259–61.
33. Chang JY, Shim JO, Ko JS, Seo JK, Lee JA, Kim HS, Choi JH, Shin S, Shin SM. Monitoring of Clostridium difficile colonization in preterm infants in neonatal intensive care units. Pediatr Gastroenterol Hepatol Nutr. 2012; 15(1):29–37.
34. el-Mohandes AE, Keiser JF, Refat M, Jackson BJ. Prevalence and toxigenicity of Clostridium difficile isolates in fecal microflora of preterm infants in the intensive care nursery. Biol Neonate. 1993;63(4):225–9.
35. Ferraris L, Butel MJ, Campeotto F, Vodovar M, Roze JC, Aires J. Clostridia in premature neonates' gut: incidence, antibiotic susceptibility, and perinatal determinants influencing colonization. PLoS One. 2012;7(1):e30594.
36. Kato H, Kato N, Watanabe K, Ueno K, Ushijima H, Hashira S, Abe T. Application of typing by pulsed-field gel electrophoresis to the study of Clostridium difficile in a neonatal intensive care unit. J Clin Microbiol. 1994; 32(9):2067–70.
37. Kim KH, Fekety R, Batts DH, Brown D, Cudmore M, Silva J Jr, Waters D. Isolation of Clostridium difficile from the environment and contacts of patients with antibiotic-associated colitis. J Infect Dis. 1981;143(1):42–50.
38. Lishman AH, Al Jumaili IJ, Elshibly E, Hey E, Record CO. Clostridium difficile isolation in neonates in a special care unit. Lack of correlation with necrotizing enterocolitis. Scand J Gastroenterol. 1984;19(3):441–4.
39. Malamou-Ladas H, O'Farrell S, Nash JQ, Tabaqchali S. Isolation of Clostridium difficile from patients and the environment of hospital wards. J Clin Pathol. 1983;36(1):88–92.
40. Phua TJ, Rogers TR, Pallett AP. Prospective study of Clostridium difficile colonization and paracresol detection in the stools of babies on a special care unit. J Hyg (Lond). 1984;93(1):17–25.
41. Tina LG, Proto N, Sciacca A. Asymptomatic intestinal colonization by Clostridium difficile in preterm neonates. Pediatr Infect Dis J. 1994; 13(12):1158–9.
42. Zedd AJ, Sell TL, Schaberg DR, Fekety FR, Cooperstock MS. Nosocomial Clostridium difficile reservoir in a neonatal intensive care unit. Pediatr Infect Dis. 1984;3(5):429–32.
43. Freifeld AG, Simonsen KA, Booth CS, Zhao X, Whitney SE, Karre T, Iwen PC, Viljoen HJ. A new rapid method for Clostridium difficile DNA extraction and detection in stool: toward point-of-care diagnostic testing. J Mol Diagn. 2012;14(3):274–9.
44. de Jong E, de Jong AS, Bartels CJ, van der Rijt-van den Biggelaar C, Melchers WJ, Sturm PD. Clinical and laboratory evaluation of a real-time PCR for Clostridium difficile toxin a and B genes. Eur J Clin Microbiol Infect Dis. 2012;31(9):2219–25.
45. Fong KS, Fatica C, Hall G, Procop G, Schindler S, Gordon SM, Fraser TG. Impact of PCR testing for Clostridium difficile on incident rates and potential on public reporting: is the playing field level? Infect Control Hosp Epidemiol. 2011;32(9):932–3.
46. Gould CV, Edwards JR, Cohen J, Bamberg WM, Clark LA, Farley MM, Johnston H, Nadle J, Winston L, Gerding DN, McDonald LC, Lessa FC, Clostridium difficile Infection Surveillance Investigators, Centers for Disease Control and Prevention. Effect of nucleic acid amplification testing on population-based incidence rates of Clostridium difficile infection. Clin Infect Dis. 2013;57(9):1304–7.
47. Koo HL, Van JN, Zhao M, Ye X, Revell PA, Jiang ZD, Grimes CZ, Koo DC, Lasco T, Kozinetz CA, Garey KW, DuPont HL. Real-time polymerase chain reaction detection of asymptomatic Clostridium difficile colonization and rising C. Difficile-associated disease rates. Infect Control Hosp Epidemiol. 2014;35(6):667–73.
48. Lyerly DM, Ball DW, Toth J, Wilkins TD. Characterization of cross-reactive proteins detected by Culturette brand rapid latex test for Clostridium difficile. J Clin Microbiol. 1988;26(3):397–400.
49. Miles BL, Siders JA, Allen SD. Evaluation of a commercial latex test for Clostridium difficile for reactivity with C. Difficile and cross-reactions with other bacteria. J Clin Microbiol. 1988;26(11):2452–5.
50. Penders J, Vink C, Driessen C, London N, Thijs C, Stobberingh EE. Quantification of Bifidobacterium spp., Escherichia coli and Clostridium difficile in faecal samples of breast-fed and formula-fed infants by real-time PCR. FEMS Microbiol Lett. 2005;243(1):141–7.
51. Vael C, Desager K. The importance of the development of the intestinal microbiota in infancy. Curr Opin Pediatr. 2009;21(6):794–800.

18

Hypertrophic pyloric stenosis following persistent pulmonary hypertension of the newborn

Shigeo Iijima*, Daizo Ueno, Toru Baba and Akira Ohishi

Abstract

Background: Although persistent pulmonary hypertension of the newborn (PPHN) and infantile hypertrophic pyloric stenosis (HPS) are both well-known diseases that occur in early infancy, PPHN complicated by HPS is rare. As nitric oxide (NO) is an important mediator of biological functions, on both the vascular endothelium and smooth muscle cells, the decreased production of NO might play a role in the pathogenesis of both PPHN and HPS. We present the case of a neonate who developed HPS following PPHN, including a detailed review on research published to date, and we discuss the pathogenesis of PPHN and HPS.

Case presentation: A female neonate born at 38 weeks of gestation, weighing 3140 g, developed PPHN due to meconium aspiration syndrome. Intensive treatment with high frequency oscillations and inhaled NO were initiated, and sildenafil and bosentan were added. She gradually recovered. At 15 days of age, the patient developed recurrent vomiting after feeding and the diagnosis of HPS was made. Intravenous atropine therapy was started at 20 days of age, but the efficacy was clinically unsatisfactory. The coadministration with transdermal nitroglycerin improved the symptoms, and oral feeding was successfully re-introduced.

Conclusions: Our patient recovered from both PPHN and HPS using NO-related medications. A decrease in NO synthesis is likely to be a common pathway for PPHN and HPS.

Keywords: Arginine, Hypertrophic pyloric stenosis, Neonate, Nitric oxide, Persistent pulmonary hypertension of the newborn, Pulmonary hypertension

Background

Persistent pulmonary hypertension of the newborn (PPHN) is a life-threatening syndrome of failed circulatory adaptation at birth with persistently increased pulmonary vascular resistance [1]. Inhaled nitric oxide (NO), which improves oxygenation through selective pulmonary vasodilation without causing systemic hypotension, is the mainstay of PPHN treatment. On the other hand, hypertrophic pyloric stenosis (HPS) is a common surgical cause of vomiting during early infancy [2]. This condition is characterized by an abnormal thickening of the pyloric sphincter muscle layer, creating an obstruction of the gastric outlet. Although the exact etiology and pathogenesis of HPS are unknown, one hypothesis is impaired function of acetylcholine and muscarinic receptors [3], and medical treatment with atropine, a cholinergic blocking agent with antimuscarinic activity, is an available alternative to pyloromyotomy [4–6]. Moreover, the increased sphincter tone is believed to be related to a decrease in NO production [7]. Recently in Japan, the efficacy of transdermal nitroglycerin, a NO donor, as a non-surgical treatment option was reported [8]. Although PPHN and HPS are well-known diseases, their co-occurrence is rare. In this report, we describe a neonate with PPHN who subsequently developed HPS and discuss the relationship between these two diseases.

* Correspondence: sige_pd@yahoo.co.jp
Department of Pediatrics, Hamamatsu University School of Medicine, 1 - 20 - 1 Handayama, Hamamatsu, Shizuoka 431 - 3192, Japan

Case presentation

The patient was a female neonate born at 38 weeks of gestation, weighing 3140g. She was delivered to a 34-year-old primigravida uncomplicated mother by emergency cesarean section due to fetal distress following idiopathic oligohydramnios which occurred during the third trimester. At birth, the infant was non-vigorous due to meconium aspiration and required resuscitation using endotracheal intubation and tracheal suctioning. The Apgar scores were 5 and 7 at 1 and 5 min, respectively. She required mechanical ventilation after transfer to the neonatal intensive care unit due to the development of respiratory insufficiency. A chest X-ray revealed bilateral diffused, grossly patchy opacities, which is a typical finding in meconium aspiration syndrome. Moreover, a > 10% difference between pre- and post-ductal saturation of peripheral oxygen, measured by pulse oximetry, persisted despite increased oxygen supplementation and ventilatory support. An echocardiogram revealed a structurally normal heart with marked tricuspid regurgitation, right-to-left shunting through the ductus arteriosus, and suprasystemic pulmonary pressures. Based on the clinical presentation and findings on imaging, a diagnosis of PPHN was made and intensive treatment with high frequency oscillations and inhaled NO were initiated. Subsequently, sildenafil, a specific phosphodiesterase type 5 inhibitor that enhances NO-mediated vasodilation, and bosentan, an endothelin receptor-inhibitor that increases internal activity of endogenous NO, were added to treatment. The symptoms gradually improved, and the infant was subsequently weaned from inhaled NO and ventilatory support, with extubation performed at 11 days of age.

Oral feeds with breast milk were started at 12 days of age. However, 3 days later, the infant developed non-bilious vomiting after feeding, which increased in frequency in the following days. The daily clinical examination was unremarkable and no mass was palpable in the abdomen. Plain abdominal X-ray at 17 and 19 days of age showed a dilated stomach. A contrast study was not performed. At 20 days of age, abdominal ultrasonography (US) revealed a hypertrophic pylorus, with a 5–6-mm mural thickening over a length of 18 mm, confirming the diagnosis of HPS. At this time, the plasma arginine level was 53.3 μmol/L (reference range: 53.6–133.6 μmol/L). The parents selected conservative treatment for their child, and atropine therapy was started. Atropine was administered intravenously at a dose of 0.1 mg/kg/day, which was divided equally by the number of oral feedings. Frequency of vomiting did not decrease in 3 days, and the dose was increased to 0.13 mg/kg/day. Subsequently, the frequency of vomiting decreased, but significant gastric residuals continued for more than 7 days after the start of atropine therapy. Hypertrophic pyloric muscle remained unchanged on repeated US. We considered the efficacy of the treatment was clinically unsatisfactory referring to previous studies [6, 9]. Then, transdermal nitroglycerin (5 mg/day) was added to the treatment at 29 days of age. Thereafter, the infant tolerated full enteral feeds, with no further vomiting, and oral feeding was successfully re-introduced. At 34 days of age, atropine was changed to oral administration at a dose of 0.2 mg/kg/day. Transdermal nitroglycerin was ceased over a day after that (the total dosing period was 7 days). Subsequently, the infant remained well and was discharged home at 43 days of age.

Discussion

PPHN occurs in 2 per 1000 live births [1], with the incidence of HPS estimated at 1–8 in 1000 live births [2]. However, to the best of our knowledge, there are only five previously reported cases in the literature on the occurrence of both conditions in a patient [10–12]. The characteristics of those cases of HPS and PPHN or PH are summarized in Table 1 [10–13]. Brouwers et al. considered that if there was no common pathophysiologic pathway between HPS and PPHN, the combination of both conditions would occur in approximately 1 per 100,000 live births, and they proposed a deficiency in NO as a common pathway [10].

NO has many physiological and pathological functions, and is endogenously synthesized from L-arginine by the family of NO synthetases (NOS) [14]. NOS is one of the most regulated enzymes in biology; in mammals, three isoforms have been identified, with two being constitutive (neuronal NOS [nNOS] and endothelial NOS [eNOS]) and the third being inducible NOS (Table 2) [14, 15]. NO is a potent vasodilator that is involved in the normal transition from fetal to neonatal circulation. In PPHN, an impairment in endothelial NO production was previously reported [1]. Hypoxia causing PPHN may reduce NO production through an uncoupling of NOS in pulmonary arterial endothelial cells [16]. On the other hand, NO has been demonstrated as a major inhibitory non-adrenergic and non-cholinergic neurotransmitter in the gastrointestinal tract, causing relaxation of the smooth muscle of the myenteric plexus upon its release [17]. There is evidence suggesting that impairment in NO synthesis contributes to HPS. Mice with reduced NOS activity developed grossly enlarged stomachs, with hypertrophy of the circular muscle wall [18]. In humans, decreases in serum NO and tissue expression of nNOS were observed in patients with HPS [7]. Therefore, NO deficiency may play a role in the pathogenesis of both PPHN and HPS. However, previous case reports have not demonstrated a substantial relationship between these two disorders and NO [10, 11]. In the case described by Brouwers et al., recovery from PPHN and HPS was obtained with treatments not associated with

Table 1 Cases of hypertrophic pyloric stenosis following persistent pulmonary hypertension of the newborn or pulmonary hypertension

Study	Gestational age	Birth weight	Sex	PPHN or PH		HPS	
				Cause	Treatment	Age at onset	Treatment
Brouwers et al. [10]	39 weeks	2990 g	Male	MAS	ECMO	13 days	Pyloromyotomy
Malwade et al. [11]	Unknown	3200 g	Male	MAS	Sildenafil[a]	21 days	Pyloromyotomy
Present case	38 weeks	3140 g	Female	MAS	Inhaled NO[a] Sildenafil[a] Bosentan[a]	15 days	Atropine[a] Nitroglycerin[a]
Robertson et al. [12]	37 weeks	3600 g	Male	CDH	Inhaled NO[a] Epoprostenol Sildenafil[a]	40 days	Pyloromyotomy
Robertson et al. [12]	38 weeks	3714 g	Female	CDH	–	47 days	Pyloromyotomy
Robertson et al. [12]	38 weeks	2800 g	Male	CDH	ECMO Prostaglandin Milrinone	73 days	Pyloromyotomy
Ravindra et al. [13]	Term	2500 g	Male	CHD	–	2 months	Pyloromyotomy

PPHN persistent pulmonary hypertension of the newborn, *PH* pulmonary hypertension, *HPS* hypertrophic pyloric stenosis, *MAS* meconium aspiration syndrome, *CDH* congenital diaphragmatic hernia, *CHD* congenital heart disease, *ECMO* extracorporeal membrane oxygenation, *NO* nitric oxide
[a] treatment associated with nitric oxide

NO. Similarly, Malwade et al. did not provide a NO-related treatment for PPHN. In contrast, the present case of PPHN and HPS was successfully treated using inhaled NO, sildenafil, bosentan, and transdermal nitroglycerin. Regarding the HPS, transdermal nitroglycerin alone was not effective; coadministration with intravenous atropine was effective. Carr et al. demonstrated in their animal study that the inhibition of myopia by atropine is dependent on production of NO [19]. This suggests that the effect of atropine for HPS might also be mediated by NO and might support the efficacy of our treatment. Therefore, the approaches provided in our case all contributed to increasing NO in the affected organs. Regarding the mechanism of NO synthesis, eNOS, associated with PPHN, and nNOS, associated with HPS, do not have an association that can be explained by a single gene abnormality because these NOSs are encoded by different genes (Table 2) [14]. As NOS requires L-arginine for the production of NO regardless of the type, an impairment in arginine metabolism is likely to play an important role in NOS dysfunction. Therefore, the association between PPHN and HPS may be explained by a decrease in plasma concentration of arginine, leading to a deficiency in NO synthesis in the affected organ systems (Fig. 1). A previous study demonstrated that infants with PPHN had a low plasma concentration of arginine [20]. In HPS, Glass et al. reported an increase in plasma arginine levels in patients with HPS after surgery [21], but, to the best of our knowledge, there is no evidence of a decreased level of plasma arginine. In our patient, the plasma level of arginine at the time of diagnosis of HPS was borderline low, and we measured the arginine level only once for HPS, without measurement for PPHN.

Table 2 Characteristics of different forms of nitric oxide synthase [14, 15]

Type	Gene(s)	Location	Function
Neuronal NOS (nNOS)	NOS 1 Chromosome 12 (12q24.22)	Nervous tissue Skeletal muscle type II	Cell communication: Neurotransmission Skeletal muscle contraction Sexual function Body fluid homeostasis
Inducible NOS (iNOS)	NOS 2 Chromosome 17 (17q11.2)	Immune system Cardiovascular system	Immune defense against pathogens: Inflammation Infection Malignant diseases Blood pressure regulation
Endothelial NOS (eNOS)	NOS 3 Chromosome 7 (7q36.1)	Endothelium	Cardiovascular homeostasis: Vasodilation Inhibition of platelet aggregation and adhesion Inhibition of vascular inflammation

NOS nitric oxide synthase

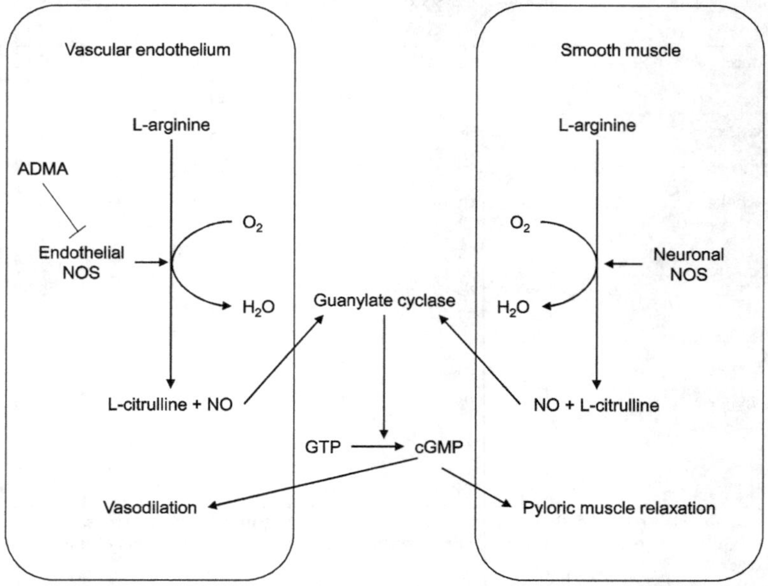

Fig. 1 Diagram showing the mechanism of nitric oxide production that mediates vasodilation and smooth muscle relaxation. ADMA, asymmetric dimethylarginine; NOS, nitric oxide synthase; NO, nitric oxide; GTP, guanosine triphosphate; cGMP, cyclic guanosine monophosphate. ADMA is an inhibitor of endothelial NOS activity

Further research is required to evaluate arginine metabolism in patients with either PPHN or HPS.

Conclusions

The present patient recovered from both PPHN and HPS using NO-related medications. A decrease in NO synthesis is likely to be a common pathway for PPHN and HPS. If an infant recovering from PPHN develops recurrent vomiting, physicians should consider HPS as a complication.

Abbreviations

CDH: Congenital diaphragmatic hernia; eNOS: Endothelial nitric oxide synthetases; HPS: Hypertrophic pyloric stenosis; nNOS: Neuronal nitric oxide synthetases; NO: Nitric oxide; NOS: Nitric oxide synthetases; PH: Pulmonary hypertension; PPHN: Persistent pulmonary hypertension of the newborn

Authors' contributions

SI wrote the first draft of the manuscript; DU, TB, and AO performed the clinical practice. All authors reviewed the manuscript for important intellectual content and approved the final version to be published.

Competing interests

The authors declare that they have no competing interests.

References

1. Nair J, Lakshminrusimha S. Update on PPHN: mechanisms and treatment. Semin Perinatol. 2014;38:78–91.
2. Chung E. Infantile hypertrophic pyloric stenosis: genes and environment. Arch Dis Child. 2008;93:1003–4.
3. Okazaki T, Yamataka A, Fujiwara T, Nishiye H, Fujimoto T, Miyano T. Abnormal distribution of nerve terminals in infantile hypertrophic pyloric stenosis. J Pediatr Surg. 1994;29:655–8.
4. Wu SF, Lin HY, Huang FK, Chen AC, Su BH, Li CI, et al. Efficacy of medical treatment for infantile hypertrophic pyloric stenosis: a meta-analysis. Pediatr Neonatol. 2016;57:515–21.
5. Kawahara H, Imura K, Nishikawa M, Yagi M, Kubota A. Intravenous atropine treatment in infantile hypertrophic pyloric stenosis. Arch Dis Child. 2002;87:71–4.
6. Nagita A, Yamaguchi J, Amemoto K, Yoden A, Yamazaki T, Mino M. Management and ultrasonographic appearance of infantile hypertrophic pyloric stenosis with intravenous atropine sulfate. J Pediatr Gastroenterol Nutr. 1996;23:172–7.
7. Huang LT, Tiao MM, Lee SY, Hsieh CS, Lin JW. Low plasma nitrite in infantile hypertrophic pyloric stenosis patients. Dig Dis Sci. 2006;51:869–72.
8. Nagita A, Kosaka Y, Sakata R, Amemoto K, Okuda M, Ogita S, et al. Coadministration of transdermal nitroglycerin and intravenous atropine sulfate for hypertrophic pyloric stenosis. J Jpn Pediatr Soc. 2006;110:1271–3. (in Japanese)
9. Meissner PE, Engelmann G, Troeger J, Linderkamp O, Nuetzenadel W, et al. Conservative treatment of infantile hypertrophic pyloric stenosis with intravenous atropine sulfate does not replace pyloromyotomy. Pediatr Surg Int. 2006;22:1021–4.
10. Brouwers AG, Waals-van de Wal CM. Hypertrophic pyloric stenosis and pulmonary hypertension in a neonate. A common mechanism? Acta Paediatr. 2009;98:1064–5.
11. Malwade S, Agarkhedkar S, Joshi H. Persistent pulmonary hypertension and infantile hypertrophic pyloric stenosis in a neonate: reduced nitric oxide levels could be a common etiological factor. Med J DY Patil Univ. 2014;7:661–4.
12. Robertson JO, Gadepalli SK. Hypertrophic pyloric stenosis following repair of congenital diaphragmatic hernia. J Pediatr Surg Case Rep. 2017;27:16–8.
13. Ravindra MN, Bhagya DV. Dobutamine infusion for complex heart disease with pulmonary hypertension in an infant posted for open pyloromyotomy. Karnataka Anaesth J. 2015;1:92–4.

14. Wang Y, Marsden PA. Nitric oxide synthases: biochemical and molecular regulation. Curr Opin Nephrol Hypertens. 1995;4:12–22.
15. Förstermann U, Sessa WC. Nitric oxide synthases: regulation and function. Eur Heart J. 2012;33:829–37.
16. Fike CD, Summar M, Aschner JL. L-citrulline provides a novel strategy for treating chronic pulmonary hypertension in newborn infants. Acta Paediatr. 2014;103:1019–26.
17. Currò D, Ipavec V, Preziosi P. Neurotransmitters of the non-adrenergic non-cholinergic relaxation of proximal stomach. Eur Rev Med Pharmacol Sci. 2008;12(1):53–62.
18. Chung E, Curtis D, Chen G, Marsden PA, Twells R, Xu W, et al. Genetic evidence for the neuronal nitric oxide synthase gene (NOS1) as a susceptibility locus for infantile pyloric stenosis. Am J Hum Genet. 1996;58: 363–70.
19. Carr BJ, Stell WK. Nitric oxide (NO) mediates the inhibition of form-deprivation myopia by atropine in chicks. Sci Rep. 2016;6:9.
20. Vosatka RJ, Kashyap S, Trifiletti RR. Arginine deficiency accompanies persistent pulmonary hypertension of the newborn. Biol Neonate. 1994;66: 65–70.
21. Glass RE, Goode AW, Houghton BJ, Rowell LW. Plasma arginine in cancer of the gastrointestinal tract: effect of surgical treatment. Gut. 1986;27:844–8.

Adherence to the neonatal resuscitation algorithm for preterm infants in a tertiary hospital in Spain

Silvia Maya-Enero[1*], Francesc Botet-Mussons[1], Josep Figueras-Aloy[1], Montserrat Izquierdo-Renau[2], Marta Thió[2] and Martin Iriondo-Sanz[2]

Abstract

Background: There is evidence that delivery room resuscitation of very preterm infants often deviates from internationally recommended guidelines. There were no published data in Spain regarding the quality of neonatal resuscitation. Therefore, we decided to evaluate resuscitation team adherence to neonatal resuscitation guidelines after birth in very preterm infants.

Methods: We conducted an observational study. We video recorded resuscitations of preterm infants < 32 weeks' gestational age and evaluated every step during resuscitation according to a score-sheet specifically designed for this purpose, following Carbine's method, where higher scores indicated that more intense resuscitation maneuvers were required. We divided the score achieved by the total possible points per patient to obtain the percentage of adherence to the algorithm. We also compared resuscitations performed by staff neonatologists to those performed by pediatricians on-call. We compared percentages of adherence to the algorithm with the Chi-square test for large groups and Fisher's exact test for smaller groups. We compared assigned Apgar scores with those given after analyzing the recordings and described them by their median and interquartile range. We measured the interrater agreement between Apgar scores with Cohen's kappa coefficient. Linear and logarithmic regressions were drawn to characterize the pattern of algorithm adherence. Statistical analysis was performed using SPSS V.20. A p-value < 0.05 was considered significant. Our Hospital Ethics Committee approved this project, and we obtained parental written consent beforehand.

Results: Sixteen percent of our resuscitations followed the algorithm. The number of mistakes per resuscitation was low. Global adherence to the algorithm was 80.9%. Ventilation and surfactant administration were performed best, whereas preparation and initial steps were done with worse adherence to the algorithm. Intubation required, on average, 2.2 attempts; success on the first attempt happened in 33.3% of cases. Only 12.5% of intubations were achieved within the allotted 30 s. Many errors were attributable to timing. Resuscitations led by pediatricians on-call were performed as correctly as those by staff neonatologists.

Conclusions: Resuscitation often deviates from the internationally recognized algorithm. Perfectly performed resuscitations are infrequent, although global adherence to the algorithm is high. Neonatologists and pediatricians need intubation training.

Keywords: Neonatal resuscitation, Video recording, Very preterm infant, Delivery room

* Correspondence: smaya1@clinic.cat
[1]Neonatology Service, Hospital Clínic, seu Maternitat, ICGON (Institut Clínic de Ginecologia, Obstetrícia i Neonatologia), Barcelona University, Sabino de Arana, 1, 08028 Barcelona, Spain

Background

Neonatal resuscitation (NR) is the most frequently performed resuscitation in hospitals [1–3]. Infants that are more immature are more likely to require support. Approximately 85% of very preterm neonates need intervention during transition after birth and their viability and prognosis greatly depend on the care they receive in the delivery room (DR) [4–6]. Most preterm infants initiate breathing after birth, but they often have a weak, insufficient respiratory drive. Guidelines recommend tactile stimulation (warming, drying and rubbing the back or soles of the feet) to stimulate breathing. Guidelines exist to standardize and optimize resuscitation. However, there is evidence that the sequence and quality of interventions during NR often deviate from guidelines [3, 7–11]. Video recording has been widely used for educational and clinical quality assessment purposes, with good acceptance by caregivers [12, 13]. It is inexpensive, it does not interfere with resuscitation, and it offers data to assess performance accurately. Video reviewing reinforces teamwork and permits identification and amendment of errors that otherwise could be neglected. Combining the recording of physiological parameters (ECG, pulse oximetry (PO), capnography and respiratory function monitoring) with video images helps audit performance [12–15]. There is a lack of information about adherence to NR guidelines in Spain. Consequently, we sought to evaluate adherence to NR guidelines in very preterm neonates at our hospital. Our main hypothesis was that resuscitation often deviates from the algorithm. A secondary hypothesis was that staff neonatologists perform better than pediatricians on-call because they work only with neonates and have more experience on average, whereas pediatricians are younger and work with children up to 18 years.

Methods

We conducted this observational study at Hospital Clínic de Barcelona, a tertiary referral center in Spain where approximately 150 babies < 32 weeks' gestational age (GA) are born every year. Our Hospital Ethics Committee approved this project. We recorded and analyzed these infants' resuscitations after obtaining written parental informed consent. We aimed to analyze as many NRs as possible. However, given the difficulties in obtaining parental consent in such moments of stress, we aimed to analyze a representative sample of at least one-third of all NRs performed. Thus, we decided to record 50 resuscitations. We had planned to obtain the data in 1 year, although it took us longer (16 months), as fewer candidates were born during the study period than expected. This study was the basis for the doctoral thesis of the main author (see link in http://www.ub.edu/medicina/doctorat/lectura.htm May 27, 2011). However, the data were never published. The authors believe that the results and conclusions may be perfectly applicable today.

Inclusion criteria: All babies < 32 weeks GA were candidates for inclusion in this study. When the pediatrician was required in the delivery room, parents were approached for consent to record the NR. After obtaining written consent, the resuscitator began recording the NR, and that case was included in the study.

All infants were resuscitated under a radiant heater equipped with a neonatal automatic ventilator (Babylog 2, Dräger Medical, Drägerwerk AG & Co. KGaA, Lübeck, Germany) that included an oxygen blender and could provide Continuous Positive Airway Pressure (CPAP) and Positive Pressure Ventilation (PPV) and with a pulse-oximeter (Nellcor™ NPB-295, Minneapolis, MN, USA). A Sony Handycam DCR-SR 32 E (Sony, Tokyo, Japan) digital video camera attached to the upper left side of the radiant warmer recorded the newborn, the hands of the resuscitators and the PO screen. The clinical team turned the recording on before the baby was born.

We designed an evaluation sheet to score 12 domains in each resuscitation (Table 1) according to the algorithm of the Spanish Society of Neonatology, adapted from the ILCOR 2005 guidelines (see Fig. 1). We assigned a numerical score to every resuscitation, following Carbine's previously described method [16]: we awarded 2 points for every correct decision and proper procedure, 1 point for delayed interventions or inadequate technique, and 0 points for indicated procedures that were omitted or for inappropriate procedures (for details of how we scored each domain, see Table 1). The total score per resuscitation ("resuscitation score") ranged from 4 to 22 points. A higher score indicated that more intense resuscitation was required. We obtained the percentage of adherence to the algorithm by dividing the score achieved (X) by the maximum possible score per patient that is, X of a potential of (4–22) points, as a percentage. We registered admission temperature and Apgar scores at 1, 5 and 10 minutes (min) as assigned by the caregiver and after video recording review.

We compared two groups of resuscitators: staff neonatologists (group N) and pediatricians on-call (group P). Neonatologists on-call performed a few of the resuscitations after-hours.

Statistic analysis

We present the characteristics of our study population and its subgroups using the median, standard deviation (SD) and range for quantitative variables (gestational age, birth weight, temperature at admission and adherence to the algorithm and resuscitation score). We

Table 1 Data collection sheet

Patient's identification:		Gestational age:	
Birth weight:		Sex:	
Twin? 1st or 2nd of 2		Time and date of birth	
C-section?			
Apgar score: assigned: 1 min: 5 min: 10 min:			
Apgar score: camera: 1 min: 5 min: 10 min:			
Admission temperature: ºC			
Analyzed aspects	0 points	1 point (any technical error in a correctly indicated maneuver is awarded 1 point; the main errors and examples are listed in every domain)	2 points
Heat loss prevention measures[a]	Not performed	No cap; baby dried with towels and then placed in a plastic wrap; if towels were used, they had to be replaced by new, preheated ones	Well done (dried and towels replaced OR plastic wrap)
Head in a "sniffing position"[a]	Not performed	Head in hyperextension or bent or to a side	Well done
Suctioning	Not performed when indicated	Done after the first 20 s; for more than 5 s; incorrect order (nasal suction before oral); incorrect suction catheter (not 8 F); excessively introduced catheter (more than 10 cm)	Well done
Stimulation	Not performed when indicated: inactive, apneic or not spontaneously breathing, or gasping, or bradycardic	Stimulation performed on other places than the back or the soles of the feet. Too aggressive (not gentle rubbing)	Well done
Preductal PO probe	Not placed in a baby who needed CPAP, PPV or oxygen	Not preductal (left hand or wrist, foot)	Preductal (right hand or wrist)
Administration of oxygen	Not used in a baby who needed it	Given free-flow oxygen; not administered with PPC or PPV; not discontinued when color or SpO_2 improved; use of initial FiO_2 other than 0.3	Well done
Administration of CPAP	Mandatory if < 28 weeks GA or ≥ 29 with a positive initial evaluation but distress	Evident mask leak; incorrect mask/cannula size	Well done
Administration of mask PPV	Not performed when needed	Initiation after the first 20 s; use of a self-inflating bag instead of an automatic or manual ventilator; incorrect mask size; incorrect rate (not 40-60 rpm); mask leak; not re-evaluated for response (HR and color) after 30 s)	Well done
Intubation	Not performed when needed	Duration of each intubation attempt (time from the introduction of the laryngoscope blade to the mouth to its removal) > 30 s); incorrect size of the endotracheal tube; position of the endotracheal tube not checked (auscultation/chest wall rise/inserted to correct depth); lack of ventilation between intubation attempts, Number of intubation attempts; Unplanned extubation	Well done
Chest compressions	Not performed when needed	Incorrect method (other than 2 thumbs or 2 fingers); incorrect area (other than lower third of the sternum); incorrect depth (not one third of the anterior-posterior diameter of the chest); incorrect rate (not 90 bpm); incorrect coordination with ventilation (not 3:1); initiation without correct ventilation; Not re-evaluated for response	Well done
Epinephrine administration	Not performed when needed	Not administered after 30 s of CC if heart rate < 60 bpm; Dose and route of administration	Well done
Surfactant administration	Not performed when indicated: intubated and < 28 or ≥ 29 weeks GA and FiO_2 ≥ 0.3	Not administered at 10 min of life; Dose	Well done
tal points			

vays mandatory
V, CC or drugs are necessary, breathing, heart rate and color must be reassessed every 30 s.
Ainutes, *PO* Pulse-Oximeter, *CPAP* Continuous Positive Airway Pressure, *PPV* Positive Pressure Ventilation, *GA* Gestational Age, *CC* Chest Compressions

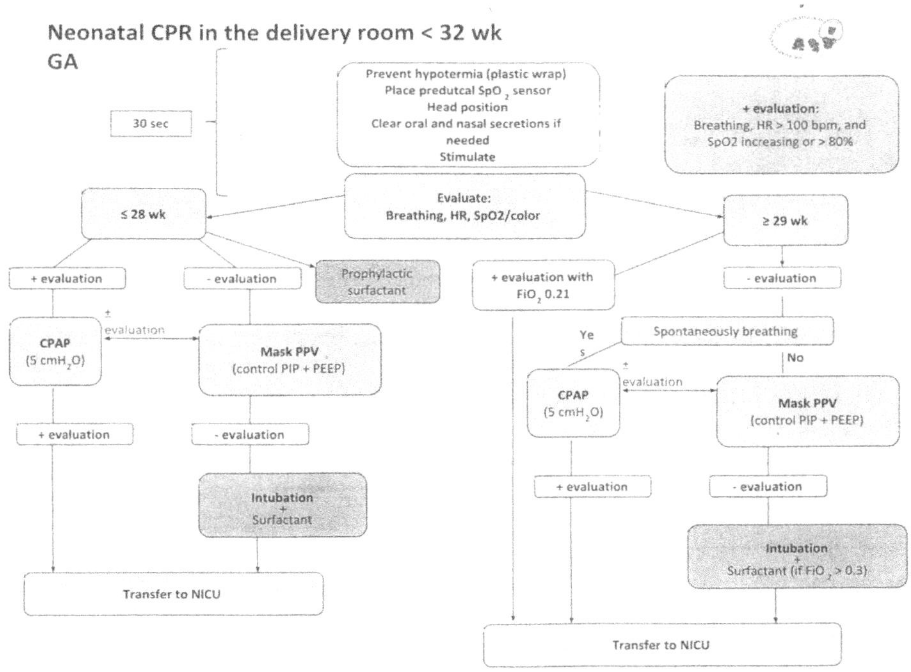

Fig. 1 Algorithm of the Spanish Society of Neonatology for the resuscitation of the very preterm infant. Spanish Society of Neonatology, 2007. Obtained from http://www.se-neonatal.es/Comisionesygruposdetrabajos/GrupodeRCPNeonatal/tabid/76/Default.aspx#Publicaciones

confirmed homogeneity of our subgroups in terms of gestational age, birth weight and resuscitation score. We used the Shapiro-Wilk test to evaluate normality in our subgroups. We compared normally distributed quantitative variables with a paired T-test between our two groups. For nonnormally distributed quantitative variables, we used the Mann-Whitney U test to compare the two groups.

We compared percentages of adherence to the algorithm for every domain with the Chi-square test for large groups and with Fisher's exact test for smaller groups (fewer than 5 cases). Linear and logarithmic regressions were drawn to characterize the pattern of adherence to the algorithm.

We compared assigned Apgar scores with those given after analyzing the recordings and described them by their median and interquartile range (IQR). We measured interrater agreement between Apgar scores with Cohen's kappa coefficient.

Statistical analysis was performed using SPSS (SPSS for Windows, V.20, Chicago, Illinois, USA). A p-value < 0.05 was considered significant.

Results

Between April 2008 and August 2009, 162 infants < 32 weeks GA were born in our center. We analyzed 50 resuscitations (30.6%), a representative sample of the population. Groups N (staff neonatologists) and P (pediatricians on-call) were homogeneous. Tables 2 and 3 show the characteristics of our population and subgroups.

Global adherence to the algorithm was 80.9 ± 14.2%, with no differences between groups N and P (81.5 ± 12.7% in group N versus 80.7 ± 15.0% in group P, P = 0.93, Mann-Whitney U), and was independent of the

Table 2 Characteristics of our population and neonates < 32 weeks GA born during the study period

Characteristic	Study patients (n = 50)	Neonates < 32 weeks GA born during the study period (n = 162)	P^c
Gestational age, SD (weeks) (range)	$29^4 \pm 2^5$ (25^5–31^6)	$29^1 \pm 2$ (24^1–31^6)	NS (0.24)[a]
Male (%)	26/50 (52%)	88/162 (54.3%)	NS (0.07)[b]
BW, SD (g) (range)	1181 ± 368 (460–2015)	1201 ± 377 (340–2475)	NS (0.75)[a]
Twins (%)	19/50 (38)	81/162 (50)	NS (0.13)[b]
BW < 1500 g (%)	42/50 (84)	131/162 (80.8)	NS (0.61)[b]
C-section (%)	33/50 (66)	94/162 (58)	NS (0.31)[b]

SD Standard Deviation, *BW* Birth Weight, *GA* Gestational Age. [a]Paired T- test, [b]Chi-square, [c]Indicates significance at the P < 0.05 level. NS: non-significant

Table 3 Subgroups in our study

Characteristic	Group N (staff neonatologists) ($n = 18$)	Group P (pediatricians oncall) ($n = 32$)	p[d]
GA (weeks, SD) (range)	$29^4 \pm 1^6$ (25^5–31^6)	$29^3 \pm 1^4$ (26^0–31^6)	NS (0.90)[a]
Male (%)	8/18 (44.4)	18/32 (56.2)	NS (0.61)[b]
BW (g, SD) (range)	1091 ± 418 (460–1900)	1232 ± 333 (720–2015)	NS (0.20)[a]
RS (possible points) (range)	12.66 ± 4.39 (6–20)	13.96 ± 3.71 (6–20)	NS (0.29)[c]

Group N Staff Neonatologists, *group P* Pediatricians On-call, *GA* Gestational Age, *SD* Standard Deviation, *BW* Birth Weight, *RS* Resuscitation Score. [a]Paired T-test, [b]Chi-square, [c]Mann-Whitney U test, [d]Indicates significance at the $P < 0.05$ level. NS: non-significant

number of interventions required. Eight resuscitations (16%) were technically correct; 15/50 (30%) failed in one domain; 12/50 (24%) in two; 5/50 (10%) in three; 6/50 (12%) in four; 2/50 (4%) in five; and 2/50 (4%) in seven. The mean (SD) resuscitation score was 13.5 (3.9) points/resuscitation (range: 6–20). Table 4 analyzes the adherence to the algorithm by domains.

Table 5 shows results from measures to prevent heat loss and its relation to admission temperature. We found no differences between the group that received correct measures to prevent hypothermia and the group that did not. Intubation differentiated intensive (16–20 total possible points) from mild resuscitation (6–16 points). Infants who did not need intubation ($n = 36$) had a mean global adherence to the algorithm of 83%. Deviations from the algorithm in this group did not correlate with the intensity of resuscitation ($R^2 = 0.0013$).

Some errors we observed

Heat loss prevention

Twelve percent of patients were placed in plastic wrap after drying. When only dried, the technique was correct in 58.1% (18/31) of cases; 22.6% (7/31) did not have the towels changed, and 19.3% (6/31) had no cap. Only 22.4% of patients (11/49) were normothermic (36.5–37.5 °C); 73.5% (36/49) were hypothermic. More critically ill patients were more likely to receive worse anti-hypothermia measures because they were being subjected to other procedures: ventilation, intubation, chest compressions (CC) and surfactant administration. Sixty-eight percent of patients (13/19) in whom heat loss prevention was incorrect had a resuscitation score ≥ 14 points, which means that they received at least ventilatory support.

Clearing the airway with a suction catheter

The following errors were observed: oral without nasal suctioning, 16.7%; undue suction (over 5 s, range 31–50 s), 8.3%; use of a larger catheter than recommended, 8.3%; delayed suctioning after 20 s, 6.2%, or after ventilation, 4.2%; incorrect suctioning order (first nasal), 2.1%; and excessive introduction of the catheter, 2.1%. We observed no episodes of severe bradycardia during suctioning.

Table 4 Adherence to the algorithm

Domain	Indicated (%)	Performed (%)	Adherence to the algorithm (%) (PO/TTPx100)			
			Global	Group N	Group P	p[3]
Heat loss prevention	100 (50/50)	100 (50/50)	62 (31/50)	66.7 (12/18)	59.4 (19/32)	NS (0.84)[2]
Head in a "sniffing" position	100 (50/50)	94 (47/50)	94 (47/50)	94.4 (17/18)	93.7 (30/32)	NS (0.71)[1]
Clearing the airway	96 (48/50)	96 (48/50)	62.5 (30/48)	55.6 (10/18)	66.7 (20/30)	NS (0.59)[2]
Stimulation	64 (32/50)	30 (15/50)	93.3[4] (14/15)	80 (4/5)	100 (10/10)	NS (0.33)[1]
Placing a preductal pulse-oximeter probe	82 (41/50)	90.2 (37/41)	63.4 (26/41)	76.9 (10/13)	57.1 (16/28)	NS (1.49)[1]
Administration of oxygen	68 (34/50)	68 (34/50)	94.1 (32/34)	100 (10/10)	91.3 (21/23)	NS (0.48)[1]
CPAP	60	60	100	100	100	–
Administration of PPV	60 (30/50)	96.7 (29/30)	79.3 (23/29)	60 (6/10)	85 (17/20)	NS (0.14)[1]
Intubation	32 (16/50)	87.5 (14/16)	0 (0/16)	0 (0/5)	0 (0/11)	–
CC	4 (2/50)	2 (1/50)	0	0	0	–
Epinephrine administration	?	4 (2/50)	0	0	0	–
Surfactant administration	24 (12/50)	20 (10/50)	100[4] (10/10) 83.3 (10/12)[5]	75 (3/4)	87.5 (7/8)	NS (0.58)[1]

PO Points Obtained, *TPP* Total Possible Points, *Group N* Staff Neonatologists, *Group P* Pediatricians On-call, *CPAP* Continuous Positive Airway Pressure, *PPV* Positive Pressure Ventilation, *CC* Chest Compressions. [1]Fisher's exact test, [2]Chi-square, [3]Indicates significance at the $P < 0.05$ level, [4]when done, [5]when indicated. NS: non-significant

Table 5 Heat loss prevention

Group	Heat loss prevention adherence to algorithm (%) (PO/TPP)	P[c]	Admission temperature (C) (range)	P[c]
Total	62 (31/50)		36.0 ± 0.6 (34.6–37.8)	
Group N	66.7 (12/18)	NS (0.84)[a]	35.8 ± 0.7 (34.6–37.6)	NS (0.09)[b]
Group P	59.4 (19/32)		36.1 ± 0.6 (35.0–37.8)	
Correct heat loss prevention measures (*n* = 31)			36.1 ± 0.7 (35.0–37.8)	NS (0.60)[b]
Incorrect heat loss prevention measures (*n* = 19)			36.0 ± 0.6 (34.6–36.9)	

[a]Chi-square
[b]Paired T-test
[c]Indicates significance at the $P < 0.05$ level. *NS* non-significant, *PO* Points Obtained, *TPP* Total Possible Points, *Group N* Staff Neonatologists, *Group P* Pediatricians On-call

Stimulating breathing

One baby was stimulated when unnecessary, and 32% (16/50) who needed stimulation did not receive it, particularly those in worse condition. One baby had his face rubbed.

Administration of PPV

One patient was intubated without previous PPV. We observed the following errors: undue delay in starting PPV (at 56, 60 and 69 s) in 10.3% of cases (3/29), use of a self-inflating bag instead of a ventilator in 6.9% of patients (2/29), ventilation without previous suctioning when airway was obstructed in 6.9% (2/29), lack of ventilation between intubation attempts in 3.4% (1/29), and face mask leak in 3.4% (1/29). We did not use a respiratory function monitor, so we could not objectively document leaks; however, in one patient, the lack of a mask seal was obvious. In some patients, more than one mistake occurred.

Intubation

All intubations deviated from the algorithm. Two of 16 (12.5%) patients could not be intubated after several attempts; their indication for intubation was respiratory distress. They were transferred to the Neonatal Intensive Care Unit (NICU) with CPAP and intubated under sedation. The mean number of intubation attempts was 2.2 (range 1–6); success on the first attempt happened in 33.3% of cases; on second attempt, 38.9%; on third attempt, 16.7%; and 11.1% needed more than three attempts (5 and 6). We analyzed 40 intubation attempts. Two unplanned extubations after surfactant administration (due to incorrect securing of the tube) required reintubation. In all intubation cases, at least one attempt took longer than recommended (30 s). Mean duration to perform intubation was 58.8 ± 23.4 s (range 17–128 s). Only 5 of 40 intubations (12.5%) were achieved within 30 s.

Chest compressions and epinephrine administration

CC technique was correct, but it was initiated late. Despite correct intubation and ventilation, one newborn was bradycardic at 3:59 min, and CCs were started at 7:22 min. One patient received epinephrine without previous CCs, and another received epinephrine when CCs were started.

The median (IQR) assigned Apgar scores at 1, 5 and 10 min were 7 (5.7–9), 9 (8–10) and 10 (8–10). The median (IQR) Apgar scores after reviewing NRs were 7 (5–9), 9 (6.7–10) and 9 (7.7–10). Agreement at the three time points was acceptable (Kappa coefficient 0.35). Interrater reliability in evaluating Apgar scores was moderate at 1, 5 and 10 min (Cohen's kappa coefficients: 0.57, 0.60 and 0.44, respectively).

Our resuscitation team obtained a median of 10 points per resuscitation (red line), regardless of the resuscitation score (blue line), which means that resuscitations with a resuscitation score above 10 were poorly done (Fig. 2). Figure 3 shows that the relationship between the resuscitation score and the points obtained was nearly logarithmic ($R^2 = 0.7053$), which means that resuscitators scored very few additional points as the resuscitation intensity increased.

Discussion

All our patients were resuscitated in our dedicated room for resuscitation, which provides a setting similar to that in the NICU. Vento [4, 6] suggested that incorporating an intensive care environment into the DR could enhance survival and reduce the morbidity of extremely low birth weight (BW) infants. Among our study population, we found a high percentage of hypothermia (73.5%), which led us to make some changes in our resuscitation room to reduce hypothermia: we increased the temperature to 26 °C by keeping the doors locked and installed a heater next to the resuscitation cot. We use heated, humidified gases for ventilation.

Several authors have proven that performance often deviates from guidelines. Our study is the first report on adherence to the neonatal resuscitation algorithm for very preterm infants in a tertiary care center in Spain.

Carbine was the first to use video recording to evaluate NR [16]. We based our study on his publication and adopted his scoring system. Carbine found deviations in 54% of NRs. We evaluated more aspects and may have detected more errors (84%). We believe

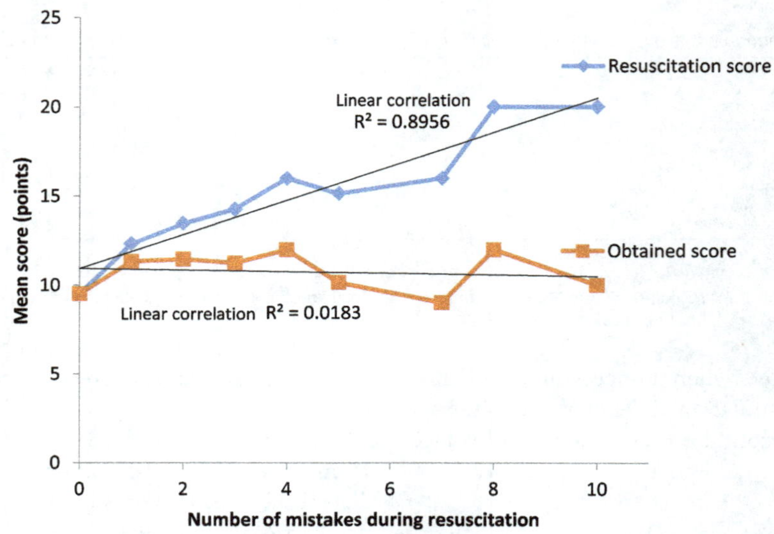

Fig. 2 Correlation between the number of errors during resuscitation and the mean obtained resuscitation score (red line) and the maximum resuscitation score (blue line). The difference between the blue and red lines was the average of virtually lost points

that our resuscitation score was higher: 22% of Carbine's patients only required stimulation (whereas 64% of ours needed stimulation); 80% required stimulation and oxygen, and only 7% needed PPV (vs our 80% respiratory support and 32% intubation). Carbine reported errors in the mask ventilation rate. We considered the use of a self-inflating bag an error, as we used an automatic ventilator. Consequently, we did not find this error. Only 28.6% of Carbine's cases involving PPV had no deviations, which is worse than our 72.7% rate of proper ventilation. Among Carbine's infants, 58.3% were intubated on the first attempt (vs our 33.3%), and only 33.3% (vs our 87.5%) were intubated within the established time limit. Like Carbine,

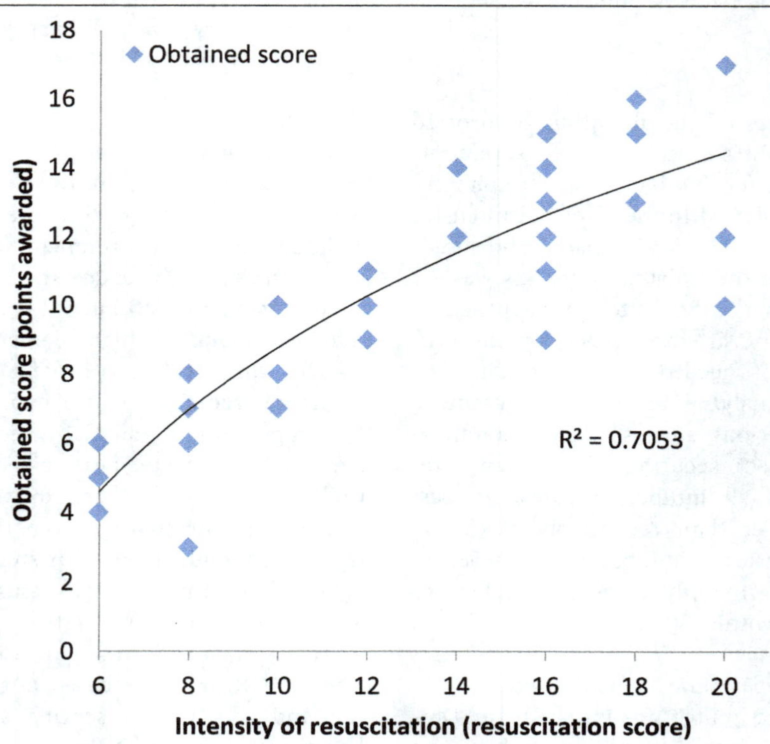

Fig. 3 Relationship between intensity of resuscitation and obtained score

we observed that perfect resuscitations were more likely for less intense interventions. None of our patients who required intubation received a perfect resuscitation.

Similar to Dekker [17], we observed that stimulation was often indicated but not performed, and when it was applied, it was most often indicated. Dekker's infants who received no stimulation required intubation more often (18 vs 7%); in our case, 62.5% of intubated infants had not been stimulated and 25% of stimulated infants did not require intubation. However, 18.7% of infants (6/32) who were stimulated were also intubated afterward.

By using video recording at a Nepalese tertiary hospital, Lindbäck [10] identified deviation from guidelines in over 50% of resuscitations. Most errors concerned the use of bag-and-mask ventilation (which we did not evaluate, as ventilating with a bag and mask was an error in our study), suction and excessive use of oxygen. Their results seem more favorable than ours. However, Lindbäck did not focus on preterm infants.

Gelbart [8] reported that the demanding technical skills scored higher than the more basic steps of resuscitation because technique is taught, whereas clinical assessment, communication skills and teamwork need practice. He found that invasive ventilation and surfactant administration were best performed, with median scores of 100%, whereas the performance of preparation and initial steps (69%) and assessment and communication of heart rate (75%) was worse. In our patients, most errors took place during the initial steps as well, whereas administration of CPAP, PPV and surfactant were performed better. Surfactant was administered in 83.3% of our cases when indicated. Technique was always correct, although two patients who required it did not receive it; the PO was not functioning, and the pediatrician preferred to administer it in the NICU with proper monitoring.

Schilleman [9] used video recording to evaluate compliance with NR guidelines in a population similar to ours, although our patients were in better conditions according to the Apgar scores. Schilleman found that deviations mainly occurred within the first 30 s because caregivers needed more time to perform the initial steps and mainly involved the way ventilation was given. As such, Schilleman suggested that 1 min be allowed for the initial evaluation, which is what the current ILCOR guidelines allow.

No intubations were perfectly performed. We analyzed 40 intubation attempts. Success occurred on the first attempt in 33.3% of cases and on the second attempt in 38.9%; more than three attempts (5 and 6) were required in only 11.1% of cases. In all intubation cases, at least one attempt took longer than recommended. Only 12.5% of intubations took place within the allotted 30 s. Other authors have reported similar deficiencies. Lane [18] reported a mean duration for successful attempts of 27.3 s; 30% infants were intubated on the first attempt, 30% on the second, 20% on the third, and 20% required more than three. Success was higher for 30 s, and no infants decompensated between 20 and 30 s; 20% of successful attempts took longer than 40 s. Finer and Rich's [3, 15] overall success rate for intubation was 33% within the allotted 20 s and 56% within 30 s. They reported an average of at least three attempts to successfully intubate infants < 1000 g. Our intubation success rate was higher than that reported by Finer and Rich. We needed, on average, 2.2 attempts to intubate infants < 1000 g (range 1–5), but unfortunately, it took longer (median (SD) 58.1 s (23.4), range 17–128 s). O'Donnell [19] analyzed intubation attempts in 31 infants (mean GA 28 weeks and BW 1227 g). Intubation attempts were often unsuccessful and successful attempts often took more than 30 s (17% were successful within 20 s, 20% between 20 and 29 s, and 25% > 30 s). Konstantelos [7] needed a median of 2 attempts, and 47 (25–60) s for intubation, and only 11% were successful within the allotted time. Wozniak [20] analyzed intubation attempts in preterm infants (795 g median BW, 25 weeks' GA) and reported a mean duration of 35 s and 2 attempts. Like Konstantelos [21], we believe that the lack of medication for intubation and surfactant administration are the reasons for the longer time needed for intubation. Because health care providers often underestimate the passage of time during NR, it is difficult to realize when the allotted time has passed. The American Academy of Pediatrics NRP used to allow 20 s for intubation, but since several studies reported that it often took longer [3, 16, 18, 19, 21] and that infants did not decompensate between 20 and 30 s, the current limit is 30 s [20].

As Fig. 2 shows, resuscitators obtained, on average, 10 points per patient regardless of the intensity of resuscitation, which means that caregivers did not score more points in more complex resuscitations. There are two reasons for the constant red line: a) some initial, common mistakes in heat loss prevention, suctioning and a postductal PO probe placement prevented most mild NRs (mean resuscitation score of 13 points) from scoring higher, and b) the points corresponding to almost all complex domains (intubation, chest compressions or epinephrine administration) were lost. The consequence is the flat line in the relationship between mistakes and the obtained score. However, the more mistakes that occur in a NR, the higher the resuscitation score (blue line, $R^2 = 0.895$), meaning that complex domains (the area above the red line) are lost in terms of obtained points. Not surprisingly, the relationship between the resuscitation score and the obtained score (Fig. 3) followed a strong logarithmic pattern ($R^2 = 0.705$). This finding means that although more points are possible, the resuscitator team would gain little benefit from those complex domains. More emphasis must be placed on the initial steps, which are common to most NRs, and especially on training for complex skills such as intubation.

This study has some limitations. Its purpose was to evaluate adherence to NR guidelines. For this reason, all mistakes counted equally, although it is obvious that not all the deviations are equally serious: some are mild and nontranscendental (for example, duration of oral suctioning) whereas others are potentially harmful (like timing and route of epinephrine administration). The same mistake could have consequences or not, depending on the patient. For example, placing a postductal PO probe in a patient who does not receive oxygen or ventilatory support has no impact on the maneuvers performed but may lead to hyperoxia in an intubated neonate. Only 16% of our resuscitations perfectly followed the algorithm, but the number of mistakes per resuscitation was low, and global adherence to the algorithm was 80.9%. We acknowledge that the value of global adherence in itself has little meaning without the proper analysis of the main and more critical errors. Another limitation of our study is the lack of feedback of our findings to the resuscitation team. We designed the study to assess adherence to the algorithm and find the most common errors. In the pilot study, we did not consider an active intervention with the resuscitation team. Sharing our findings with them would probably improve performance. In most cases, the resuscitation team consisted of two neonatologists or two pediatricians on-call. All of them are trained in neonatal resuscitation, although their expertise varies from more than 30 years to only a few months after completing a residency. However, 38% of our patients were twins, which may worsen performance, as in some cases, there was only one caregiver per patient [22]. All our medical staff was aware of this study when it started, and we periodically reminded them about it. All the neonatologists and pediatricians who work at our hospital participated in this study. The medical staff turned the video camera on, automatically consenting to be recorded, when they were called to the DR. Recording usually began minutes before the neonate was born but sometimes began when the newborn arrived at the resuscitation room.

Similar to many other previous studies, our study demonstrated that deviations from the algorithm exist. Many of the errors have to do with timing: some maneuvers take longer than allotted, and personnel are not aware of this [23].

We compared performance of staff neonatologists with pediatricians on-call. We thought that the neonatologists would perform better since they work with only newborns and are subspecialized in neonatology, whereas after-hour on-call pediatricians who cover this shift often do not work with only newborns. We observed no differences between these two groups, which means that we have a good team of pediatricians who perform as well as neonatologists. This is a positive aspect to consider. Although global adherence to the algorithm was high, mistakes were common despite our staff's training.

In line with other authors [8, 22–25], we found a discrepancy in Apgar scores, particularly when the Apgar was not 9/10/10, and the staff attending the delivery commonly overestimated the score. It is easy to score 9/10/10 if no resuscitation is necessary, whereas it is difficult to remember the patient's situation at 5 and 10 min when resuscitation is required. Video recording scores tended to be lower than scores given by neonatologists (47.1% at 1 min, 73.3% at 5, 88.9% at 10). Gelbart [8] also found overestimation of Apgar scores by a median value of 2 points at 1 and 5 min. As other authors suggest, we believe that memories of a stressful past event can be inaccurate, and Apgar scores are usually calculated afterward [24].

Finally, we are aware that our study sample was small. We aimed to analyze 50 resuscitations due to the difficulty in obtaining written consent before resuscitation started. Nonetheless, we managed to record one-third of our potential cases, which is a significant sample. The ILCOR guidelines have changed twice since we conducted this study, and some actions that we considered mistakes would now be correct, for example, supporting transition rather than keeping timing strict or not suctioning routinely. While it is true that our data are old, and a few aspects are outdated, our aim was to assess our performance in terms of adherence to the algorithm, that is, if our physicians performed according to the written rules, not the appropriateness of the algorithm. Our results would probably be similar today. Even though only one person reviewed the recordings, the camera was in a good position, and the scoring system was clear, so this bias is likely minimal. There was no feedback given to the resuscitation team during the study period, but our findings could serve as both a starting point for further studies and a teaching tool. As far as we know, there are no similar studies published in Spain to date.

Conclusions

Resuscitation of very preterm newborns often deviates from guidelines. Perfectly performed resuscitations are infrequent, although global adherence to the algorithm is high. Resuscitations led by pediatricians on-call and neonatologists are performed equally correct. Intubation training may improve complex resuscitations the most.

Abbreviations

bpm: Beats Per Minute; BW: Birth Weight; C: Celsius; CC: Chest Compressions; CPAP: Continuous Positive Airway Pressure; DR: Delivery Room; GA: Gestational Age; ILCOR: International Liaison Committee on Resuscitation; min: Minute; NICU: Neonatal Intensive Care Unit; NR: Neonatal Resuscitation; NRP: Neonatal Resuscitation Program; PO: Pulse-Oximeter; PPV: Positive Pressure Ventilation; s: Second; SD: Standard Deviation; Temp: Temperature

Acknowledgements

We would like to thank the medical and nursing NICU staff for participating and taking ownership during the realization of this project. We thank all the neonatologists and pediatricians on-call for supporting this study.

Authors' contributions

SM conceptualized and designed the study, carried out the initial analyses, drafted the initial manuscript and approved the final manuscript as submitted. FB helped to conceptualize and design the study, reviewed and revised the manuscript, and approved the final manuscript as submitted. JF helped to design the study, helped to carry out the statistical analyses, reviewed and revised the manuscript, and approved the final manuscript as submitted. MI-R helped to carry out the initial analyses, reviewed and revised the manuscript, and approved the final manuscript as submitted. MT helped to conceptualize and design the study, helped to develop the neonatal resuscitation algorithm for very preterm infants (2007), reviewed and revised the manuscript, and approved the final manuscript as submitted. MI-S helped to conceptualize and design the study, helped to develop the neonatal resuscitation algorithm for very preterm infants (2007), reviewed and revised the manuscript, and approved the final manuscript as submitted.

Competing interests

The authors have no financial relationships relevant to this article to disclose. I declare that I have no competing interests.

Author details

[1]Neonatology Service, Hospital Clínic, seu Maternitat, ICGON (Institut Clínic de Ginecologia, Obstetrícia i Neonatologia), Barcelona University, Sabino de Arana, 1, 08028 Barcelona, Spain. [2]Neonatology Service, Hospital Sant Joan de Déu, BCNatal (Centre de Medicina Maternofetal i Neonatal de Barcelona, Hospital Sant Joan de Déu, Hospital Clínic), Barcelona University, Passeig de Sant Joan de Déu, 2, 08950 Esplugues de Llobregat, Barcelona, Spain.

References

1. Perlman JM, Wyllie J, Kattwinkel J, Wyckoff MH, Aziz K, Guinsburg R, et al. Part 7: Neonatal Resuscitation: 2015 International Consensus on Cardiopulmonary Resuscitation and Emergency Cardiovascular Care Science With Treatment Recommendations. Pediatrics. 2015. https://doi.org/10.1542/peds.2015-3373D.
2. https://data.unicef.org/topic/child-survival/neonatal-mortality/ (accessed 2017 July 25).
3. Finer N, Rich W. Neonatal resuscitation for the preterm infant: evidence versus practice. J Perinatol. 2010. https://doi.org/10.1038/jp.2010.115.
4. Vento M, Cheung PY, Aguar M. The first golden minutes of the extremely-low-gestational-age neonate: a gentle approach. Neonatology. 2009. https://doi.org/10.1159/000178770.
5. Izquierdo-Renau M, Gómez-Robles C, Pino-Vázquez A. Lección 12. El recién nacido muy prematuro (<32 semanas). In: Sociedad Española de Neonatología. Manual de Reanimación Neonatal. 4th edition. Editorial Ergon. Madrid 2017. Pages 167-180. ISBN: 9788416732494. Spanish.
6. Vento M, Aguar M, Leone TA, Finer NN, Gimeno A, Rich W, et al. Using intensive care technology in the delivery room: a new concept for the resuscitation of extremely preterm neonates. Pediatrics. 2008. https://doi.org/10.1542/peds.2008-1422
7. Konstantelos D, Ifflaender S, Dinger J, Rüdiger M. Suctioning habits in the delivery room and the influence on postnatal adaptation - a video analysis. J Perinat Med. 2015. https://doi.org/10.1515/jpm-2014-0188.
8. Gelbart B, Hiscock R, Barfield C. Assessment of neonatal resuscitation performance using video recording in a perinatal centre. J Paediatr Child Health. 2010. https://doi.org/10.1111/j.1440-1754.2010.01747.x.
9. Schilleman K, Siew ML, Lopriore E, Morley CJ, Walther FJ, Te Pas AB. Auditing resuscitation of preterm infants at birth by recording video and physiological parameters. Resuscitation. 2012. https://doi.org/10.1016/j.resuscitation.2012.01.036.
10. Lindbäck C, KC A, Wrammert J, Vitrakoti R, Ewald U, Målqvist M. Poor adherence to neonatal resuscitation guidelines exposed; an observational study using camera surveillance at a tertiary hospital in Nepal. BMC Pediatr. 2014. https://doi.org/10.1186/1471-2431-14-233.
11. Finer NN, Rich W. Neonatal resuscitation: toward improved performance. Resuscitation. 2002;53(1):47–51.
12. Murphy MC, O'Donnell CPF, McCarthy LK. Attitudes of staff members towards video recording in the delivery room. Arch Dis Child Fetal Neonatal Ed. 2018. https://doi.org/10.1136/archdischild-2017-313789.
13. den Boer MC, Houtlosser M, van Zanten HA, Foglia EE, Engberts DP, Te Pas AB. Ethical dilemmas of recording and reviewing neonatal resuscitation. Arch Dis Child Fetal Neonatal Ed. 2018. https://doi.org/10.1136/archdischild-2017-314191.
14. Van Vonderen JJ, van Zanten HA, Schilleman K, Hooper SB, Kitchen MJ, Witlox RS, et al. Cardiorespiratory Monitoring during Neonatal Resuscitation for Direct Feedback and Audit. Front Pediatr. 2016. https://doi.org/10.3389/fped.2016.00038.
15. Rich WD, Leone T, Finer NN. Delivery room intervention: improving the outcome. Clin Perinatol. 2010. https://doi.org/10.1016/j.clp.2010.01.011.
16. Carbine DN, Finer NN, Knodel E, Rich W. Video recording as a means of evaluating neonatal resuscitation performance. Pediatrics. 2000;106:654–8.
17. Dekker J, Martherus T, Cramer SJE, van Zanten HA, Hooper SB, Te Pas AB. Tactile stimulation to stimulate spontaneous breathing during stabilization of preterm infants at birth: a retrospective analysis. Front Pediatr. 2017;5:61. https://doi.org/10.3389/fped.2017.00061.
18. Lane B, Finer N, Rich W. Duration of intubation attempts during neonatal resuscitation. J Pediatr. 2004. https://doi.org/10.1016/j.jpeds.2004.03.003.
19. O'Donnell CP, Kamlin CO, Davis PG, Morley CJ. Endotracheal intubation attempts during neonatal resuscitation: success rates, duration, and adverse effects. Pediatrics. 2006. https://doi.org/10.1542/peds.2005-0901.
20. Wozniak M, Arnell K, Brown M, Gonzales S, Lazarus D, Rich W, et al. The 30 second rule: the effects of prolonged intubation attempts on oxygen saturation and heart rate in preterm infants in the delivery room. Minerva Pediatr. 2018. https://doi.org/10.23736/S0026-4946.16.04469-8.
21. Konstantelos D, Dinger J, Ifflaender S, Rüdiger M. Analyzing video recorded support of postnatal transition in preterm infants following a c-section. BMC Pregnancy Childbirth. 2016. https://doi.org/10.1186/s12884-016-1045-2.
22. Layouni I, Danan C, Durrmeyer X, Dassieu G, Azcona B, Decobert F. Video recording of newborn resuscitation in the delivery room: technique and advantages. Arch Pediatr 2011; doi: https://doi.org/10.1016/S0929-693X(11)71094-6. French.
23. Trevisanuto D, De Bernardo G, Res G, Sordino D, Doglioni N, Winer G, et al. Time Perception during Neonatal Resuscitation. J Pediatr. 2016. https://doi.org/10.1016/j.jpeds.2016.07.003.
24. McCarthy LK, Morley CJ, Davis PG, Kamlin CO, O'Donnell CP. Timing of interventions in the delivery room: does reality compare with neonatal resuscitation guidelines? J Pediatr. 2013. https://doi.org/10.1016/j.jpeds.2013.06.007.
25. Schilleman K, Witlox RS, van Vonderen JJ, Roegholt E, Walther FJ, te Pas AB. Auditing documentation on delivery room management using video and physiological recordings. Arch Dis Child Fetal Neonatal Ed. 2014. https://doi.org/10.1136/archdischild-2014-306261.

Case report: acute clinical presentation and neonatal management of primary hyperparathyroidism due to a novel CaSR mutation

Manuela Capozza[1,7*], Iolanda Chinellato[2], Vito Guarnieri[3], Natascia Di Iorgi[4], Maria Accadia[3], Cristina Traggiai[5], Girolamo Mattioli[6], Antonio Di Mauro[1] and Nicola Laforgia[1]

Abstract

Background: Neonatal severe primary hyperparathyroidism (NSHPT) is a rare autosomal recessive disorder of calcium homeostasis, characterized by striking hyperparathyroidism, marked hypercalcemia and hyperparathyroid bone disease. We report the case of a newborn with a novel homozygous mutation of the CaSR, treated by successful subtotal parathyroidectomy, who had an acute presentation of the disease, i.e. out-of hospital cardiorespiratory arrest. .

Case presentation: A 8-day-old female newborn was admitted to the NICU of University of Bari "Aldo Moro" (Italy) after a cardiorespiratory arrest occurred at home. Severe hypercalcemia was found and different drug therapies were employed (Furosemide, Cinacalcet and bisphosphonate), as well as hyperhydration, until subtotal parathyroidectomy, was performed at day 32. Our patient's mutation was never described before so that a strict and individualized long-term follow-up was started.

Conclusions: This case of NSHPT suggests that a near-miss event, labelled as a possible case of SIDS, could also be due to severe hypercalcemia and evidentiates the difficulties of the neonatal management of NSHPT. Furthermore, the identification of the specific CaSR mutation provides the substrate for prenatal diagnosis.

Keywords: Hypercalcemia, Calcium sensing receptor, Neonatal severe primary hyperparathyroidism, Out-of-hospital cardiorespiratory arrest, Parathyroidectomy

Background

Neonatal severe primary hyperparathyroidism (NSHPT) is a rare autosomal recessive disorder of calcium homeostasis that presents shortly after birth, characterized by striking hyperparathyroidism, marked hypercalcemia and hyperparathyroid bone disease [1].

NSHPT patients shows hypotonia, respiratory distress, bone fractures, intestinal dysmotility and failure to thrive [1] and their neurological development can be significantly affected. If NSHPT is not diagnosed and treated it can be fatal [2]. NSHPT is caused by a loss of function of the calcium-sensing receptor CaSR, whose gene is encoded in the long arm of chromosome 3 (3p-13.3- 21) [3]. More than 250 different CaSR inactivating mutations have been described. The type of mutation can affect both clinical severity and response to treatment. CaSR is a G-protein-coupled receptor found in many tissues throughout the body, but its action is best understood in the parathyroid gland and in the kidney, where parathyroid hormone (PTH) synthesis and secretion and calcium reabsorption and excretion are regulated, respectively [4]. PTH is the main regulator of serum calcium levels and its secretion from the parathyroid is regulated by signals from CaSR [5]. Different treatment options have been proposed for NSHPT, such as drug therapies or surgical removal of the hyperplastic parathyroids [6, 7]. Recently calcimimetics (Cinacalcet) have been used

* Correspondence: manuelacapozza26@gmail.com; manuela.capozza@uniba.it
[1]Neonatology and Neonatal Intensive Care Unit, Department of Biomedical Science ad Human Oncology, University of Bari "Aldo Moro", Bari, Italy
[7]Policlinico Hospital, Piazza Giulio Cesare n. 11, 70124 Bari, Italy

to increase the calcium-responsiveness of mutated CaSR proteins with significant and lasting effect [8]. Medical treatment of NSHPT includes also intravenous hyper-hydration, diuretics and bisphosphonates. However, total or subtotal parathyroidectomy is still the treatment of choice often needed even if very difficult in newborns [9]. We report the case of a newborn with NSHPT due to a homozygously inherited mutation not previously described, treated first medically and then by subtotal parathyroidectomy.

Presenting concerns

A full-term AGA neonate, by third-degree cousins, born at 38 weeks by spontaneous vaginal delivery, after a normal pregnancy, with no significant obstetric and family history was discharged at the 3rd DOL home.

At 8 days of age, because of poor feeding and lethargy, paediatrician was called at home. During her visit, the neonate had a cardiorespiratory arrest. Immediately high quality cardiopulmonary resuscitation (30:2, single rescuer) was initiated and maintained for 3 minutes with reappearance of vital signs. The neonate was immediately brought to the Neonatal Intensive Care Unit of the Department of Biomedical Science and Human Oncology, of "Aldo Moro" University of Bari, Italy .

Clinical findings

On physical examination, lethargy, hypotonia and absent deep tendon reflexes were evident and a weight loss of 465 g since birth was recorded.. Blood pressure was 68/40 mmHg and SaO_2 = 97% on room air. Initial laboratory evaluation revealed severe hypercalcemia (serum calcium level = 28.7 mg/dl; RR: 8.6 ± 11.8 mg/dl). High serum alkaline phosphatase activity (663 U/L; RR: 105÷410 U/L), hyperparathyroidism (PTH 465 pg/ml; RR: 6.5÷36.8 pg/ml) and hypophosphatemia (2 mg/dl; RR: 3.1÷7.7 mg/dl) with normal magnesium (2.2 mg/dl; RR 1.8–2.4 mg/dl) and 25-hydroxyvitamin D (33.1 pg/ml; RR: 19.8 ± 79.3 pg/ml) were also found. Urine calcium was 35.8 mg/dl, urine creatinine 15.4 mg/dl with a spot urinary calcium/creatinine ratio of 2.3. During the following days, hypercalcemia persisted: the peak of serum calcium was 29.3 mg/dl with serum-ionized calcium of 14.9 mg/dl (RR: 4.6 ± 5.3 mg/dl).

The following graph reports calcium and phosphate values in comparison with qualitative data provided (Fig 1).

Total body X-rays revealed generalized skeletal undermineralization and subperiosteal bone resorption. Abdominal, cerebral and cardiac ultrasound were normal. "QT stretching" were found at the ECG as sign of hypercalcemia.

Both parents had calcium levels within normal range.

Timeline

Table 1 shows the timeline that includes specific dates and times of the patient.

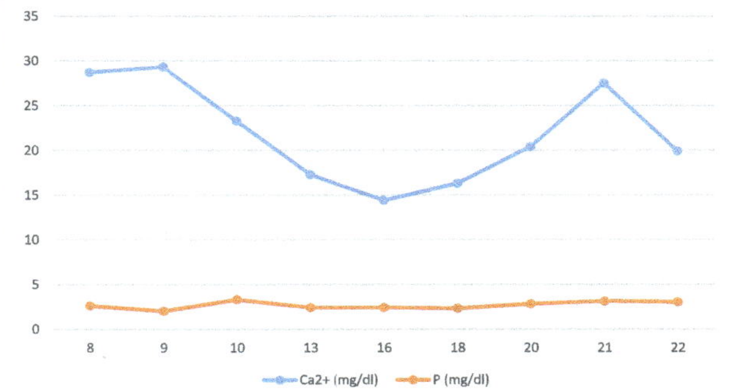

Fig. 1 Calcium and phosphate levels from 8 to 22 DOL

Diagnostic focus and assessment

The differential diagnosis for hyperparathyroidism is wide and includes parathyroid adenoma/hyperplasia, PTH-like peptide secondary to malignancy, CaSR mutation, PTH receptor mutation and Vitamin D excess.

Considering the early onset, life-threatening hypercalcemia and the biochemical findings in the patient, genetic studies of CASR gene were performed revealing NSHPT secondary to a CaSR gene mutation. NSHPT is often discovered during the first days of life because of severe, symptomatic, PTH-dependent hypercalcemia, polyuria, dehydration, hypotonia, bone changes and failure to thrive. Untreated NSHPT can be letal or have devastating neurodevelopmental effects [10].

CaSR is a seven transmembrane G-protein coupled receptor essential for normal calcium homeostasis, located in organs involved with calcium metabolism, such as the parathyroid cells, the parafollicular thyroid-C cells, the kidney epithelium and cells in bone and intestine [11]. It is encoded by chromosome 3p-13.3- 21 loci [12]. Heterozygous mutations of CaSR gene cause mild forms of asymptomatic hypercalcemia while homozygous mutations cause a rare form of NSHPT [13].

After written informed consent of the parents, genomic DNA of proband and parents was extracted from peripheral blood leukocytes and molecular screening of the 7 exons including intron-exon boundaries of the CASR gene was performed as previously described [14] at the Medical Genetics, IRCCS "Casa Sollievo della Sofferenza" Hospital in San Giovanni Rotondo, Foggia, Italy.

NSHPT was confirmed by the finding of a novel autosomal recessive mutation of the CaSR gene, causing the loss of receptor's function. Sequence analysis revealed a previously undefined mutation of the donor splicing site of the intron 5, namely c.1608 + 1G > A –IVS5 + 1G > A, in homozygosity (Fig. 2).

Segregation analysis of parents evidentiated CaSR variant in heterozygosity, confirming the autosomal recessive inheritance of NSHPT and the familial

Table 1 Timeline

Dates	Relevant Past Medical History and Interventions		
13/11/2016	A full-term AGA neonate, by third-degree cousins, born by spontaneous vaginal delivery, after a normal pregnancy. No remarkable obstetric and family history. Discharged home at the 3rd DOL.		
Dates	Summaries from Initial and Follow-up Visits	Diagnostic Testing (including dates)	Interventions
21/11/2016	During paediatrician's visit because of poor feeding and lethargy, the neonate had a cardiorespiratory arrest.		High quality cardiopulmonary resuscitation (30:2, single rescuer) for 3 minutes with reappearance of vital signs.
21/11/2016	Admission at NICU-Policlinico of Bari (Italy): significant weight loss, lethargy, hypotonia and absent tendon reflexes.	Severe hypercalcemia (28.7 mg/dl; RR: 8.6 ± 11.8 mg/dl), high serum alkaline phosphatase activity (663 U/L; RR: 105÷410 U/L), hyperparathyroidism (PTH 465 pg/ml; RR: 6.5÷36.8 pg/ml), hypophosphatemia (2 mg/dl; RR: 3.1÷7.7 mg/dl), normal magnesium (2.2 mg/dl; RR 1.8–2.4 mg/dl), normal 25-hydroxyvitamin D (33.1 pg/ml; RR: 19.8 ± 79.3 pg/ml).	Low calcium intake (85 mg/day), intravenous fluid hyperhydration (glucose solution 8% with aminoacids and physiologic solution - 220 ml/kg/day), Furosemide (2 mg/kg/day), Clodronate (1 mg/kg/day): No response (after 7 days of therapy)
26/11/2016	Persistent severe hypercalcemia, polyuria, dehydration, hypotonia, bone changes and failure to thrive.	Total body X-rays (skeletal undermineralization, subperiosteal bone resorption). ECG (anomalies of the recovery phase,"QT stretching"). Abdominal, cerebral and cardiac ultrasound (normal). Parathyroid glands Ultrasound: glands not detectable.	Cinacalcet (0.4 mg/kg/day): No response (after 2 weeks of treatment). No adverse reactions.
05/12/2016	Both parents were clinically and biochemically normal.	Genomic DNA of proband and parents extracted from peripheral blood leukocytes and molecular screening of the Calcium-sensing receptor (CASR) gene (Sanger sequencing).	Proband: a novel autosomal recessive mutation in the CaSR gene: (c.1608 + 1G > A –IVS5 + 1G > A in homozygosity). Parents: presence of the CaSR variant in heterozygosity (FHH clinical state).
13/12/2016	She was transferred to the NICU department of the G. Gaslini Institute of Genova (Italy).	Total calcium level stabilized around 6 mEq/L (equal to 12 mg/dl).	Increasing doses of Cinalcalcet (up to 4 mg/kg/day), low orally calcium intake (45 mg/day), intravenous fluid hyperhydration (up to 220 ml/kg/day).
20/12/2016	She was transferred to the Pediatric Surgery Unit of the G. Gaslini Institute of Genova (Italy).	Parathyroid glands Ultrasound: glands detectable by only the day before surgery.	Subtotal parathyroidectomy: three-excised hyperplastic parathyroid glands (5 × 3, 1.5 × 1.4 and 1.4 × 1.2 mm, respectively).
22/12/2016	Two days after surgery: transient asymptomatic hypocalcemia appeared (hungry bone syndrome).	X-rays of the right arm: pathological fracture of the humerus neck.	Daily Calcium gluconate replacement (0,5 ml/kg) and α-Calcidol (0,05 mcg/kg) for 40 days.
31/01/2017	Slow and progressive improvement of clinical conditions and hypocalcaemia.		Stop-therapy 40 days post-surgery (Calcium gluconate and α-Calcidol).
	A longer and personalized follow up started in order to confirm if the partial parathyroidectomy was sufficient for calcium balance or a second surgical approach is needed.		

hypocalciuric hypercalcemia (FHH) clinical state of the parents, although asymptomatic (Fig. 3).

Minigene-based functional approach

The CASR gene is expressed in the parathyroids, bone, kidneys and neural cells but it is not expressed into the blood. Thus, in absence of a source of these tissues, we verified the mutation by an in-vitro assay that artificially reproduced the splicing process on a chimeric gene. The presumed altered mRNA splicing of this novel variant was tested by an "in vitro minigene-based assay" [14]. Briefly, the exon 5 of the CaSR gene along with 150 intronic flanking bases was PCR amplified with primers containing the HindIII and XhoI restriction sites. The amplicon was cloned into the HindIII/XhoI digested pCDNA3.1 vector containing a "chimeric" genetic sequence between the exon 1 of the PTHR1 gene and the exons 2 and 3 of the RAB1 gene. Sequencing of the vector confirmed the correctness of the construct that was further modified in order to introduce the splicing mutation (IVS5 + 1G > A) by a site-specific mutagenesis approach [14]. Both the vectors (hereafter named Mini-WT and Mini-Mut) were transfected in (700 thousands) HEK293 cells seeded in six well plates with Fugene Transfection reagent (Promega, Madison, WI, USA), following manufacturer's instructions. After 48 h, RNA was extracted with Trizol (Qiagen, Hilden, Germany), retrotranscribed with the Superscript III

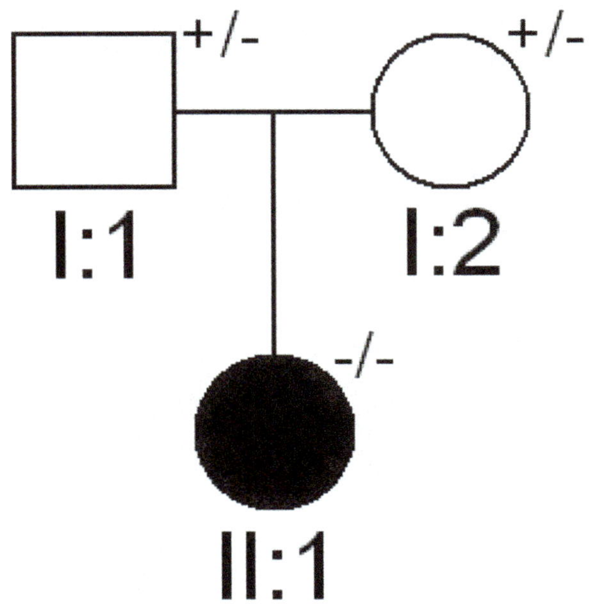

Fig. 2 Electropherograms showing the heterozygous mutation in the father and mother and the homozygosity in the proband. On the bottom the control

(ThermoFisher, Whaltam, MA, USA), PCR amplified with specific primers annealing on the chimera gene (mutagenesis and PCR primer sequence, annealing temperatures and size of the amplicons are available upon request). Finally amplicons were loaded on an ethydium bromide (1%, Sigma Aldrich) stained 1,5% agarose gel; they were purified (ExoSap-IT, Thermo-Fisher, Whaltam, MA, USA) and directly sequenced (Big Dye Terminator Cycle Sequencing Kit v.1.1, ThermoFisher, Whaltam, MA, USA).

The mini-gene assay proved the complete skipping of the exon 5 of the CaSR gene (Fig. 4a-c-d), thus leading to an in-frame deletion of 77 residues and thus to a shorter, but presumably expressed, receptor.

Moreover, a different reverse primer specifically designed on the 3′ end of the exon 5, was used to amplify the WT and mutated cDNAs. In both the cases, an amplicon was obtained thus proving that the mutated vector was able to read-through the splicing mutation, giving a (not quantified) amount of WT CaSR RNA form (Fig. 4b). This is can be also confirmed by the higher "faint" band present in the lane of mutated cDNA, having the same size of the correct WT cDNA amplicon (Fig. 4).

Therapeutic focus and assessment

For the management of hypercalcemia, the newborn received very low calcium intake, intravenous hyper-hydration (total

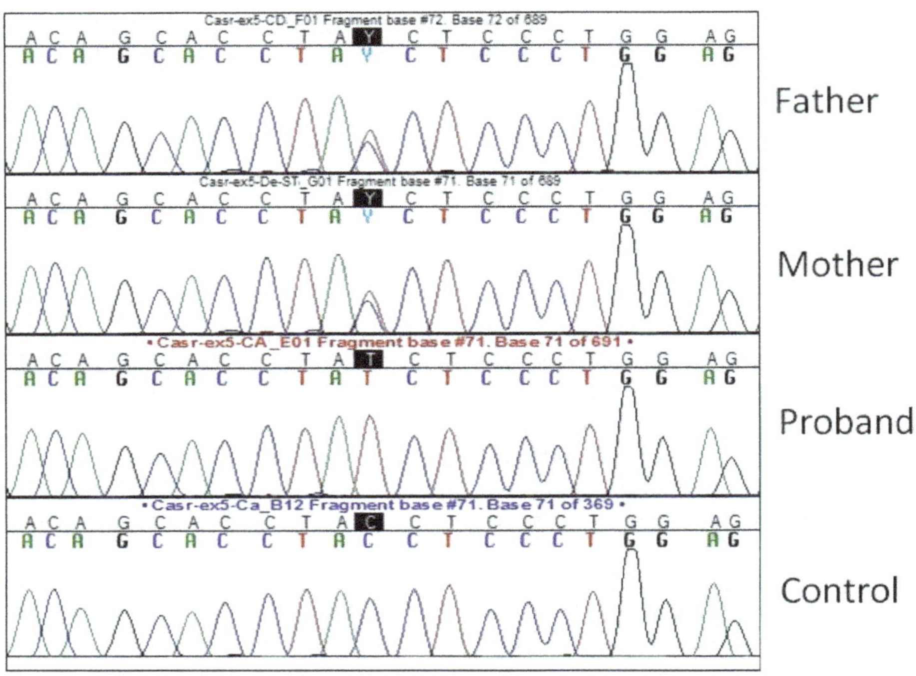

Fig. 3 Pedigree of the family under study. Filled symbol indicates the affected proband. Clear symbols indicate the unaffected status; +/− = presence/absence of the mutation

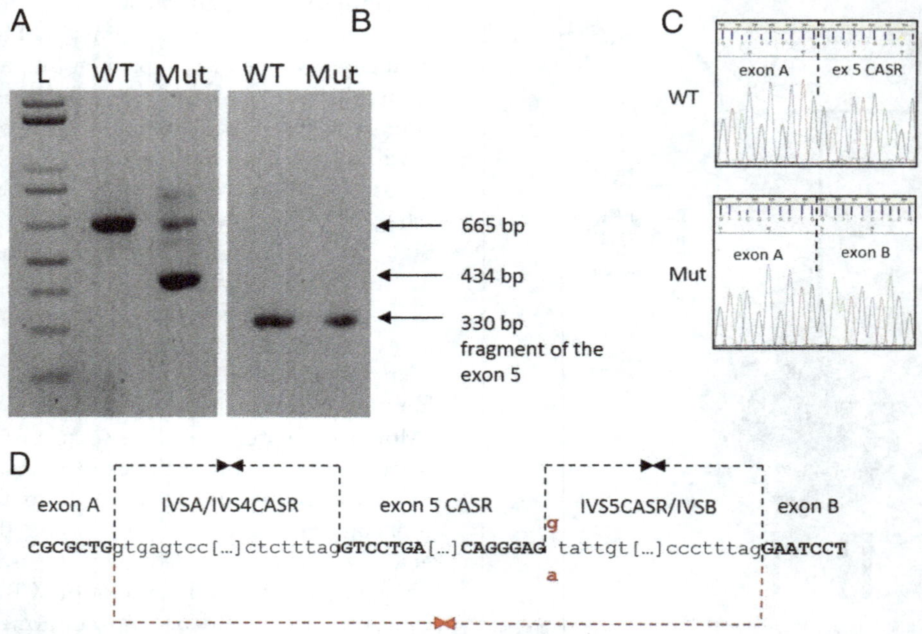

Fig. 4 Schematic showing the effect of the splicing mutation. **a**. The retrotranscription of RNA extracted from HEK293 cells transfected with WT/ Mutated minigene vectors (see the methods) leads to amplicons of different size: a full chimeric amplicon (665 bp) and a shorter chimeric cDNA fragment (434), both sequenced in **c**; **b**. cDNA amplification with an internal primer designed on the exon 5, shows that both the WT and the mutated RNA produce a normal amplicon (here not quantified): this is partially confirmed by the "faint" band in the lane of mutated cDNA; **d**: diagram showing the exon skipping mechanism induced by the presence of the IVS5 + 1G > A mutation

intake 220 ml/kg/day) and Furosemide (2 mg/kg/day), without significant reduction of calcium levels. Ten days after, Cinacalcet (0,4 mg/kg/day), a type 2 calcimimetic agent that increases CaSR affinity for calcium, leading to parathormone suppression and increasing calcium renal excretion, after a written informed consent obtained from his parents, was started [15]. She initially responded, but 10 days after start therapy serum calcium raised up to 27.5 mg/dl, with a serum ionized calcium of 14.9 mg/dl. Bisphosphonates (Clodronate 1 mg/kg for 3 days) were then associated to Cinacalcet and Furosemide [16], but hypercalcemia did not resolve.

Finally, at 1 month of life, she was transferred to the NICU department of the Giannina Gaslini Institute, Genova, Italy, where the child was stabilized to a total calcium level around 12 mg/dl with increasing doses of Cinalcalcet (up to 4 mg/kg/day), low orally calcium/free vitamin D formula, and hyper-hydratation before undergoing an exploratory surgery of the neck. Parathyroid glands were repeatedly undetectable by ultrasound up to the day before surgery. Subtotal parathyroidectomy was then performed with removal of three (two left and one right) hyperplastic parathyroid glands (5 × 3, 1.5 × 1.4 and 1.4 × 1.2 mm, respectively). Baseline PTH level was 1339 pg/ml and intraoperative PTH by bilateral jugular sampling of blood demonstrated 30 min after excision a bilateral PTH reduction of 75% from baseline, and at 70 min a further reduction on the left side (202 pg/ml) and an increase on the right side (658 pg/ml). The surgeons looked for any other areas of the neck region excluding any visible nodes.

It is not yet clear whether subtotal parathyroidectomy or total parathyroidectomy with reimplantation would be best. Some studies highlight they have similar rates of complications, readmission, and 30-day mortality, but subtotal parathyroidectomy is less likely to have extended hospital stay. [17]

Follow-up and outcomes

Two days after surgery, the patient developed transient asymptomatic hypocalcemia (Ca^{2+} 5 mg/dl) that required daily Calcium gluconate replacement (0,5 ml/kg) and α-Calcidol (0,05 mcg/kg) for 40 days. The X-rays of the right arm showed fracture of the humerus neck and severe osteoporosis.

Hypocalcemia is a common problem after parathyroidectomy because of reduction in bone reabsorption and increase in bone formation. The hypocalcemia is generally transient but it could be severe and prolonged because of a chronic increase in bone resorption induced by previous high levels of PTH ("hungry bone syndrome") [18].

One month post-surgery, her calcium and α-Calcidol requirements decreased, and 10 days later, these medications were suspended.

She began the follow up with controls of serum calcium levels, which at the time were always normal. We believe that in our NSHPT case, due to a novel homozygous inherited intronic mutation of the CaSR, a longer and personalized follow up is warranted in order to confirm if the partial parathyroidectomy was sufficient for calcium balance or a second surgical approach is needed to remove the fourth gland or any residual.

Discussion

NSHPT is a rare life-threatening disease characterized by marked hypercalcemia, diffuse parathyroid hyperplasia and skeletal demineralization, due to the biallelic inactivation (homozygous or compound heterozygous mutations) of the CaSR gene.

NSHPT-related mutations have been identified throughout the coding sequence and result in PTH-hyperproduction. The overproduction of PTH leads to hypercalcemia and hypocalciuria due both to significant calcium release from bones and increase of renal calcium reabsorption [19]. De novo heterozygous missense mutations, compound heterozygous missense mutations, frameshift and nonsense mutations have been reported in patients with NSHPT [3, 20, 21].

Our patient shows a homozygous novel mutation of the splicing donor site of the intron 5 in homozygosity. Both asymptomatic FHH parents were found to be heterozygous for this novel mutation, suggesting an autosomal recessive pattern of transmission.

In vitro functional assay proved that this novel mutation leads to an altered splicing process with the skipping of the exon 5, thus presumably giving a short CASR protein, lacking 77 residues of the extracellular domain, previously reported to be a not functional but normally expressed in keratinocytes [22]. Interestingly, it has been proved that this alternatively spliced transcript has a dominant-negative effect on the wild type copy making it less sensible to calcium concentrations and inducing its decrease during keratinocyte differentiation [22]. However, it has to be noted, that this alternative transcript naturally occurs in specified peripheral tissues, in absence of any mutational event. In our clinical case, a different landscape of the mutation could be deduced. We provided evidence that the splicing machinery is able to read through the mutation to give an amount of correct transcript that, however, at this stage, we were not able to quantify. We can hypothesize that in the proband, homozygous for this mutation, this amount of correct mRNA was not enough to compensate the overall huge loss of protein function. In the parents, who already had the 50% of WT protein, the presence of this additional amount of correct mRNA coming from the mutated allele, may have contributed to making them asymptomatic. However, although our results have been obtained "in vitro" and with a cellular system that could not reproduce entirely the in vivo state, our hypothesis would explain why the parents are clinically and biochemically normal. Further studies on mRNAs extracted from the fibroblasts of the parents and proband would clarify this issue.

Moreover, we confirm that the use of Cinacalcet could be indicated provided that the CASR mutation does not induce a premature truncation or a structural conformation change of the protein. In our case, although in absence of a specific functional proof, but taking into account of the positive effect of the Cinacalcet in the first weeks of treatment, we might presume that the deletion of 77 residues located in the ECD did not compromise the binding of the drug with the ICD. In our patient, a trial of Cinacalcet was initiated at 20 days of life resulting in escaping responses of calcemia with increasing doses of calcimimetic [23]. This is consistent with Soblechero et al. that reported a case of neonatal hypercalcemia due to a homozygous deletion/frameshift mutation in the *CaSR* in which there was therapeutic failure of Cinacalcet [1]. The success or failure in response to therapy with Cinacalcet can depend on the CASR genotype [24]. In all cases of NSHPT, a trial with Cinacalcet could be attempted but, if ineffective, definitive surgical treatment is necessary. If not treated by parathyroidectomy, fully developed NSHPT can have a devastating effect on the psychomotor development and it can be fatal, because of complications of hypercalcemia [3]. Respiratory failure, extreme hypercalcemia or failure to thrive are all indications for early total or subtotal parathyroidectomy, which can significantly improve prognosis and quality of life of infants with NSHPT.

Conclusions

The management of patients with NSHPT can be very challenging. This case of NSHPT suggests that a near-miss event, as well as a case of SIDS, could be due to severe hypercalcemia and also presents the difficulties of medical management.

The identification of the specific CaSR mutation is useful not only for prenatal diagnosis, but also because could explain the response to Cinacalcet.

In most cases, surgical treatment remains the gold standard treatment of NSHPT. There are cases of subtotal parathyroidectomy followed for 10 years of follow-up, without need for a second surgical treatment [25].

Abbreviations

AGA: Appropriate for gestational age; CaSR: Calcium sensing receptor; DOL: Day of life; FHH: Familial hypocalciuric hypercalcemia; NSHPT: Neonatal severe primary hyperparathyroidism; PTH: Parathyroid hormone.

Funding
Not applicable.

Authors' contributions
MC and NL analyzed and interpreted the patient data and reviewed the initial manuscript. VG and MA performed the genetic examinations. GM performed surgical treatment of the infant. ND and CT made substantial contributions to data interpretation and reviewed and revised the manuscript. IC and AD drafted the initial manuscript and revised the final manuscript. All authors read and approved the final manuscript.

Competing interests
The authors declare that they have no competing interests.

Author details
[1]Neonatology and Neonatal Intensive Care Unit, Department of Biomedical Science ad Human Oncology, University of Bari "Aldo Moro", Bari, Italy. [2]S.C. Pediatria, P.O.C. SS. Annunziata Hospital, Taranto, Italy. [3]Medical Genetics, IRCCS Casa Sollievo della Sofferenza Hospital, San Giovanni Rotondo, Foggia, Italy. [4]Department of Pediatrics, Endocrine, Diabetes and Metabolic Unit, Istituto Giannina Gaslini, University of Genova, Genoa, Italy. [5]Neonatology and Neonatal Intensive Care Unit, Istituto Giannina Gaslini, Genoa, Italy. [6]Pediatric Surgery Unit, Istituto Giannina Gaslini, University of Genoa, Genoa, Italy. [7]Policlinico Hospital, Piazza Giulio Cesare n. 11, 70124 Bari, Italy.

References
1. García Soblechero E, Ferrer Castillo MT, Jiménez Crespo B, Domínguez Quintero ML, González Fuentes C. Neonatal hypercalcemia due to a homozygous mutation in the calcium-sensing receptor: failure of cinacalcet. Neonatology. 2013;104:104–8.
2. Ward DT. Calcium receptor-mediated intracellular signalling. Cell Calcium. 2004;35:217–28.
3. Hendy GN, D'Souza-Li L, Yang B, Canaff L, Cole DE. Mutations of the calcium-sensing receptor (CASR) in familial hypocalciuric hypercalcemia, neonatal severe hyperparathyroidism, and autosomal dominant hypocalcemia. Hum Mutat. 2000;16:281–96.
4. Lu JYL, Yang Y, Gnacadja G, Christopoulos A, Reagan JD. Effect of the calcimimetic R-568 [3-(2-chlorophenyl)-N-((1R)-1-(3-methoxyphenyl) ethyl)-1-propanamine] on correcting inactivating mutations in the human calcium-sensing receptor. J Pharmacol Exp Ther. 2009;331:775–86.
5. Chen RA, Goodman WG. Role of the calcium-sensing receptor in parathyroid gland physiology. Am J Physiol Renal Physiol. 2004;286:F1005–11.
6. Reh CMS, Hendy GN, Cole DEC, Jeandron DD. Neonatal hyperparathyroidism with a heterozygous calcium-sensing receptor (CASR) R185Q mutation: clinical benefit from cinacalcet. J Clin Endocrinol Metab. 2011;96:E707–12.
7. Wilhelm-Bals A, Parvex P, Magdelaine C, Girardin E. Successful use of bisphosphonate and calcimimetic in neonatal severe primary hyperparathyroidism. Pediatrics. 2012;129:e812–6.
8. Gannon AW, Monk HM, Levine MA. Cinacalcet monotherapy in neonatal severe hyperparathyroidism: a case study and review. J Clin Endocrinol Metab. 2014;99:7–11.
9. García-García E, Domínguez-Pascual I, Requena-Díaz M, Cabello-Laureano R, Fernández-Pineda I, Sánchez-Martín MJ. Intraoperative parathyroid hormone monitoring in neonatal severe primary hyperparathyroidism. Pediatrics. 2014;134:e1203–5.
10. Ismail A, Abbas TO, Al-Khalaf F. Needle in a haystack-parathyroid gland in a 10-day old infant: a case report and literature review. ISRN Pediatr. 2011; 2011:678070.
11. Egbuna OI, Brown EM. Hypercalcaemic and hypocalcaemic conditions due to calcium-sensing receptor mutations. Best Pract Res Clin Rheumatol. 2008; 22:129–48.
12. Nesbit MA, Hannan FM, Howles SA, Babinsky VN, Head RA, Cranston T, et al. Mutations affecting G-protein subunit α11 in hypercalcemia and hypocalcemia. N Engl J Med. 2013;368:2476–86.
13. Diaz-Thomas A, Cannon J, Iyer P, Al-Maawali A, Fazalullah M, Diamond F, et al. A novel CASR mutation associated with neonatal severe hyperparathyroidism transmitted as an autosomal recessive disorder. J Pediatr Endocrinol Metab JPEM. 2014;27:851–6.
14. Guarnieri V, Canaff L, Yun FHJ, Scillitani A, Battista C, Muscarella LA, et al. Calcium-sensing receptor (CASR) mutations in hypercalcemic states: studies from a single endocrine clinic over three years. J Clin Endocrinol Metab. 2010;95:1819–29.
15. Fisher MM, Cabrera SM, Imel EA. Successful treatment of neonatal severe hyperparathyroidism with cinacalcet in two patients. Endocrinol Diabetes Metab Case Rep. 2015;2015:150040.
16. Sebestyen JF, Srivastava T, Alon US. Bisphosphonates use in children. Clin Pediatr (Phila). 2012;51:1011–24.
17. Anderson K, Ruel E, Adam MA, Thomas S, Youngwirth L, Stang MT, et al. Subtotal vs. total parathyroidectomy with autotransplantation for patients with renal hyperparathyroidism have similar outcomes. Am J Surg. 2017;214:914–9.
18. Atay Z, Bereket A, Haliloglu B, Abali S, Ozdogan T, Altuncu E, et al. Novel homozygous inactivating mutation of the calcium-sensing receptor gene (CASR) in neonatal severe hyperparathyroidism-lack of effect of cinacalcet. Bone. 2014;64:102–7.
19. D'Souza-Li L. The calcium-sensing receptor and related diseases. Arq Bras Endocrinol Metabol. 2006;50:628–39.
20. Pearce SH, Trump D, Wooding C, Besser GM, Chew SL, Grant DB, et al. Calcium-sensing receptor mutations in familial benign hypercalcemia and neonatal hyperparathyroidism. J Clin Invest. 1995;96:2683–92.
21. Kobayashi M, Tanaka H, Tsuzuki K, Tsuyuki M, Igaki H, Ichinose Y, et al. Two novel missense mutations in calcium-sensing receptor gene associated with neonatal severe hyperparathyroidism. J Clin Endocrinol Metab. 1997;82:2716–9.
22. Oda Y, Tu CL, Pillai S, Bikle DD. The calcium sensing receptor and its alternatively spliced form in keratinocyte differentiation. J Biol Chem. 1998; 273:23344–52.
23. null N, null F. Calcimimetic compounds: a direct approach to controlling plasma levels of parathyroid hormone in hyperparathyroidism. Trends Endocrinol Metab TEM. 1999;10:66–71.
24. Murphy H, Patrick J, Báez-Irizarry E, Lacassie Y, Gómez R, Vargas A, et al. Neonatal severe hyperparathyroidism caused by homozygous mutation in CASR: a rare cause of life-threatening hypercalcemia. Eur J Med Genet. 2016; 59:227–31.
25. Alagaratnam S, Brain C, Spoudeas H, Dattani MT, Hindmarsh P, Allgrove J, et al. Surgical treatment of children with hyperparathyroidism: single Centre experience. J Pediatr Surg. 2014;49:1539–43.

21

A retrospective study of neonatal case management and outcomes in rural Rwanda post implementation of a national neonatal care package for sick and small infants

Merab Nyishime[1*], Ryan Borg[1], Willy Ingabire[1], Bethany Hedt-Gauthier[1,3], Evrard Nahimana[1], Neil Gupta[1,4], Anne Hansen[5], Michelle Labrecque[5], Fulgence Nkikabahizi[2], Christine Mutaganzwa[1], Francois Biziyaremye[1], Claudine Mukayiranga[2], Francine Mwamini[2] and Hema Magge[1,4,5,6]

Abstract

Background: Despite worldwide efforts to reduce neonatal mortality, 44% of under-five deaths occur in the first 28 days of life. The primary causes of neonatal death are preventable or treatable. This study describes the presentation, management and outcomes of hospitalized newborns admitted to the neonatal units of two rural district hospitals in Rwanda after the 2012 launch of a national neonatal protocol and standards.

Methods: We retrospectively reviewed routinely collected data for all neonates (0 to 28 days) admitted to the neonatal units at Rwinkwavu and Kirehe District Hospitals from January 1, 2013 to December 31, 2014. Data on demographic and clinical characteristics, clinical management, and outcomes were analyzed using median and interquartile ranges for continuous data and frequencies and proportions for categorical data. Clinical management and outcome variables were stratified by birth weight and differences between low birth weight (LBW) and normal birth weight (NBW) neonates were assessed using Fisher's exact or Wilcoxon rank-sum tests at the $\alpha = 0.05$ significance level.

Results: A total of 1723 neonates were hospitalized over the two-year study period; 88.7% were admitted within the first 48 h of life, 58.4% were male, 53.8% had normal birth weight and 36.4% were born premature. Prematurity (27.8%), neonatal infection (23.6%) and asphyxia (20.2%) were the top three primary diagnoses. Per national protocol, vital signs were assessed every 3 h within the first 48 h for 82.6% of neonates ($n = 965/1168$) and 93.4% ($n = 312/334$) of neonates with infection received antibiotics. The overall mortality rate was 13.3% ($n = 185/1386$) and preterm/LBW infants had similar mortality rate to NBW infants (14.7 and 12.2% respectively, $p = 0.131$). The average length of stay in the neonatal unit was 5 days.

Conclusions: Our results suggest that it is possible to provide specialized neonatal care for both LBW and NBW high-risk neonates in resource-limited settings. Despite implementation challenges, with the introduction of the neonatal care package and defined clinical standards these most vulnerable patients showed survival rates comparable to or higher than neighboring countries.

Keywords: Neonatal mortality, Neonate, Low birth weight, Prematurity, Quality of care, Mortality rate

* Correspondence: nymerab@gmail.com
[1]Partners In Health/Inshuti Mu Buzima (PIH/IMB), P.O. Box 3432, Kigali, Rwanda

Background

Despite efforts to reduce neonatal mortality globally, in 2015, nearly half of the 5.9 million under-five deaths occurred in the first 28 days of life [1] and eight of the 10 countries with the highest neonatal mortality rates are in sub-Saharan Africa (SSA) [2]. The main clinical causes of death include prematurity, infection, inadequate management of complications of pregnancy and delivery, and lack of quality care immediately after birth [1–4]. The majority of these deaths are preventable through evidence-based clinical interventions, such as antibiotic administration [5], oxygen therapy, continuous positive airway pressure [6] and caffeine treatment [7, 8]. However, implementing these interventions in resource-limited settings can be challenging due to health system constraints, including limited equipment, lack of standardized protocols to guide neonatal management, insufficient training and support for clinical staff, and the shortage of pediatricians and neonatologists [9, 10].

In Rwanda, there has been a tremendous reduction in under-five mortality, which fell from 196 per 1000 live births in 2000 to 50 per 1000 live births in 2015, making the country one of the few in SSA to achieve the Millennium Development Goals for child mortality [11–14]. In addition, the neonatal mortality rate significantly declined from 41 per 1000 live births in 1990 to 17 per 1000 live births in 2016 [2]. Although national surveillance systems are able to provide population level data on neonatal survival [15], little data exists on the treatment and quality of care provided to high-risk newborns at health facilities, as well as predictors of clinical success in Rwanda or other countries in SSA. One study conducted in a rural Rwandan district hospital reported that over 60% of neonatal deaths occurred at presentation or shortly after admission and could be attributed in part to the lack of trained staff and lack of standard care practice supported by protocols [16]. Subsequently, the researchers identified the need for training staff and establishing protocols as vital for improving neonatal care.

The Rwanda Ministry of Health (MOH) developed a national neonatal care protocol and standards in partnership with a number of organizations, including Partners In Health/Inshuti Mu Buzima (PIH/IMB) - an international non-profit organization committed to improving health services in impoverished communities - and specialists from Boston Children's Hospital in Boston, USA. The neonatal care package was nationally adopted in 2012 with the goal of providing quality care to sick and preterm/low birth weight infants in rural district hospitals which lack specialist physicians [17, 18]. The protocol was initially implemented and tested in the neonatal units of two rural PIH/IMB supported MOH district hospitals in 2010–2011. Details on the development and implementation of the newborn medicine program have been reported previously in Hansen et al's 2015 study [18]. The protocol implementation included roll-out of standardized medical records, quality indicators, and corresponding training materials. Here, we describe the presentation, clinical management, and outcomes of neonates after approximately 2 years of implementation of the neonatal care package. Neonates admitted between January 2013 and December 2014 to the neonatal units of the two rural district hospitals where the care package was first introduced were included. We also compared outcomes between low birth weight (LBW) and normal birth weight (NBW) neonates to detect any differences that may exist in the delivery of care to these patients. We aimed to highlight successes and gaps in the implementation of the national neonatal care package that could support quality care provision for neonates in Rwanda and similar settings.

Methods

Study design and setting

This retrospective cross-sectional study included neonates admitted to the neonatal units of PIH/IMB supported MOH Rwinkwavu and Kirehe District Hospitals (RDH, KDH). Both hospitals are located in rural areas of the Eastern Province of Rwanda and serve a total population of approximately 550,000 [19]. The initial roll-out involved international neonatal physician and nurse specialist support. After introduction, routine technical support has included support for training and ongoing mentorship of general practitioners and nurses working in the neonatal units by PIH/IMB-employed Rwandan nurse mentors. Visiting specialist physicians supporting PIH/IMB's medical education mission provided intermittent support. Additionally, PIH/IMB provided targeted support for essential equipment and consumables as part of health system strengthening.

At either of these two district hospitals, about 2700 to 2800 deliveries per year are recorded and roughly over 90% are referrals from health centers in the district hospitals' catchment areas. The average facility delivery rate in the Eastern Province is 88.8% [15]. When neonates are born in clinical distress or exhibit risk factors such as LBW, prematurity, sepsis or birth asphyxia, they are transferred to a neonatal unit for ongoing clinical management.

Neonatal unit structure and function

At the time of this study, seven to ten certified nurses or midwives staffed each neonatal unit. During the day shift, two nurses/midwives worked in the neonatology unit and one general practitioner (GP) supervised both the pediatric and neonatal units. Overnight, one to two GPs staffed the hospital and nurses/midwives in the neonatal units called them if in need of assistance. On average, there were 10 to 15 neonates in the neonatal unit at each hospital per day.

Training and on-site mentorship were provided intermittently throughout the study period by an expert physician and nurse trainers to the physicians and nurses staffing the units. Available equipment in the neonatal units included beds for kangaroo mother/skin-to-skin care, syringe pumps, incubators, radiant warmers and phototherapy units since 2011 and bubble continuous positive airway pressure (bCPAP) machines had recently been introduced in January 2013.

Study population, sources of data and analysis

All neonates aged 0 to 28 days and admitted to the hospitals between January 1, 2013, and December 31, 2014 were included in our analysis. Data was extracted from patients' medical files using a standardized neonatal data collection form and entered into an electronic database by hired and trained non-clinical data officers supporting hospital monitoring and evaluation. Before data collection the officers completed a two-day orientation and training that focused on specific clinical terms used in the neonatal units and how to read patients' medical files and abstract data from the file to the data collection form. The data were extracted over a one-month period of time.

We analyzed a subset of data that contained neonatal demographic and clinical characteristics, clinical management and outcome information. The clinical management variables are based on the quality indicators, which were originally drafted for the protocol according to expert opinion and literature review and later modified to address topics identified as challenging by hospital clinical staff. The indicators aim to monitor key aspects of neonatal care provision per protocol, with a focus on the needs of sick, LBW and preterm neonates [17, 18]. The indicators tracked the monitoring of vital signs, thermoregulation, hypoglycemia, administration of antibiotics for infectious diseases, fluid electrolytes and nutrition, and respiratory distress and included targets for high quality (Table 1). Cut-off point for hypoglycemia changed during the study period. Originally, low blood sugar was defined as less than 40 mg/dl. The definition was eventually changed to be less than 45 mg/dl in order to support more cautious clinical management. It took time for the new definition to be applied, so for the purposes of our analysis we used the range of less than 40 or less than 45 mg/dl to define low blood sugar.

For this study, the antibiotic indicator is limited to antibiotics provided in the first 24 h of therapy. For routine monitoring and evaluation, it was most feasible to assess all charts with antibiotic provision, rather than algorithmic exclusions of those who were ruled out within 72 h. Additionally, medication safety is a critical issue, particularly when introducing treatments in a neonatal population which can require dilution calculations. Therefore, the routinely monitored indicator was adapted to the version included here. Correct dose and interval for the first 24 h of therapy was determined according to the national neonatal protocol [17]. The actual dose administered was compared to the calculated correct dose using the

Table 1 Quality indicators definitions and targets

Category	Indicator Definitions	Targets
Vital signs	Percent of patient records in which vital signs are documented on average every 3 h within the first 48 h of admission	*15 (every 3 h × 48 h with possibility of one less on day of admission) per patient and 80% overall.*
Thermoregulation	Percent of neonates who have first temperature documented within 30 min of admission to neonatal unit	*80%*
	Percent of neonates with documented first temperature after admission < 36.0 °C having temperature improve to > 36.0 °C in ≤2 h	*80%*
Hypoglycemia[a]	Percent of neonates with documented blood sugar < 40- < 45 mg/dL who had blood sugar level improve to > 40- > 45 mg/dL within 1 h	*80%*
Infectious disease	Percent of neonates who received antibiotics (ampicillin and gentamicin) at correct dose and interval for first 24 h of therapy	*80%*
Fluid electrolytes and nutrition	Percent of neonates admitted to neonatal unit within first 48 h of life and remain in unit until at least 2 weeks of age who regain their birth weight by < 2 weeks of age	*80%*
Respiratory	Percent of neonates with BW < 1.5 kg or GA < 33 weeks for whom methylxanthine treatment (caffeine or aminophylline) is prescribed	*80%*
	Percent of preterm/LBW neonates eligible for CPAP who are started on CPAP within 2 h of life (eligibility criteria: BW < 2 kg or GA < 33 weeks and any degree of respiratory distress - O_2 saturation ≤ 90% oxygen requirement and/or RR ≥50 and/or grunting/flaring/retractions)	*90%*

°C degrees centigrade, *mg/dL* milligrams per deciliter, *BW* birth weight, *LBW* low birth weight, *kg* kilogram, *GA* gestational age, *O2* Oxygen, *RR* respiratory rate, *CPAP* continuous positive airway pressure

[a]Cut-off point for hypoglycemia changed during the study period. Originally, low blood sugar was defined as less than 40 mg/dl. The definition was eventually changed to be less than 45 mg/dl. It took time for the new definition to be applied, so for the purposes of our analysis we used the range of less than 40 or less than 45 mg/dl to define low blood sugar

neonate's birth weight, and administration interval was calculated using the time of medication administration as documented. In the two participating hospitals, the quality indicators were reviewed quarterly to monitor progress and inform quality improvement initiatives. All extracted data was verified for accuracy and completeness during routine audits performed by the MOH's and PIH/IMB's monitoring and evaluation teams.

We report demographic and clinical characteristics, clinical management and outcome variables using frequencies and proportions for categorical data and medians with interquartile ranges (IQR) for continuous data. We stratified the data by birth weight and used Fisher's exact tests for categorical variables and Wilcoxon rank-sum tests for continuous variables to compare clinical management and outcomes variables between LBW and NBW neonates at the $\alpha = 0.05$ significance level. NBW included neonates with a birth weight of ≥2500 g. LBW included neonates with a birth weight < 2500 g, with the sub-categories of extremely LBW neonates (< 1000 g), very LBW neonates (1000 to 1499 g) and LBW neonates (1500 to 2499 g). Although not used for stratification, gestational age is reported for some variables and was categorized as term (≥37 weeks) and preterm (<37 weeks). Outcomes included the number of neonates discharged, transferred, absconded (defined as leaving against medical advice) and deceased at the end of the study period, as well as weight at discharge and length of stay in the neonatal unit. Missing data were analyzed using a pairwise deletion for the missing data at random. Data were analyzed using Stata v13 (College Station, TX: StataCorp LP).

Results

A total of 1723 neonates were admitted to the two district hospital neonatology units; 49.7% ($n = 856$) to Kirehe and 50.3% ($n = 867$) to Rwinkwavu (Table 2), respectively. Admission age was recorded for 1684 neonates; 88.7% ($n = 1493$) were admitted within the first 48 h of life and 58.4% ($n = 949$ of 1624) were males. Birth weight was recorded for 1518 neonates and gestational age recorded for 1528; 46.2% ($n = 501$) were LBW and 53.8% ($n = 817$) were NBW, and 36.4% ($n = 556$) were preterm and 63.6% ($n = 972$) were term. The top three primary diagnoses (among the 1663 neonates with recorded diagnoses) were prematurity (27.8%, $n = 463$), neonatal infection (23.6%, $n = 392$), and asphyxia (20.2%, $n = 336$).

For clinical management during a hospital stay, 82.6% ($n = 965$ of 1168) of neonates had their vital signs checked and documented at least 15 times within the first 48 h of their hospital admission (Table 3). For thermoregulation, 55.0% ($n = 812$ of 1476) of neonates had their initial temperature measured within 30 min of admission; 29.4% ($n = 435$ of 1480) had an initial

Table 2 Socio-demographic and clinical characteristics of neonates admitted to neonatology units at two rural district hospitals in Rwanda ($N = 1723$)

	n	%
Hospital		
Kirehe	856	49.7
Rwinkwavu	867	50.3
Age at admission (days)	$N = 1621$	
< 1	1140	70.3
1–3	310	19.1
4–7	54	3.3
8–28	117	7.2
Admitted in first 48 h of life	$N = 1684$	
Yes	1493	88.7
No	191	11.3
Gender	$N = 1624$	
Male	949	58.4
Female	675	41.6
Birth weight (grams)	$N = 1518$	
Low birth weight (< 2500)	701	46.2
LBW (≥1500- < 2500)	528	34.8
Very LBW (≥1000- < 1500)	139	9.2
Extremely LBW (< 1000)	34	2.2
Normal birth weight (≥2500)	817	53.8
Gestational age (weeks)	$N = 1528$	
Preterm (<37)	556	36.4
Preterm (≥33 to < 37)	391	25.6
Very preterm (< 33)	165	10.8
Term (≥37)	972	63.6
Primary diagnosis	$N = 1663$	
Prematurity	463	27.8
Neonatal infection	392	23.6
Asphyxia at birth/low APGAR score/HIE	336	20.2
Respiratory distress/apnea	113	6.8
Low birth weight	95	5.7
Poor feeding	51	3.1
Malformation	36	2.2
Convulsion	28	1.7
Pneumonia	21	1.3
Jaundice	13	0.8
Hypothermia	10	0.6
Hypoglycemia	8	0.5
Others	97	5.8

LBW Low birth weight, *APGAR* A measurement of Appearance, Pulsation, Grimace, Activity and Respiration, *HIE* Hypoxic Ischemic Encephalopathy

Table 3 Clinical management and interim outcomes of neonates with birth weight recorded upon admission to neonatology units at two rural district hospitals in Rwanda ($N = 1518$)

	All neonates ($N = 1518$)		Low birth weight (< 2500 g) ($N = 701$)		Normal birth weight (≥2500 g) ($N = 817$)		*p*-value
	n	%	n	%	n	%	
Vital signs							
Vital signs checked every 3 h for the first 48 h of admission	$N = 1168$		$N = 556$		$N = 612$		
Yes (≥15 times)	965	82.6	478	86.0	487	79.6	0.004
No (< 15 times)	203	17.4	78	14.0	125	20.4	
Thermoregulation							
Initial temperature measured within 30 min of admission	$N = 1476$		$N = 683$		$N = 793$		
Yes	812	55.0	367	53.7	445	56.1	0.373
No	664	45.0	316	46.3	348	43.9	
Initial temperature < 36 °C	$N = 1480$		$N = 684$		$N = 796$		
Yes	435	29.4	249	36.4	186	23.4	< 0.001
No	1045	70.6	435	63.6	610	76.6	
If initial temperature < 36 °C, temperature improved from < 36 °C to > 36 °C within 2 h	$N = 402$		$N = 234$		$N = 168$		
Yes	156	38.8	99	42.3	57	33.9	0.097
No	246	61.2	135	57.7	111	66.1	
Hypoglycemia							
Low blood sugar (< 40/< 45 mg/dl)	$N = 871$		$N = 418$		$N = 453$		
Yes	31	3.6	21	5.0	10	2.2	0.028
No	840	96.4	397	95.0	443	97.8	
If blood sugar low, improved to > 40/> 45 mg/dl within 1 h	$N = 12$		$N = 7$		$N = 5$		
Yes	2	16.7	1	14.3	1	20	> 0.999
No	10	83.3	6	85.7	4	80	
Infectious diseases							
Received antibiotics (ampicillin and gentamicin)[a]	$N = 334$		$N = 69$		$N = 265$		
Yes	312	93.4	68	98.6	244	92.1	0.053
No	22	6.6	1	1.4	21	7.9	
Ampicillin received at correct dose and interval	$N = 301$		N = 66		$N = 235$		
Yes	204	67.8	36	54.6	168	71.5	0.009
No	97	32.2	30	45.4	67	28.5	
Gentamicin received at correct does and interval	$N = 286$		$N = 64$		$N = 222$		
Yes	146	51.0	23	35.9	123	55.4	0.006
No	140	49.0	41	64.1	99	44.6	
Fluid electrolytes and nutrition							
Regained birth weight within 2 weeks[b]	$N = 225$		$N = 169$		$N = 56$		
Yes	126	56.0	88	52.1	38	67.9	0.044
No	99	44.0	81	47.9	18	32.1	
Respiratory distress							
Received caffeine[c]			$N = 548$				
Yes			206	37.6			
No			342	62.4			

Table 3 Clinical management and interim outcomes of neonates with birth weight recorded upon admission to neonatology units at two rural district hospitals in Rwanda ($N = 1518$) *(Continued)*

	All neonates ($N = 1518$)		Low birth weight (< 2500 g) ($N = 701$)		Normal birth weight (≥2500 g) ($N = 817$)		*p*-value
	n	%	n	%	n	%	
Received oxygen therapy	$N = 1491$		$N = 690$		$N = 801$		
Yes	603	40.4	278	40.3	325	40.6	0.916
No	888	59.6	412	59.7	476	59.4	
Method of oxygen therapy	$N = 540$		$N = 247$		$N = 293$		
Mask/nasal cannula	449	83.1	185	74.9	264	90.1	< 0.001
bCPAP	91	16.9	62	25.1	29	9.9	
If eligible, received bCPAP[d]			$N = 107$				
Yes			13	12.2			
No			94	87.8			
Duration of oxygen therapy in hours	Median	IQR	Median	IQR	Median	IQR	
Mask/nasal cannula	24	20, 96	48	24, 120	24	14, 72	0.050
bCPAP	60	24, 120	72	24, 144	48	24, 72	0.093

[a]For neonates with primary diagnosis of infection; [b]Restricted to neonates that were hospitalized for at least 2 weeks; [c]Restricted to preterm neonates (< 33 weeks) or LBW (< 1500 g); [d]Restricted to preterm (< 33 weeks) or LBW (< 1500 g) neonates with any sign of respiratory distress
°C degrees centigrade, *gm/dl* grams per decilitre, *bCPAP* bubble continuous positive airway pressure, *IQR* inter-quartile range

temperature below 36 °C recorded, and 38.8% ($n = 156$ of 402) had an initial temperature below 36 °C improve to be greater than 36 °C within 2 h of the time the initial temperature was taken. Hypoglycemia was also assessed; 3.6% (31 of 871) of neonates had low blood sugar levels (either < 40 or < 45 mg/dl) and 16.7% ($n = 2$ of 12) neonates with low blood sugar improved to have a blood sugar measurement of either > 40 or > 45 mg/dl documented within the hour.

Of the 334 neonates with a primary diagnosis of infection, 93.4% ($n = 312$) received antibiotics. Among the 301 neonates who had data recorded on ampicillin administration and the 286 neonates who had data recorded on gentamicin administration, 67.8% ($n = 204$) and 51.0% ($n = 146$) received the correct dose at the correct time interval, respectively. Of 225 neonates who stayed in the hospital for at least 14 days, 56.0% ($n = 126$) regained their birth weight within the 2 weeks. With regard to respiratory support, 40.4% ($n = 603$) of 1491 neonates received oxygen therapy. Of 540 neonates with oxygen therapy method documented, 83.1% ($n = 449$) received mask or nasal cannula and 16.9% ($n = 91$) received bCPAP. Of the 107 preterm/low birth weight neonates meeting eligibility criteria for bCPAP (born < 1500 g or < 33 weeks and showing any signs of respiratory distress), 12.2% ($n = 13$) received bCPAP. Among the 548 neonates born < 1500 g or < 33 weeks (meeting eligibility criteria), 37.6% ($n = 206$) received caffeine citrate.

When results were stratified by birth weight, there was no evidence of differences in clinical management between LBW and NBW neonates for the following variables: initial temperature measured within 30 min of admission ($p = 0.373$), improvement in initial temperature from < 36 °C to > 36 °C ($p = 0.097$), improvement in low blood sugar levels to normal levels ($p > 0.999$), and administration of oxygen therapy ($p = 0.916$) (Table 3).

However, we observed significant differences in the clinical management of LBW and NBW neonates for a number of variables. Vital signs were checked at least 15 times within the first 48 h of admission for 86.0% ($n = 478$ of 556) of LBW neonates and 79.6% ($n = 487$ of 612) of NBW neonates ($p = 0.004$). Antibiotics were administered to 98.6% ($n = 68$ or 69) of LBW neonates with infection and 92.1% ($n = 244$ of 265) of NBW neonates with infection ($p = 0.053$). Correct dosage and interval of ampicillin was provided to 54.6% ($n = 36$ of 66) LBW neonates and 71.5% ($n = 168$ of 235) NBW neonates ($p = 0.009$), and to 35.9% ($n = 23$ of 64) LBW neonates and 55.4% ($n = 123$ of 222) NBW neonates for gentamicin ($p = 0.006$). Approximately half (52.1%, $n = 88$ of 169) of LBW neonates regained birth weight within 2 weeks, compared to 67.9% ($n = 38$ of 56) of NBW neonates ($p = 0.044$). For method of oxygen therapy, LBW neonates were more likely to receive bCPAP compared to NBW neonates (25.1%, $n = 62$ of 247 and 9.9%, $n = 29$ of 293, respectively, $p < 0.001$). LBW neonates received oxygen for a longer duration, whether on mask/nasal cannula (median = 48 h, IQR: 24–120, $p = 0.050$) or bCPAP (median = 72 h, IQR: 24–144, $p = 0.093$) compared to NBW neonates, who used mask/nasal cannula for a median of 24 h (IQR 14–72) and bCPAP for a median of 48 h (IQR 24–72, $p = 0.093$).

Overall, 83.3% ($n = 1162$) of the neonates were discharged, 13.3% ($n = 185$) died, 2.3% ($n = 32$) transferred and 0.5% (n = 7) absconded (Table 4). The top three primary diagnoses among the 183 deceased neonates with primary diagnosis recorded were asphyxia (36.1%, $n = 66$), prematurity (29.5%, $n = 54$), and respiratory distress (13.1%, $n = 24$). There was no evidence of differences in outcomes between LBW and NBW neonates ($p = 0.131$). The overall median length of stay in the neonatal unit was 5 days (IQR: 2–10). The length of stay was significantly longer for LBW neonates (median = 7 days, IQR: 2–14) compared to NBW neonates (median = 4 days, IQR: 2–7, $p < 0.001$). This remained true when stratified by those who survived to discharge (median = 8 days, IQR: 3–18 vs. median = 5, IQR: 2–8, $p < 0.001$) and those who did not (median = 2 days, IQR: 0–2 vs median = 1 day, IQR: 0–2, $p = 0.003$). Of the neonates who were discharged, 477 were low birthweight at admission, and 94.1% ($n = 449$) remained under 2500 g when they were discharged, while of the 536 neonates of normal birthweight at admission, 12.3% ($n = 66$) were under 2500 g at discharge ($p < 0.001$).

Discussion

Neonatal care provision in rural resource-limited settings is a challenge for many countries in SSA and in the early stages of introduction [18–25]. Hansen et al. (2015) showed that while neonatal care may be considered a specialized clinical service, it can be standardized and implemented in rural district hospitals in Rwanda [18]. Here, we show clinical management and quality of neonatal care in two rural district hospitals that were guided by this neonatal care package. Our study had a number of key results.

First, we found that the demographic and clinical characteristics of our neonatal sample were similar to those reported in other studies. Consistent with studies showing higher and earlier hospital admission rates for neonates within the first 7 days of birth and higher morbidity rates among male neonates [2, 20, 26, 27], most neonates in our study were admitted to the neonatal units within the first 48 h after birth and were males. Prematurity, infection and asphyxia were the top three causes of infant illnesses, mirroring findings reported in other parts of SSA [1, 20, 27, 28]. These patterns show that more research into the underlying causes of neonatal illness in resource-limited settings is needed, as are interventions that can address these persistent challenges.

Second, our assessment of clinical management and outcome variables shows that it is possible to provide care to high-risk neonates in this setting with reasonable patient outcomes, particularly when compared to those of other countries in the region [27]. A study on the use of medicines in 104 developing and transitional countries from 1990 to 2009 found that the percentage of patients receiving antibiotics increased from 45 to 54% over this 20-year period [29] and the management of prematurity-related complications using antibiotics was only 50% [27]. Additionally, the majority of LBW neonates, who are at the highest risk of morbidity, were more likely to receive care according to protocol compared to

Table 4 Outcomes of neonates with birth weight recorded upon admission to neonatology units at two rural district hospitals in Rwanda ($N = 1518$)

	All neonates ($N = 1518$)		Low birth weight (< 2500 g) ($N = 701$)		Normal birth weight (≥2500 g) ($N = 817$)		*p*-value
	n	%	n	%	n	%	
Outcome	$N = 1386$		$N = 626$		$N = 760$		
Discharged	1162	83.3	522	83.4	640	84.2	0.131
Transferred	32	2.3	11	1.8	21	2.8	
Absconded	7	0.5	1	0.2	6	0.8	
Died	185	13.3	92	14.7	93	12.2	
Length of stay[a]	Median	IQR	Median	IQR	Median	IQR	
All neonates	5	2, 10	7	2, 14	4	2, 7	< 0.001
Discharged	6	2, 11	8	3, 18	5	2, 8	< 0.001
Transferred	3	0.5, 9.5	3.5	0, 11	2.5	0.5, 7.5	0.722
Absconded	7	1, 15	21	21, 21	5	1, 8	0.134
Died	1	0, 3	2	1, 4	1	0, 2	0.003
Weight at discharge (grams)[b]	$N = 1013$		$N = 477$		$N = 536$		
< 2500	515	50.8	449	94.1	66	12.3	< 0.001
≥ 2500	498	49.2	28	5.9	470	87.7	

[a]Only reported for neonates that had an admission date and outcome date or age at admission and age at discharge; [b]Limited to neonates who were discharged

NBW neonates in a number of clinical domains, including close monitoring (vital sign measurement) and duration on oxygen therapy, which are important interventions to reduce clinical deterioration in this population [5, 30]. LBW neonates also stand to gain the greatest impact from bCPAP for the treatment of respiratory distress syndrome [5, 21] and their higher rates of bCPAP use and longer duration on oxygen therapy showed possible prioritization of their needs by health care workers, particularly in a staff-constrained environment. The transfer rate for neonates was low and impressively similar to a study conducted at a Rwandan provincial hospital (which is supposed to have a higher level of care than district hospitals) which reported a drop-in neonate transfer rates from 50 to 2% in 1 year after a series of quality improvement interventions were implemented, including introduction of standardized treatment procedures [16].

Finally, and most importantly, the overall neonatal unit survival rate for both LBW and NBW neonates was higher than results reported from similar settings and did not differ across birth weight categories [23, 26, 31]. This study is descriptive and limits any assessment of causality; however, given that no standardized care for sick and preterm infants was provided before the establishment of the neonatal care unit and these infants were previously being referred to the one national referral hospital in the country, it demonstrates that neonatal care can be provided in a decentralized manner with the appropriate investment in neonatal unit establishment, vastly improving population access to this essential service. Availability and ease of protocol use, presence of essential equipment and medications, along with intermittent training and mentorship for providers likely influenced the quality of care for high-risk neonates in these hospitals [32, 33]. Asphyxia was a leading diagnosis among those who died, which could indicate a greater need to target improvement efforts during delivery and immediately after birth and underscore the need for interdepartmental coordination within the hospital across maternity, delivery, and neonatal units. Further research assessing the impact of the neonatal care package on population level neonatal mortality, as well as assessment of the optimal content and level of complexity for rural district hospitals is warranted.

Despite these successes, there is still a need to improve treatment practices to meet quality indicator targets and further improve neonatal outcomes. These targets were intentionally set high to serve as a goal for quality improvement efforts. Based on our results, management of vital signs measurement, weight gain, administration of antibiotics and thermoregulation measurement of temperature within the first 30 min of admission were close to the targets, while other indicators, such as improved temperature within 2 h of admission, caffeine administration, improved blood sugar levels and weight gain were not. These results can be used to inform the design and goals of quality improvement initiatives so they can be most effective. For example, while LBW infants had relatively strong outcomes, a low percentage of the bCPAP-eligible LBW/preterm neonates received bCPAP therapy, indicating further potential gains in neonatal outcomes that could be made. While this gap could be exaggerated due to the fact that bCPAP was introduced in first month of the study period and may have improved with increasing health care worker comfort and practice over time during the study period, a gap in bCPAP implementation was also noted by a second bCPAP-focused study from an overlapping time period [34]. Therefore, this area has been targeted for quality improvement since the completion of this study.

In addition, while antibiotics were administered to neonates diagnosed with infections, there is room for improvement in the timing and dosage of these antibiotics. As these data were used for quarterly data review with the clinical teams, quality improvement problem analyses found a number of challenges with hospital level neonatal antibiotic administration. The dose has to be selected based on gestational age/birth weight and a weight-based dose had to be correctly calculated. Some providers new to neonatal care, or not providing neonatal care routinely, found this selection challenging, and more NBW neonates received correct administration of gentamicin. Staff shortages and high patient volume could be challenges to administering antibiotics on-time. There is also room for improvement around documentation and recordkeeping. Further exploration into the issue should be pursued by asking the neonatal nurses about the documentation processes they follow and challenges they face. Observation of documentation practices can also be done if possible. Strategies for improving documentation should be designed and implemented as a collaborative effort between nurses and researchers to better support uptake and sustainability.

Our results also show that quality improvement efforts need to be directed at NBW neonates as well. We found that 12% of neonates admitted to the hospital with a normal birthweight were discharged weighing less than 2500 g. While this could be focused among neonates born just above the LBW cut-off experiencing normal weight loss in the first few days of life with short-course hospitalizations, this may indicate that supporting neonatal growth and nutrition was challenging. Taking the full context into consideration, this may be due to a family's inability to pay for the costs of hospitalization or because parents are unable to leave other children at home or be absent from work to be in the hospital. Therefore, this finding warrants further investigation into how to support families comprehensively, and more interventions, such as social support packages that can address financial challenges, are needed to ensure these high-risk vulnerable neonates get the treatment they need to thrive.

Health systems challenges may have also influenced the ability to reach certain indicator targets. Not being able to apply to full protocol due to staffing shortages, high turnover of trained staff, misaligned rotations where providers not trained in neonatal care are assigned to the neonatal unit and stock outs of drug and laboratory reagents may have impacted the quality of care provided in the neonatal units [4, 28]. We recommend implementation of quality improvement projects that target the national indicators, accurate and timely documentation of management and outcomes, revision of the rotation system to ensure the nurses staffing the neonatal unit have necessary training and skills for neonatal management and harmonizing internal transfers of neonates to ensure continuity of care as activities that can address the challenges we see in our neonatal units [35].

It is important to note that the care protocol was not introduced as an isolated document – when first introduced, it was paired with medical record introduction, quality indicators, and institutionalized training and mentorship. More broadly, will-building across hospital leadership and health care providers to establish a neonatal unit with designated physician and nursing staff and management was critical to providing a setting in which this introduction could have any measure of success. The district hospitals have both adopted district-based quality improvement initiatives in response to these data which were reviewed quarterly, including projects aimed at accurate and timely documentation of management and outcomes, revision of the rotation system to ensure the nurses staffing the neonatal unit have necessary training and skills for neonatal management, and coordination of internal transfer processes of neonates to ensure continuity of care [36].

This study has several limitations. First, as a retrospective cross-sectional study over a two-year time period, we were unable to assess variations in quality across time and potential relationships with intervening variables such as those related to constrained health systems and timing of introduction of new initiatives such as bCPAP listed previously. We do not have data for year-to-year variations in the indicators. Data variation over a longer period would have to take issues like staffing and policy changes into consideration, which were outside the scope of this study. Along the same vein, we chose not to examine trends in performance on the quality indicators because we chose to focus on the current level of performance. Trends in performance in relation to specific quality improvement interventions could be the subject of future studies. Additionally, some of the diagnoses, such as infection and asphyxia, require laboratory evaluations for definitive diagnosis that were not available at this district hospital level [22]. However, we believe the clinical management to be appropriate if the provider closely followed the guidance for clinical management of a given suspected diagnosis, as they are designed to leverage the diagnostic resources available in these low-resource settings. Finally, another limitation was missing data, which we believe was due to the high documentation burden placed on the nurses and physicians staffing the neonatal units. Approximately 12% of the records were missing data and not included in the analysis of clinical management and interim outcomes shown in Table 3. Results were reported only for neonates who had a birth weight recorded upon admission to the neonatology unit. While missing data limited the ability to which we were able to generalize our study findings, we are still able to present outcomes and discuss our experiences of treating small and sick neonates in accordance with a national neonatal care package. Periodic data quality checks and training with an emphasis on the importance of proper documentation in clinical charts could improve data quality. In addition, future plans to implement electronic medical record systems in the hospital units could also help address these data quality gaps.

Conclusions

This study demonstrates the feasibility of specialized neonatal care in resource-limited settings supported by a standardized national package of services including infrastructure, training and supplies, as well as the implementation of a national neonatal protocol. LBW neonates received higher quality care compared to NBW and overall mortality rates were lower or comparable to other urban and tertiary hospital settings among both categories. However, gaps in care management remain that should be addressed in order to achieve further gains in morbidity and mortality. We recommend quality improvement efforts to address lagging indicators as well as continuous training and mentorship to ensure new providers are empowered with the tools necessary to provide high quality care to these vulnerable newborns and families.

Abbreviations

bCPAP: Bubble continuous positive airway pressure; GP: General practitioner; IQR: Interquartile range; KDH: Kirehe District Hospital; LBW: Low birth weight; NBW: Normal birth weight; °C: Degrees centigrade; PIH/IMB: Partners In Health/ Inshuti Mu Buzima; RDH: Rwinkwavu District Hospital; MOH: Ministry of Health; SSA: Sub-Saharan Africa

Acknowledgements

This study was developed under the Partners In Health/Inshuti Mu Buzima Intermediate Operational Research Training Program, developed and facilitated by Bethany Hedt-Gauthier and Neil Gupta. We thank Hari Iyer, Evariste Bigirimana and Jackline Odhiambo for their support in the data cleaning, analysis and manuscript editing. We also thank Janet Umuhoza and Liliose Mukantaganzwa for their help with data collection. We would like to acknowledge the Rwanda Ministry of Health for its leadership, and the doctors and nurses at Kirehe and Rwinkwavu District Hospitals who work tirelessly to improve the lives of newborns in their communities.

Funding
We acknowledge Partners In Health/Inshuti Mu Buzima and the IMB Innovation Grants for the support of this work. We acknowledge the PIH/IMB Doris Duke Charitable Foundation funds that supported data collection. The funding used for data collection for this study was part of a larger support by the Doris Duke Charitable Foundation. The funder had no direct role in any technical or intellectual aspect of this work.

Authors' contributions
MN led all aspects of the study from study design, data analysis and interpretation of results, and manuscript writing. BHG, NG and RB supported study design, analysis, and results interpretation and critically reviewed the manuscript. EN, WI, FN, FB, ChM, FM, CIM, ML and AH supported study design, and critically reviewed manuscript. HM supervised the study and supported design, results interpretation, and provided constructive feedback on the manuscript. All authors approved the final manuscript.

Competing interests
The authors declare that they have no competing interests.

Author details
[1]Partners In Health/Inshuti Mu Buzima (PIH/IMB), P.O. Box 3432, Kigali, Rwanda. [2]Ministry of Health, Kigali, Rwanda. [3]Department of Global Health and Social Medicine, Harvard Medical School, Boston, USA. [4]Brigham and Women's Hospital, Boston, USA. [5]Boston Children's Hospital, Boston, USA. [6]Institute for Healthcare Improvement, Addis Ababa, Ethiopia.

References
1. Liu L, Oza S, Hogan D, Chu Y, Perin J, Zhu J, et al. Global, regional, and national causes of under-5 mortality in 2000-15: an updated systematic analysis with implications for the sustainable development goals. Lancet. 2016;388(10063):3027–35. https://doi.org/10.1016/S0140-6736(16)31593-8.
2. UNICEF. Every Child Alive: The urgent need to end newborn deaths. Genève: United Nation's Children's Fund, UNICEF; 2016. available at https://www.unicef.org/publications/files/Every_Child_Alive_The_urgent_need_to_end_newborn_deaths.pdf. Accessed 7 Nov 2018.
3. Rüegger C, Hegglin M, Adams M, Bucher HU. Population based trends in mortality, morbidity and treatment for very preterm- and very low birth weight neonates over 12 years. BMC Pediatr. 2010;12(1):17.
4. Kinney MV, Kerber KJ, Black RE, Cohen B, Nkrumah F, Coovadia H, et al. Sub-Saharan Africa's mothers, newborns, and children: where and why do they die? PLoS Med. 2010;7(6):e1000294.
5. Zaidi AK, Tikmani SS, Sultana S, Baloch B, Kazi M, Rehman H, Karimi K, et al. Simplified antibiotic regimens for the management of clinically diagnosed severe infections in newborns and young facilities neonates in first-level in Karachi, Pakistan. Pediatr Infect Dis J. 2013;32(Suppl 1):S19–25. https://doi.org/10.1097/INF.0b013e31829ff7aa.
6. Martin S, Duke T, Davis P. Efficacy and safety of bubble CPAP in neonatal care in low and middle income countries: a systematic review. Arch Dis Child. 2014;99(6):F495–504.
7. Aranda JV, Gorman W, Bergsteinsson H, Gunn T. Efficacy of caffeine in treatment of apnea in the low-birth-weight infant. J Pediatrics. 1977;90(3):467–72.
8. Schmidt B, Roberts RS, Davis P, Doyle LW, Barrington KJ, Ohlsson A, et al. Caffeine therapy for apnea of prematurity. N Engl J Med. 2006;354:2112–21. https://doi.org/10.1056/NEJMoa054065
9. Bhutta ZA, Das JK, Bahl R, Lawn JE, Salam RA, Paul VK, et al. Can available interventions end preventable deaths in mothers, newborn babies, and stillbirths, and at what cost? Lancet. 2014;384(9940):347–70. https://doi.org/10.1016/S0140-6736(14)60792-3.
10. Darmstadt GL, Kinney MV, Chopra M, Cousens S, Kak L, Paul VK, Martines J, Bhutta ZA, Lawn JE. Who has been caring for the baby? Lancet. 2014; 384(9938):174–88. https://doi.org/10.1016/S0140-6736(14)60458.
11. Millennium Development Goals Rwanda Final Progress Report: 2013. Availabile at: http://www.rw.undp.org/content/rwanda/en/home/presscenter/articles/2015/03/31/millennium-development-goals-rwanda-final-progress-report-2013.html. Accessed 28 Aug 2016.
12. National Institute of Statistics of Rwanda. Rwanda Demographic and Health Survey 2014–2015: Final Report. Kigali: NISR; 2015. Available at: https://dhsprogram.com/publications/publication-fr316-dhs-final-reports.cfm. Accessed 28 Aug 2016
13. Winter R, Thomas P, Langston A, Ndicunguye V, Mivumbi PC, Rutayisire DN, et al. Trends in neonatal mortality in Rwanda, 2000–2010. DHS Further Analysis Reports. Calverton, Maryland: ICF International; 2013. p. 88. Available at: http://www.dhsprogram.com/pubs/pdf/FA88/FA88.pdf. Accessed 7 Nov 2018.
14. Farmer PE, Nutt CT, Wagner CM, et al. Reduced premature mortality in Rwanda: lessons from success. Br Med J. 2013;346:65 doi: 10/1136/bmj.f65.
15. Health Management Information Systems. National Institute of Statistics of Rwanda. Available at: http://statistics.gov.rw. Accessed 28 Aug 2016.
16. Kayinamura AM, Serubibi Y, Kakoma JB. Benefits of a neonatology service in a rural district hospital: case study of Rwamagana District hospital, Eastern Province of Rwanda. Rwanda Medical Journal. 2010;68:4.
17. Rwanda Ministry of Health. National neonatal care protocol. Kigali: MOH; 2012.
18. Hansen A, Magge H, Labrecque M, Munyaneza RBM, Nahimana E, Nyishime M, et al. The development and implementation of a newborn medicine program in resource- limited setting. Public Health Action. 2015;5(1):17–22.
19. National Institute of Statistics of Rwanda. 2012 Population and Housing Census. Kigali: NISR; 2012. Available at: http://www.statistics.gov.rw/publication/rphc4-atlas. Accessed 7 Nov 2018.
20. Hoque M, Kwadabeba CHC. Causes of neonatal admissions and deaths at a rural hospital in KwaZulu-Natal, South Africa. South Afr J Epidemiol Infect. 2011;26(1):26–9.
21. Ballot DE, Potterton J, Chirwa T, Hilburn N, Cooper PA. Developmental outcome of very low birth weight neonates in a developing country. BMC Pediatr. 2012;12(1):11.
22. Padayachee N, Ballot DE. Outcomes of neonates with perinatal asphyxia at a tertiary academic hospital in Johannesburg, South Africa. South Afr J Child Health. 2013;7(3):89–94.
23. Ike E, Modupe OO. Pattern of diseases and care outcomes of neonates admitted in special care baby unit of university college hospital, Ibadan, Nigeria from 2007 to 2011. IOSR journal of nursing and health. Science. 2015;4(3):2320–1959.
24. Lawn JE, Blencowe H, Oza S, You D, Lee ACC, Waiswa P, Lalli M, Bhutta ZA, Barros AJD, Christian P, Mathers C, Cousens SN. Progress, priorities, and potential beyond survival. Lancet. 2014;384(9938):189–205.
25. Arcury TA, Gesler WM, Preisser JS, Sherman J, Spencer J, Perin J. The effects of geography and spatial behavior on health care utilization among the residents of a rural region. BMC Health Serv Res. 2005;40(1):135–55.
26. Parkash J, Das N. Pattern of admissions to neonatal unit. J Coll Physicians Surg Pak. 2005;15(6):341–4.
27. Seale AC, Blencowe H, Manu AA, Nair H, Bahl R, Qazi AS, et al. Estimates of possible severe bacterial infection in neonates in sub-Saharan Africa, South Asia, and Latin America for 2012: a systematic review and meta-analysis. Lancet Infect Dis. 2014;14:731–41.
28. Vergnano S, Sharland M, Kazembe P, Mwansambo C. Neonatal sepsis: an international perspective. Arch Dis Child. 2005;90:F220–4.
29. Holloway KA, Ivanovska V, Wagner AK, Vialle-Valentine C, Ross-Degnan D. Have we improved the used of medicines in developing and transitional countries and do we know how to? Two decades of evidence. Tropical Med Int Health. 2013;18(6):656–64. https://doi.org/10.1111/tmi.12123.

30. Bancalari E, Claure N. Advances in respiratory support for high risk newborn infants. Matern Health Neonatol Perinatol. 2015;1:13 doi.org/10.1186/s40748-015-0014-5.
31. Chow S, Chow R, Popovic M, Lam M, Popovic M, Merrick J, Stashefsky M, Lam H, Milakovic M, Chow E, Popovic J. A selected review of the mortality rates of neonatal intensive care units. Front Public Health. 2015;3:225. https://doi.org/10.3389/fpubh.2015.00225.
32. Magge H, Manzi A, Rwabukwisi Cyamatare F, Mezzacappa C, Nkikabahizi F, Niyonzima S, Drobac PC, Ngabo F, Hirschhorn LR. Mentoring and quality improvement strengthen integrated management of childhood illness implementation in rural Rwanda. Arch Dis Child. 2014;0:1–6.
33. Manzi A, Magge H, Hedt-Gauthier BL, Michaelis AP, Cyamatare FR, Nyirazinyoye L, et al. Clinical mentorship to improve pediatric quality of care at the health centers in rural Rwanda: a qualitative study of perceptions and acceptability of health care workers. BMC Health Serv Res. 2014;14(1):275.
34. Nahimana E, Ngendahayo M, Magge H, Odhiambo J, Amoroso CL, Muhirwa E, Uwilingiyemungu JN, Nkikabahizi F, Habimana R, Hedt-Gauthier BL. Bubble CPAP to support preterm neonates in rural Rwanda: a retrospective cohort study. BMC Pediatr. 2015;15:135. https://doi.org/10.1186/s12887-015-0049-x.
35. Odhiambo J, Rwabukwisi FC, Rusangwa C, Rusanganwa V, Hirschhorn LR, Nahimana E, Ngamije P, Hedt-Gauthier BL. Health worker attrition at a rural district hospital in Rwanda: a need for improved placement and retention strategies. Pan Afr Med J. 2017;27:168.
36. Ingabire W, Reine PM, Hedt-Gauthier BL, Hirschhorn LR, Kirk CM, Nahimana E, Uwiringiyemungu JN, Ndayisaba A, Manzi A. Roadmap to an effective quality improvement and patient safety program implementation in a rural hospital setting. Healthcare. 2015;3:277–82. https://doi.org/10.1016/j.hjdsi.2015.10.010.

22

Can echocardiographic screening in the early days of life detect critical congenital heart disease among apparently healthy newborns?

Miyuki Kondo*, Akira Ohishi, Toru Baba, Tomoka Fujita and Shigeo Iijima

Abstract

Background: Delayed diagnosis of critical congenital heart disease (CCHD) carries a serious risk of mortality, morbidity, and handicap. As echocardiography is commonly used to diagnose congenital heart disease (CHD), echocardiographic investigations in newborns may be helpful in detecting CCHD earlier and with higher sensitivity than when using other screening methods. The present study aimed to evaluate the effectiveness of echocardiographic screening for CCHD in a tertiary care center.

Methods: A retrospective chart review was conducted among newborns delivered at Hamamatsu University Hospital between June 2009 and May 2016. The study included consecutive newborns who underwent early echocardiographic screening (within the first 5 days of life) performed by pediatric cardiologists, were born at ≥36 weeks of gestation, had a birthweight ≥2300 g, and were cared for in the well-baby nursery. Newborns admitted to the neonatal intensive care unit, as well as those with prenatal diagnosis of CHD and/or clinical symptoms or signs of CHD were excluded. Four CHD outcome categories were defined: critical, serious, clinically significant, and clinically non-significant.

Results: A total of 4082 live newborns were delivered during the study period. Of 3434 newborns who met the inclusion criteria and had complete echocardiography data, 104 (3.0%) were diagnosed as having CHD. Among these, none was initially diagnosed as having critical or serious CHD. Of the 95 newborns who continued follow-up with a cardiologist, 61 (64%) were determined to have non-significant CHDs that resolved within 6 months of life. Review of excluded newborns revealed nine cases of critical or serious CHD; among these newborns, six were diagnosed prenatally and three had some clinical signs of CHD prior to hospital discharge.

Conclusions: In our tertiary care center, echocardiography screening within the first 5 days of life did not help improve CCHD detection rate in newborns without prenatal diagnosis or clinical signs of CHD. Echocardiographic screening may be associated with increased rate of false-positives (defects resulting in clinically non-significant CHDs) in newborns without prenatal diagnosis or suspicion of CHD.

Keywords: Critical congenital heart disease, Echocardiography, Screening, Newborn

* Correspondence: mulberry714@gmail.com
Department of Pediatrics, Hamamatsu University School of Medicine, 1 – 20 – 1 Handayama, Hamamatsu, Shizuoka 431 – 3192, Japan

Background

Heart defects are the most common congenital malformations, with an incidence of approximately eight per 1000 live births [1], while the incidence of critical congenital heart disease (CCHD) is one or two per 1000 newborn babies [2]. In general, CCHD is defined as congenital heart disease (CHD) that leads to death or requires surgery or catheter intervention within 28 days of life [3]. Delayed detection of CCHD increases the risk of acute cardiovascular collapse and death, and is associated with worse outcomes of interventions [2, 4]. As the preference for early discharge after delivery is becoming more prevalent, newborns with CCHD are more likely to develop symptoms at home rather than during their stay in the newborn nursery. Screening for CCHD has previously relied on prenatal ultrasound and postnatal clinical examination, but both such approaches are known to have a relatively low detection rate; it is estimated that up to a third of newborns may be discharged with undiagnosed critical defects [5]. For more than a decade, many studies have assessed the usefulness of pulse oximetry for improving the detection of CCHD in newborns before hospital discharge (typically, in the newborn nursery); evidence from such studies indicates that pulse oximetry screening is highly effective in detecting CCHD in newborns with hypoxemia [6, 7] but not in those without hypoxemia [3, 8]. Echocardiography, especially when performed by pediatric cardiologists, is commonly used for diagnosing CHD, and thus may be helpful in detecting CCHD in newborns earlier and with higher sensitivity than when using other screening methods. However, few studies have assessed the effectiveness of hospital-wide echocardiography screening for CHD in newborns [9–11]. The objective of the present study was to evaluate the effectiveness of echocardiographic screening for CCHD when evaluations are performed by pediatric cardiologists in a tertiary care center.

Methods

Study population

A retrospective chart review was conducted among newborns delivered at Hamamatsu University Hospital, Japan, to identify those who underwent echocardiographic screening between June 2009 and May 2016. Hamamatsu University Hospital is a tertiary care birthing center that provides extensive prenatal screening and serves as a referral hospital for pregnant women whose fetuses have been diagnosed with congenital anomalies at other medical facilities. In this hospital's well-baby nursery, neonatologists conduct clinical examinations of newborns on the 1st and 4th day of life; echocardiographic screening is performed by a pediatric cardiologist in each live newborn, with written informed consent from the parents.

This study included consecutive newborns delivered at ≥36 weeks of gestation, having a birthweight ≥2300 g, and cared for in the well-baby nursery. Newborns admitted to the neonatal intensive care unit (NICU), as well as those prenatally diagnosed with CHD and/or with clinical signs or symptoms indicative of CHD before discharge were excluded. The study was approved by the ethics committee of our institution (Approval No: 17–277).

Screening protocol

The newborns underwent echocardiographic screening within the first 5 days of life. The echocardiographic examination was performed by one of three well-experienced pediatric cardiologists, using the same echocardiography machine (Vivid i; GE Healthcare, Tokyo, Japan) with a 12-MHz transducer. The examination protocol included two-dimensional and color Doppler imaging in the parasternal, suprasternal, subxiphoid, apical, and, when necessary, modified views. All echocardiographic examinations were recorded and reviewed by another pediatric cardiologist, who served as a second observer blinded to the patient identity. Sedation was not required in any newborn because echocardiographic screening was performed during natural sleep. In newborns who had a ductal shunt at the time of the initial screening, echocardiography was performed again upon hospital discharge; the diagnosis of patent ductus arteriosus (PDA) was only made in newborns with a ductal shunt that persisted at the time of discharge. Atrial septal defect was defined as the presence of an intra-atrial communication ≥5 mm in diameter, with an enlarged right atrium and right ventricle. An intra-atrial defect ≤4 mm in size at the fossa ovalis was considered to represent patent foramen ovale. For the purpose of the present study, echocardiographic follow-up of patients with CHD was considered complete upon spontaneous resolution of all cardiac lesions, surgery, catheter intervention, or death. On the basis of the CHD severity classification proposed by Ewer and colleagues [3], four CHD outcome categories were defined in this study: (i) critical CHD, which was defined in infants with hypoplastic left heart syndrome, pulmonary atresia (PA) with intact ventricular septum, simple transposition of the great arteries, or interruption of the aortic arch (IAA), as well as in infants who died or required surgery within the first 28 days of life for coarctation of the aorta (CoA), aortic valve stenosis, pulmonary valve stenosis, tetralogy of Fallot (TOF), PA with ventricular septal defect, or total anomalous pulmonary venous connection (TAPVC); (ii) serious CHD, which was defined in infants with non-critical cardiac lesions requiring intervention (cardiac catheterization or surgery) within the first year of life; (iii) significant CHD, defined as any cardiac lesion persisting longer than 6 months of life but not classified as serious or critical; and (iv) non-significant CHD, defined as any defects not clinically appreciable (e.g., with spontaneous resolution) and not persisting after 6 months of life.

Results

During the study period, 4082 live newborns were delivered at ≥36 weeks of gestation and with a birthweight of ≥2300 g. The flow diagram showing the progress of newborns included in the present study is shown in Fig. 1. Newborns with prenatal diagnosis of CHD ($n = 6$), those admitted to the NICU ($n = 455$), and those who had signs or symptoms of CHD prior to hospital discharge ($n = 130$) were excluded. Of the remaining 3491 newborns, 41 were not screened due to lack of parental consent. Among the 3434 newborns with complete echocardiography data, 104 (3.0%) were diagnosed as having CHD, of whom nine were lost to follow-up because of dropping out or moving away. Of the remaining 95 newborns diagnosed as having CHD during the initial echocardiographic screening, 34 (36%) and 61 (64%) were determined to have significant and non-significant CHD, respectively; no cases of critical or serious CHD were noted. A summary of the types of cardiac lesions and the duration of follow-up for these 95 newborns with CHD is provided in Table 1. Of the 34 newborns diagnosed as having significant CHD, 18 (53%) experienced spontaneous resolution of cardiac lesions during the course of the 2-year follow-up period.

Among the excluded newborns, nine (0.22% of all live births) were diagnosed as having critical ($n = 2$) or serious CHD ($n = 7$). The clinical characteristics of these nine newborns are summarized in Table 2. In six of these nine newborns, CHD had been diagnosed by fetal ultrasound; on the initial echocardiogram screening performed by a pediatric cardiologist immediately after birth, two newborns were found to have TOF, one had PA, one had single ventricle, one had CoA, and one had atrial ventricular septal defect. The remaining three newborns (one with TAPVC and two with TOF) screened negative for CHD on fetal ultrasound but exhibited heart murmur and/or cyanosis at 12–24 h after birth, though none had cardiovascular collapse.

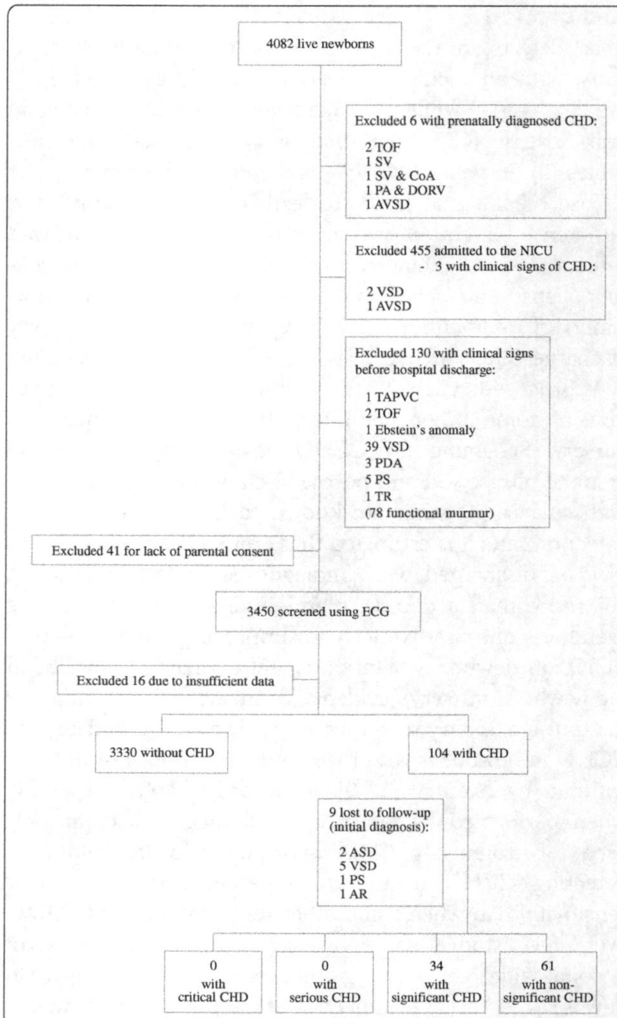

Fig. 1 Study population and flow diagram showing the progress of newborns included in the study CHD, congenital heart disease; NICU, neonatal intensive care unit; TOF, tetralogy of Fallot; SV, single ventricle; CoA, coarctation of the aorta; PA, pulmonary atresia; DORV, double-outlet right ventricle; AVSD, atrial ventricular septal defect; TAPVC, total anomalous pulmonary venous connection; ASD, atrial septal defect; VSD, ventricular septal defect; PDA, patent ductus arteriosus; MR, mitral regurgitation; AR, aortic regurgitation; TR, tricuspid regurgitation; PS, pulmonary stenosis; ECG, echocardiography

Discussion

Efficacy of postnatal echocardiographic screening for CCHD

In this study, postnatal echocardiographic screening did not help improve the detection rate of critical or serious CHD in newborns without prenatal diagnosis or clinical signs. Moreover, such early echocardiographic screening detected non-significant CHDs, which were not associated with clinical manifestations and which resolved spontaneously within the first 6 months of life.

Fetal ultrasound screening allows for early detection of CHD [12–14], especially when conducted routinely in tertiary care centers [15–17]. In our hospital, fetal ultrasound screening is routinely conducted for all pregnant women. When fetal CCHD is recognized by an obstetrician, the pregnant woman is referred for detailed fetal assessment by a pediatric cardiologist. Previous studies have also suggested that collaboration with a pediatric cardiologist may improve the sonographic detection rate of fetal CHD [18, 19]. In this setting, postnatal echocardiographic screening may not significantly improve the early detection rate of CCHD. However, the detection rate of CHD by prenatal ultrasound can be limited by fetal gestational age or position, maternal obesity, and operator experience [3, 16, 20]. In fact, of the newborns delivered during the

Table 1 Number of newborns with significant and non-significant congenital heart disease, stratified according to follow-up period

CHD	Follow-up period			
	< 1 month	1–6 months	6 months to 2 years	> 2 years
Significant				
ASD			3	3
VSD			12	2
PDA			1	4
MR			1	1
AR			1	3
PS				3
Non-significant				
VSD	2	11		
PDA	31	4		
MR	3	4		
AR	2	4		

CHD congenital heart disease, *ASD* atrial septal defect, *VSD* ventricular septal defect, *PDA* patent ductus arteriosus, *MR* mitral regurgitation, *AR* aortic regurgitation, *PS* pulmonary stenosis

study period, all except six screened negative for CHD on prenatal ultrasound, while three were postnatally diagnosed as having critical or serious CHD despite having screened negative on prenatal ultrasound; these three newborns had clinical signs indicative of CHD postnatally, including heart murmur and/or cyanosis. However, in newborns with CCHD, murmurs do not always manifest prior to hospital discharge, due to specific anatomic features, elevated pulmonary vascular resistance, or reduced contractility [21, 22]. Cyanosis may also be difficult to detect in newborns with mild desaturation or with dark or anemic skin color, as well as when lighting in the room is poor [8, 23]. Because of these problems, routine neonatal examination fails to detect CHD in about half of cases [24, 25].

Although postnatal echocardiography is the gold standard for diagnosing CHD, it has serious limitations when used as a screening tool, as we demonstrated in the present study. Moreover, while echocardiographic screening could be implemented in our hospital relatively easily (around 600 newborns delivered every year), implementing such a screening strategy is not feasible in large-volume facilities, as it would lead to an unacceptable increase in workload for pediatric cardiologists. In addition, employing experienced pediatric cardiologists to perform screening echocardiography for all newborns and to follow up all test positives would incur prohibitive costs. Upon evaluating the effectiveness and costs of several current strategies for CCHD screening of newborns, Knowles et al. found that echocardiographic screening was the most costly strategy, concluding that such a screening strategy is unlikely to be cost-effective [26, 27]. In addition, our present results confirm the fact that this screening strategy has a high rate of false-positives, which may induce adverse psychological effects in parents. To minimize the rate of false-positives, echocardiographic screening could be conducted later (e.g., at a few months from birth); however, some newborns with unsuspected CCHD may experience sudden manifestations such as cardiovascular collapse or

Table 2 Clinical characteristics of critical and serious congenital heart disease

CHD	Screening method	Clinical findings	Age at intervention		Outcome
			Cardiac catheterization	Surgery	
Critical CHD					
SV	FUS	Cyanosis (SpO_2: 30%)	-	4 days	Alive
SV & CoA	FUS	No	-	15 days	Alive
Serious CHD					
TAPVC	PE	Heart murmur Cyanosis (SpO_2: 91–94%)	-	29 days	Alive
PA & DORV	FUS	Heart murmur	-	1 month	Alive
AVSD	FUS	No	2 months	3 months	Alive
TOF	PE	Heart murmur	-	6 months	Alive
TOF	FUS	Heart murmur	4 months	10 months	Alive
TOF	PE	Heart murmur	6 months	10 months	Alive
TOF	FUS	No	7 months	11 months	Alive

CHD congenital heart disease, *FUS* fetal ultrasound, *PE* physical examination, *SV* single ventricle, *CoA* coarctation of aorta, *TAPVC* total anomalous pulmonary venous connection, *PA* pulmonary atresia, *DORV* double-outlet right ventricle, *AVSD* atrial ventricular septal defect, *TOF* tetralogy of Fallot, *SpO_2* oxygen saturation

death within 2 months of birth, and would thus not have the opportunity to be screened for CCHD.

Strengths and limitations of the study

One important strength of the present study is that echocardiographic screening was conducted by experienced pediatric cardiologists, who evaluated thousands of neonates both before and during the study period. Another strength is that the study included almost 3500 newborns. On the other hand, our study has several potential limitations. First, similar studies regarding postnatal echocardiographic screening were performed previously [9–11]. Such studies investigated the prevalence of CHD and the efficacy of screening for CHD, but not the efficacy of screening for CCHD. Moreover, these previous studies only analyzed data pertaining to short follow-up periods, which makes it difficult to assess the prognosis of most patients. In our study, the follow-up period of patients with clinically significant CHD was at least 2 years. Among these previous studies, one was conducted at our institution and covered the period between 2005 and 2010, reporting a high prevalence of CHD in an unselected series of consecutive newborns, including those with significant prematurity, chromosomal or genetic abnormality, prenatally diagnosed CHD, and/or clinical signs or symptoms of CHD [10]. On the contrary, in the present study, we evaluated the efficacy of postnatal echocardiography for detecting unsuspected CCHD in a well-baby population and found a low incidence of CHD. Another potential limitation is that our study was conducted at a single tertiary hospital, and thus selection bias could not be excluded. In fact, the incidence of CCHD in this population was lower than previously reported [2, 3]. Finally, we did not have data regarding the outcomes of newborns who screened negative on postnatal echocardiography and physical examination.

Alternative screening strategy for CCHD

Current evidence supports the introduction of pulse oximetry screening for CCHD in asymptomatic newborns before hospital discharge [6, 7], suggesting that pulse oximetry should be used as a non-invasive, inexpensive, and less time-consuming screening tool [5, 6]. However, there are technical limitations associated with oximetry measurements in newborns, resulting in a high rate of false-negatives; specifically, approximately a quarter of newborns with CCHD will not be identified by this method. The lesions most commonly missed on pulse oximetry evaluations are those causing obstruction of the aortic outflow (e.g., CoA and IAA), which may not necessarily be associated with hypoxemia [3, 8]. Such lesions are also frequently missed on prenatal ultrasound and routine physical examination [28]. Thus, in newborns with such lesions, echocardiographic screening may be the only tool suitable for early diagnosis.

Conclusions

In our tertiary care hospital, echocardiographic screening did not help improve the detection rate of CCHD in newborns without prenatal diagnosis or clinical signs of CHD, and was moreover associated with a high rate of false-positives. In light of these findings, as well as considering the high cost and increase in workload for pediatric cardiologists, we conclude that echocardiography might not represent a feasible routine screening strategy for CCHD. Instead, it may be useful to employ pulse oximetry in conjunction with fetal ultrasound and postnatal physical examination. Our institution is planning to introduce such a screening strategy, although further research is warranted in order to inform policy.

Abbreviations

AR: Aortic regurgitation; ASD: Atrial septal defect; AVSD: Atrial ventricular septal defect; CCHD: Critical congenital heart disease; CHD: Congenital heart disease; CoA: Coarctation of the aorta; DORV: Double-outlet right ventricle; IAA: Interruption of the aortic arch; MR: Mitral regurgitation; NICU: Neonatal intensive care unit; PA: Pulmonary atresia; PDA: Patent ductus arteriosus; PS: Pulmonary stenosis; SV: Single ventricle; TAPVC: Total anomalous pulmonary venous connection; TOF: Tetralogy of Fallot; TR: Tricuspid regurgitation; VSD: Ventricular septal defect

Acknowledgements

The authors would like to express their gratitude to Dr. Takamichi Ishikawa, Dr. Keigo Seki, and Dr. Satoru Iwashima, the pediatric cardiologists who conducted echocardiographic examinations at the Perinatal Center of Hamamatsu University Hospital.

Funding

The authors received no specific funding for this research.

Authors' contributions

MK performed data analysis, interpreted the data, and prepared the first draft of the manuscript. SI conceived the study and was responsible for data collection. TB, TF, and AO made substantial contributions to acquisition of data. All authors reviewed the manuscript for important intellectual content and approved the final version to be published.

Competing interests

The authors declare that they have no competing interests.

References

1. van der Linde D, Konings EE, Slager MA, Witsenburg M, Helbing WA, Takkenberg JJ, et al. Birth prevalence of congenital heart disease worldwide: a systematic review and meta-analysis. J Am Coll Cardiol. 2011;58:2241–7.
2. Chang RK, Gurvitz M, Rodriguez S. Missed diagnosis of critical congenital heart disease. Arch Pediatr Adolesc Med. 2008;162:969–74.
3. Ewer AK, Middleton LJ, Furmston AT, Bhoyar A, Daniels JP, Thangaratinam S, et al. Pulse oximetry screening for congenital heart defects in newborn infants (pulse ox): a test accuracy study. Lancet. 2011;378:785–94.

4. Ng B, Hokanson J. Missed congenital heart disease in neonates. Congenit Heart Dis. 2010;5:292–6.
5. Ewer AK, Furmston AT, Middleton LJ, Deeks JJ, Daniels JP, Pattison HM, et al. Pulse oximetry as a screening test for congenital heart defects in newborn infants: a test accuracy study with evaluation of acceptability and cost-effectiveness. Health Technol Assess. 2012;16:1–184.
6. Mahle WT, Newburger JW, Matherne GP, Smith FC, Hoke TR, Koppel R, et al. Role of pulse oximetry in examining newborns for congenital heart disease: a scientific statement from the American Heart Association and American Academy of Pediatrics. Circulation. 2009;120:447–58.
7. Plana MN, Zamora J, Suresh G, Fernandez-Pineda L, Thangaratinam S, Ewer AK. Pulse oximetry screening for critical congenital heart defects. Cochrane Database Syst Rev. 2018;3:CD011912.
8. de-Wahl Granelli A, Wennergren M, Sandberg K, Mellander M, Bejlum C, Inganäs L, et al. Impact of pulse oximetry screening on the detection of duct dependent congenital heart disease: a Swedish prospective screening study in 39,821 newborns. BMJ. 2009;338:a3037.
9. Sands A, Craig B, Mulholland C, Patterson C, Dornan J, Casey F. Echocardiographic screening for congenital heart disease: a randomized study. J Perinat Med. 2002;30:307–12.
10. Ishikawa T, Iwashima S, Ohishi A, Nakagawa Y, Ohzeki T. Prevalence of congenital heart disease assessed by echocardiography in 2067 consecutive newborns. Acta Paediatr. 2011;100:e55–60.
11. Zhao QM, Ma XJ, Jia B, Huang GY. Prevalence of congenital heart disease at live birth: an accurate assessment by echocardiographic screening. Acta Paediatr. 2013;102:397–402.
12. Berkley EM, Goens MB, Karr S, Rappaport V. Utility of fetal echocardiography in postnatal management of infants with prenatally diagnosed congenital heart disease. Prenat Diagn. 2009;29:654–8.
13. Chung ML, Lee BS, Kim EA, Kim KS, Pi SY, Oh YM, et al. Impact of fetal echocardiography on trends in disease patterns and outcomes of congenital heart disease in a neonatal intensive care unit. Neonatology. 2010;98:41–6.
14. Bensemlali M, Stirnemann J, Le Bidois J, Lévy M, Raimondi F, Hery E, et al. Discordances between pre-natal and post-natal diagnoses of congenital heart diseases and impact on care strategies. J Am Coll Cardiol. 2016;68:921–30.
15. Liu H, Zhou J, Feng QL, Gu HT, Wan G, Zhang HM, et al. Fetal echocardiography for congenital heart disease diagnosis: a meta-analysis, power analysis and missing data analysis. Eur J Prev Cardiol. 2015;22:1531–47.
16. Friedburg MK, Silverman NH, Moon-Grady AJ, Tong E, Nourse J, Sorenson B, et al. Prenatal detection of congenital heart disease. J Pediatr. 2009;155:26–31.
17. Levy DJ, Pretorius DH, Rothman A, Gonzales M, Rao C, Nunes ME, et al. Improved prenatal detection of congenital heart disease in an integrated health care system. Pediatr Cardiol. 2013;34:670–9.
18. Cuneo BF, Curran LF, Davis N, Elrad H. Trends in prenatal diagnosis of critical cardiac defects in an integrated obstetric and pediatric cardiac imaging center. J Perinatol. 2004;24:674–8.
19. Meyer-Wittkopf M, Cooper S, Sholler G. Correlation between fetal cardiac diagnosis by obstetric and pediatric cardiologist sonographers and comparison with postnatal findings. Ultrasound Obstet Gynecol. 2001;17:392–7.
20. American Institute of Ultrasound in Medicine. AIUM practice guideline for the performance of fetal echocardiography. J Ultrasound Med. 2013;32:1067–82.
21. Brunetti ND, Rosania S, D'Antuono C, D'Antuono A, De Gennaro L, Zuppa AA, et al. Diagnostic accuracy of heart murmur in newborns with suspected congenital heart disease. J Cardiovasc Med (Hagerstown). 2015;16:556–61.
22. Hoffman JIE. It is time for routine neonatal screening by pulse oximetry. Neonatology. 2011;99:1–9.
23. O'Donnell CP, Kamlin CO, Davis PG, Carlin JB, Morley CJ. Clinical assessment of infant colour at delivery. Arch Dis Child Fetal Neonatal Ed. 2007;92:F465–7.
24. Ainsworth S, Wyllie JP, Wren C. Prevalence and clinical significance of cardiac murmurs in neonates. Arch Dis Child Fetal Neonatal Ed. 1999;80:F43–5.
25. Wren C, Richmond S, Donaldson L. Presentation of congenital heart disease in infancy: implications for routine examination. Arch Dis Child Fetal Neonatal Ed. 1999;80:F49–53.
26. Knowles R, Griebsch I, Dezateux C, Brown J, Bull C, Wren C. Newborn screening for congenital heart defects: a systematic review and cost-effectiveness analysis. Health Technol Assess. 2005;9:1–152.
27. Griebsch I, Knowles RL, Brown J, Bull C, Wren C, Dezateux CA. Comparing the clinical and economic effects of clinical examination, pulse oximetry, and echocardiography in newborn screening for congenital heart defects: a probabilistic cost-effectiveness model and value of information analysis. Int J Technol Assess Health Care. 2007;23:192–204.
28. Ewer AK. Review of pulse oximetry screening for critical congenital heart defects in newborn infants. Curr Opin Cardiol. 2013;28:92–6.

Necrotizing enterocolitis leads to disruption of tight junctions and increase in gut permeability in a mouse model

Srikanth Ravisankar[1,4], Rodney Tatum[2], Parvesh M. Garg[1,5], Maja Herco[2], Prem S. Shekhawat[3*] and Yan-Hua Chen[2*]

Abstract

Background: Necrotizing enterocolitis (NEC) is a leading cause of death in preterm infants. Neonates weighing <1500 grams are at the highest risk for acquiring NEC, with a prevalence of nearly 7-10%, mortality up to 30%, and several long-term complications among survivors. Despite advancements in neonatal medicine, this disease remains a challenge to treat. The aim of this study is to investigate the effect of NEC on gut epithelial tight junctions and its barrier function using a NEC mouse model.

Methods: Three-day old C57BL/6 mouse pups were fed with Esbilac formula every 3 hours and then subjected to hypoxia twice daily followed by cold stress. Dam fed pups from the same litters served as controls. Pups were observed and sacrificed 96 hours after the treatments and intestines were removed for experiments. The successful induction of NEC was confirmed by histopathology. Changes in tight junction proteins in NEC intestines were studied by western blotting and immunofluorescent microscopy using specific protein markers. The gut leakage in NEC was visualized using biotin tracer molecules.

Results: Our study results demonstrate that we induced NEC in >50% of experimental pups, pups lost nearly 40% of weight and their intestines showed gross changes and microscopic changes associated with NEC. There were inflammatory changes with loss of tight junction barrier function and disruption of tight junction claudin proteins in the intestines of NEC mouse model. We have demonstrated for the first time that NEC intestines develop increased leakiness as visualized by biotin tracer leakage.

Conclusions: NEC leads to breakdown of epithelial barrier due to changes in tight junction proteins with increased leakiness which may explain the transmigration of microbes and microbial products from the gut lumen into the blood stream leading to sepsis like signs clinically witnessed.

Keywords: Necrotizing enterocolitis, Tight junctions, Claudin proteins, Biotin tracer molecules, Epithelial barrier function

Background

Necrotizing enterocolitis (NEC) is a common condition seen in premature neonates born with birth weight <1500g and leads to high morbidity, mortality and long-term complications. The incidence of NEC as reported in the literature varies between 7 to 10% with a high mortality of up to 30% [1]. Survivors of this condition suffer from neurodevelopmental delays [2], poor growth, and cholestasis due short bowel syndrome and may require gut transplantation in rare cases [3].

The cardinal traits considered in the pathogenesis of NEC include prematurity, microbial colonization, genetic predisposition, intestinal immaturity, role of intestinal barriers and response to inflammation by the premature intestine. There is a direct correlation between gestational age and incidence of NEC with highest incidence seen in the most premature neonates [4]. Premature neonates have poorly organized and immature intestinal absorption, digestion and motility patterns [5–9]. Intestinal microbial colonization in these premature neonates is a critical factor and has been

* Correspondence: pshekhawat@metrohealth.org; cheny@ecu.edu
[3]Department of Pediatrics, MetroHealth Medical Center, Case Western Reserve University, Cleveland, OH 44109, USA
[2]Department of Anatomy and Cell Biology, Brody School of Medicine, East Carolina University, Greenville, NC 27834, USA

demonstrated from early descriptions of this disease from almost four decades ago by Santulli et al [10].

Several animal studies have demonstrated the role of Toll-like receptor 4 (TLR4) in NEC. TLR4 is known to gradually increase in expression in the intestine until term gestation at which point its expression is actively down regulated. It has been reported that TLR4 senses lipopolysaccharides and activation of TLR4 results in local inflammation leading to destruction of the epithelial barrier [11, 12].

Tight junction (TJ) proteins bind the epithelial and endothelial cells together and form a barrier between the intestinal lumen and blood stream [13]. They regulate passage of ions, water and small molecules through the paracellular pathway and thereby maintain distinct body compartments and cellular function [13]. They were first identified in 1986 [14]. Three distinct proteins were identified, Occludin [15], Claudins [16] and junctional adhesion molecules (JAM) [17]. Since then, in addition to discovery of newer TJ proteins, various animal models have helped understand their presence in different organs such as brain, intestines, etc. and demonstrated their critical functions depending on their location in the tissues. Fujita et al. demonstrated the differential expression and localization of various claudins in the intestine of a mouse model [18]. There has been progressively better understanding of the role of TJ proteins in various diseases and the genes [19, 20] encoding for these TJ proteins.

Intestinal permeability is tightly regulated by several TJ proteins, especially the claudins. Claudins are a family of TJ integral membrane proteins with at least 24 members [21]. Claudin proteins are small molecules with ~22 kDa in molecular weight and express different isoforms depending on the tissue and cell type [22]. Claudins show a tissue-specific distribution pattern and are expressed on epithelial linings of the GI tract [18].

It is known that preterm infants have higher intestinal permeability than older children and adults because of various mechanical and nonmechanical factors including TJs that maintain the connections between adjacent cells. The integrity of gut epithelial barrier is absolutely essential for health of GI tract and any disease process which leads to increased permeability to toxins, foreign proteins or translocation of gut bacteria into the circulation starts the process which eventually leads to NEC [23]. Thus, maintenance of gut epithelial barriers by claudins and other barrier function proteins remains central in prevention of NEC. Claudins are known to form pores which are size and charge-selective for various molecules and their normal expression is critical for preservation of epithelial lining. Claudins play a key role in maintaining the epithelial barrier and protecting newborns from development of NEC. The aim of this study is to examine the integrity of the TJs and its barrier function in a NEC mouse model. The gut leakage in NEC intestines was visualized for the first time by biotin tracer molecules, demonstrating the loss of epithelial barrier function in NEC intestines.

Methods

Neonatal NEC mouse model

Our animal use protocol was reviewed and approved by the Animal Care and Use Committee of East Carolina University (AUP#A182). All animals were housed in the facility maintained by East Carolina University, which provides in-house veterinary care. The animals were kept in rooms at 22°C with a 12-h light-dark cycle. We performed the animal experiments according to the guidelines of East Carolina University and the National Institute of Health on animal care and use. These guidelines are very similar to ARRIVE guidelines practiced by investigators in the European Union [24]. Every effort was made to minimize the pain and discomfort to the animals during the experiments.

The 3-day old C57BL/6 pups were divided into 2 groups: dam fed control group (n=13) and experimental group (n=13). The latter group was fed with 30-50 μl 33% Esbilac formula (Pet-Ag, New Hampshire, IL) every 3 hours for 96 hours using a 1.9 Fr feeding tube, subjected to hypoxia (100% N_2 for 60 seconds) and cold stress (4°C for 10 min) twice a day for four days. Pups were nursed in an incubator (37°C) during the 4-day period and provided high calorie formula. Both the experimental and dam fed control pups were euthanized at 96 hours after start of the experiment. The gastrointestinal tract was carefully dissected and visually evaluated for signs of NEC (areas of bowel necrosis, intestinal hemorrhage). NEC was confirmed by histopathology using published tissue injury guidelines in mice [25, 26]. Intestinal samples were collected for histopathological and immunofluorescent studies.

Histology examinations

Intestinal tissues isolated from control and NEC pups were fixed in 10% formalin solution. After washed with phosphate buffered saline (PBS), the fixed tissues were processed through graded ethanol solutions. The 5 μm tissue sections were cut using a cryostat. Hematoxylin & Eosin (H&E) staining was performed according to the published methods [27].

Western blot analysis

Intestinal tissues from control and NEC pups were minced on ice, homogenized in RIPA buffer (1% Triton X-100, 0.5% sodium deoxycholate, 0.2% SDS, 150 mM NaCl, 10 mM Hepes, pH7.3, 2 mM EDTA, 10 μg/ml each of chymostatin, leupeptin and pepstatin A) by passing 10 times through a 22-gauge needle, and centrifuged at 15,000 g for 30 minutes at 4°C to obtain tissue lysates. The total protein concentration of each sample was measured using the BCA protein assay kit (Pierce, Rockford, IL, USA) and adjusted to equal concentration (2 mg/ml). Proteins in the SDS sample buffer were separated by SDS-PAGE and transferred to nitrocellulose membranes. After blocking by 5% nonfat dry milk, the membranes were incubated with primary and secondary antibodies, respectively. The signals were detected by enhanced chemiluminescence (Amersham, Arlington Heights, IL, USA).

Immunofluorescence microscopy

Intestinal tissues isolated from control and NEC pups were frozen in liquid nitrogen. The 5 μm frozen sections were cut using a cryostat. The frozen sections were fixed in 100% acetone and blocked with 5% BSA. The primary and secondary antibodies were applied to the intestinal tissues, respectively. The immunofluorescent signals were analyzed using a Zeiss Axio Imager M2 microscope (Carl Zeiss, Thornwood, NY).

Tight junction permeability assay *in vivo*

This TJ *in vivo* permeability assay using biotin has been published previously [28]. Biotins are small water-soluble molecules. They are membrane impermeable reagents and allow efficient labeling of proteins and primary amine - containing macromolecules on the cell surface. Biotin reagents will not diffuse through the intercellular space if TJ is intact. However, if TJ structure is disrupted, the biotin molecule will penetrate into the intercellular space.

To examine the TJ barrier function, the pups were anesthetized by intraperitoneal injection with 0.05ml/10g body weight of Ketamine (18mg/ml) and Xylazine (2mg/ml) at the end of NEC experiments. After ensuring the pup was in deep anesthesia with paw pinch, the abdominal cavity was opened by a surgical scissor. The Sulfo-NHS-Biotin (MW: 556.59) diluted in 1 mg/mL PBS was injected into the lumen of control and NEC small intestines using a low-pressure syringe pump (Harvard Apparatus). The injection was conducted at a rate of 50 μl/min through a 25G needle connected to a polyethylene tubing. Ten minutes after biotin injection, intestines were dissected and embedded in O.C.T. compound, then processed for immunofluorescence light microscopy [28]. Biotin was detected by Texas red-conjugated streptavidin.

After the tissue collection, pups were euthanized by decapitation while under anesthesia. All these procedures were approved by the East Carolina University (ECU) Animal Care and Use Committee and conducted in compliance with guidelines from the National Institute of Health and ECU on laboratory animal care and use.

Statistical analysis

Statistical analysis was performed using either Origin8 (OriginLab, MA) or SIGMAPLOT (Systat Software, Inc. CA) softwares. The differences between two groups were analyzed using the unpaired Student's *t*-test. The *p*-value of < 0.05 will be considered significant.

Results

Gross and histological examinations of intestines

After 4 days of treatments, about 50% of thirteen-treated pups developed NEC compared to none in the dam fed group. The NEC pups were smaller in size and had an average of 42% reduction of the weight compared to the control pups at the end of the treatment (Fig. 1a). The NEC intestines showed the clinical sign of the disease and were inflamed and swollen in appearance (Fig. 1b). Grossly necrotic bowel was seen mainly in the small intestines, and part of the large intestine was also involved (Fig. 1c). On microscopic examination, NEC intestines showed the clear evidence of bloody necrotic changes as indicated by the arrows when compared to the controls (Fig. 1c). The NEC phenotype was confirmed by histopathology examinations using a standard histopathological grading established to diagnose NEC [26]. Control intestines showed the intact villus structure and submucosa (Fig. 2a) while NEC intestines had a disrupted villous mucosal structure. Some NEC villi displayed complete sloughing of epithelial cells with breach of epithelium barrier (Fig. 2b and c).

Altered expression and localization of TJ proteins and elevation of inflammation marker proteins in NEC intestines

Western blot analysis showed an altered expression of TJ claudin proteins. There was an increased expression level of claudin-2 and decreased expression levels of claudin-3, -4, and -7 in NEC intestines compared to those of controls (Fig. 3a). In addition, the expression levels of PARP, a protein that can induce a programmed cell death, as well as inflammatory marker proteins NF-kB and TGF-β were all up-regulated in the NEC intestines compared to the control intestines (Fig. 3b).

Immunofluorescent microscopy results indicated reduced immunostaining signals for claudin-3, -4, and -7 as indicated by arrows in NEC intestines (Fig. 4, arrows, NEC) compared to those of control intestines (Fig. 4, arrows, CON). In addition, the aggregated signals of claudin-3, -4, and -7 could be clearly observed in NEC intestinal tissues (Fig. 4, arrowheads in NEC).

Disruption of TJ barrier function in NEC intestines

To study whether NEC intestines have a leaky TJ or not, biotin *in vivo* detection assay was employed. The biotin staining signal was examined under the immunofluorescent light microscope. We found that NEC intestines displayed a diffusion of biotin signal through the intercellular

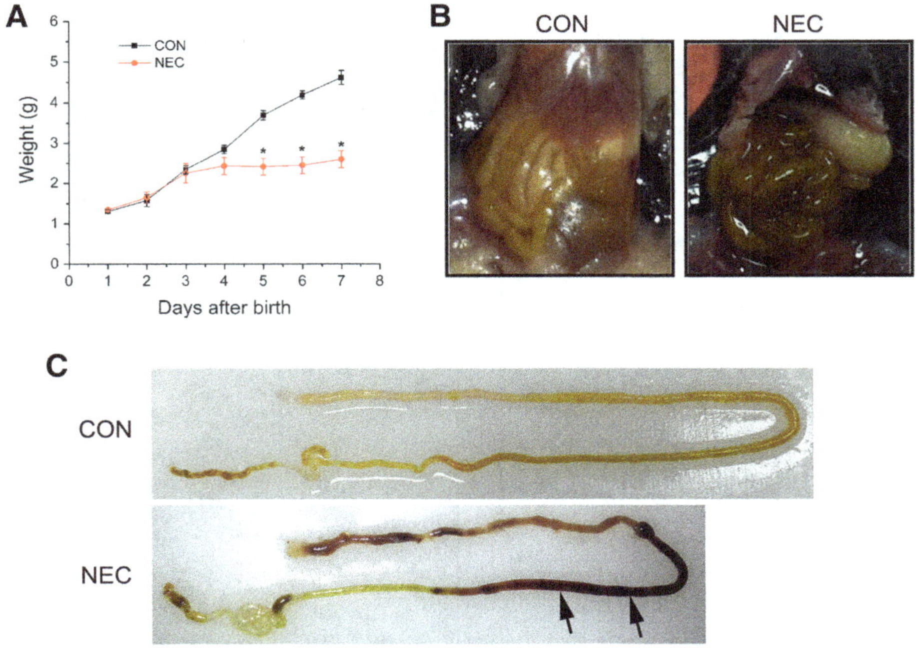

Fig. 1 Establishment of necrotizing enterocolitis (NEC) mouse model. **a**: Weight measurement of dam-fed (CON) or NEC-treated (NEC) pups. The treatment started at day 3 and was continued for 4 days. The data represent means ± s.e.m. from three independent experiments. Student's *t*-test was used for statistical analysis. A *P* value of < 0.05 was considered significant (*). N=10 pups for each group. **b**: Comparison of control and NEC intestines *in situ* at the end of the experiments. The NEC intestine showed the swollen and discolored appearance. **c**: The control and NEC intestines after removal from the body. The NEC intestine displayed the severe hemorrhage as indicated by arrows

space (Fig. 5, arrows in NEC). On the other hand, the control intestines showed no sign of leakage of TJ barrier. The biotin molecules were kept at the intestinal surface facing the lumen where biotin was applied (Fig. 5, arrowhead, CON). The strong biotin staining signal marked by asterisk reflected the accumulation of biotin molecules into the intestinal tissue (Fig. 5, asterisk in NEC).

Discussion

The conundrum of NEC will continue to be an important challenge both for the practicing clinician and the basic

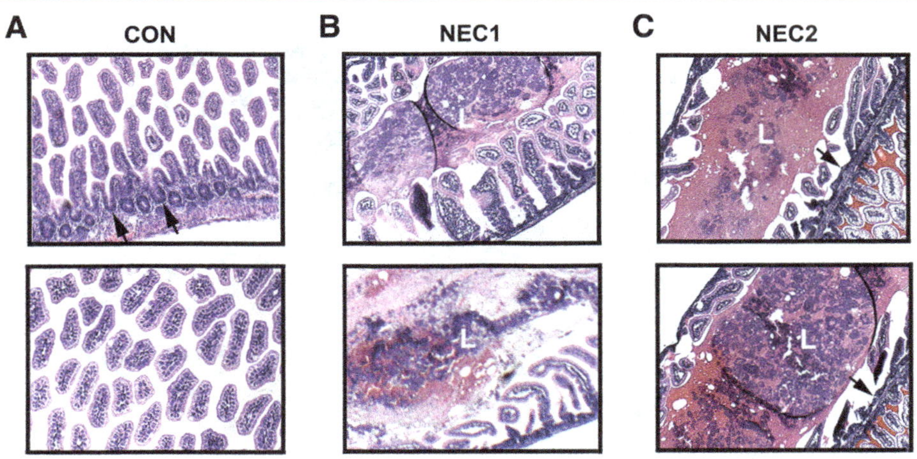

Fig. 2 H& E staining of control and NEC intestines. **a**: Tissue sections from representative control intestines shows the normal villous structure with intact crypt region (arrows). **b** and **c**: Tissue sections from representative NEC intestinal samples. The induction of NEC led to stunting of villi and disrupted villous structure with sloughing of epithelial cells into the lumen (L). The hemorrhage is evident in both B and C NEC intestinal samples. Original magnification: 200×

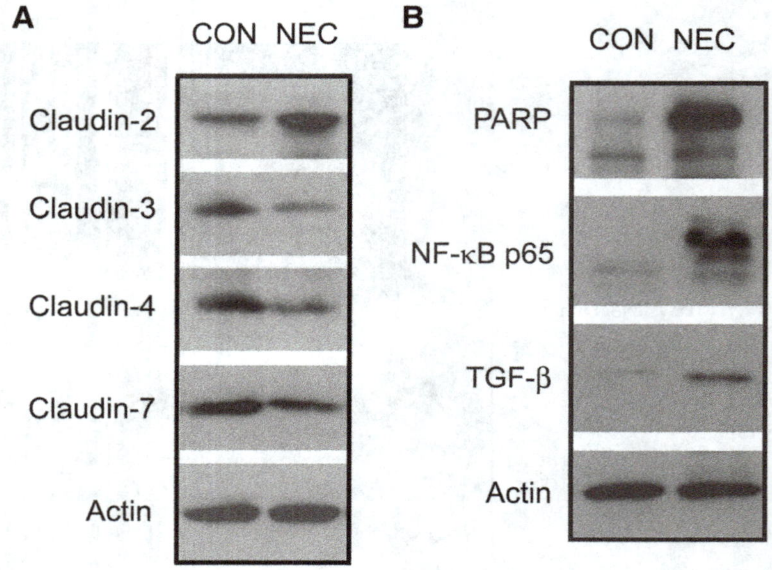

Fig. 3 Protein expression levels of control and NEC intestines. **a**: Representative western blot membrane showing claudin-2, -3, -4 and -7 expression levels in control (CON) and NEC intestines. Intestinal tissues from 7-day control and NEC pups were collected at the end of experiments. Tissue lysates were solubilized in RIPA buffer and subjected to western blotting. **b**: PARP, NF-κB and TGF-β expression levels in control (CON) and NEC intestines. A total of 30 μg protein for each sample were loaded on the SDS-polyacrylamide gel. Membranes were blotted against specific antibodies. Actin served as a loading control. Three independent experiments were performed

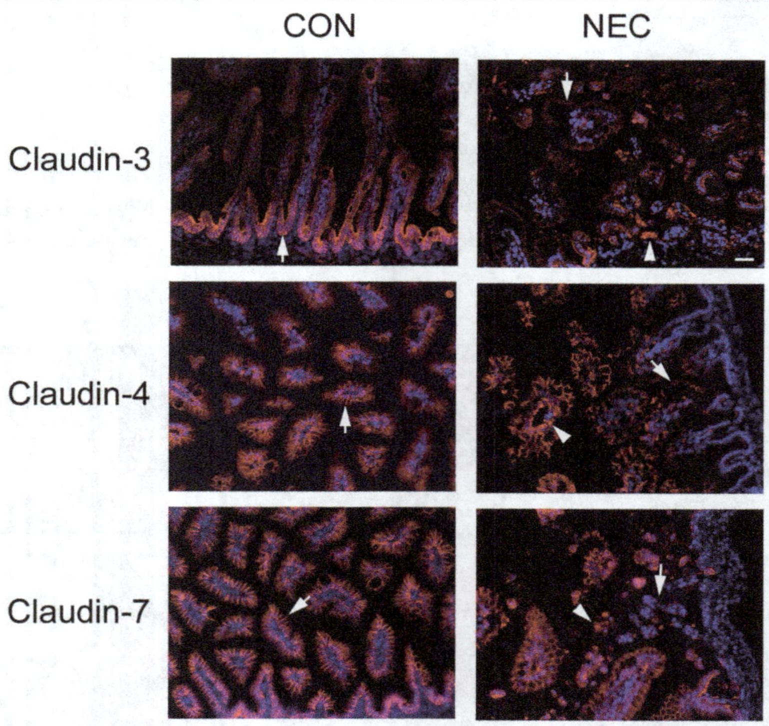

Fig. 4 Immuno-localization of claudin proteins in control and NEC intestines. Representative images of intestines from 7-day control and NEC pups were dissected from the body and frozen in liquid nitrogen. Frozen sections were immunostained with anti-claudin-3, or -4, or -7 antibodies and detected by Cy3-conjugated secondary antibody. Nuclei were stained with DAPI (blue). The claudin signals were localized at cell-cell contact area as indicated by arrows in controls (CON). Arrows were pointed to the reduced signals in NEC samples and arrowheads in NEC showed the aggregated staining pattern. Scale bar: 50 μm

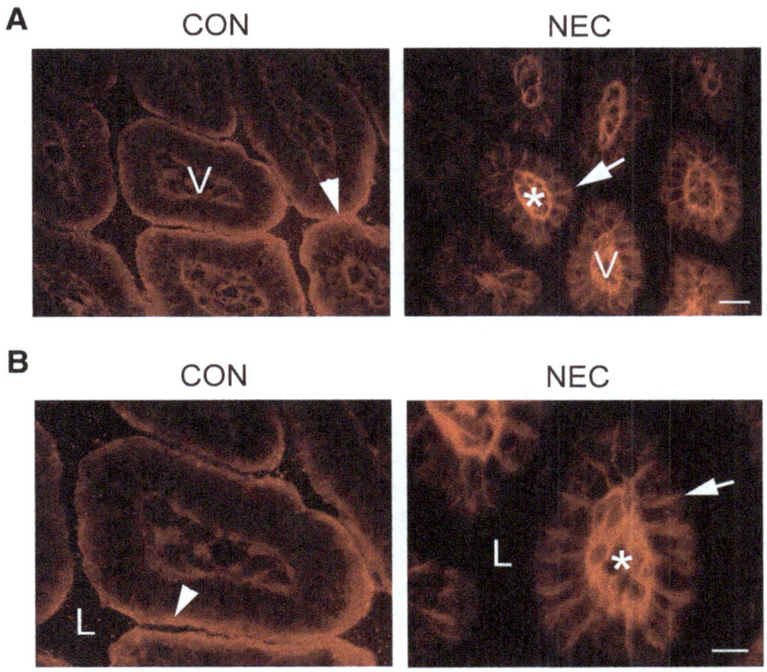

Fig. 5 Biotin permeability assays in control and NEC intestines. **a**: Sulfo-NHS-LC-Biotin was injected into the intestinal lumen of 7-day old control (CON) or NEC pups. The tissue sections were stained with Texas red-conjugated streptavidin. Biotin was mainly kept at the epithelial surface of control intestines (arrowhead) due to the intact epithelial barriers. No barrier leakage was observed in control intestines. In contrast, the leakage was clearly detected in NEC intestines. Biotin stained the intercellular space (arrow) and connective tissue (Asterisk). V: Villus. **b**: The higher magnification of the images. L: Lumen. Scale bar: 50 μm in A and 20 μm in B

science scientists. Though numerous studies have contributed to various aspects of pathogenesis of NEC, the fundamental etiopathogenesis remains a big unanswered question. This study focused on the role of TJ integral membrane protein claudins which play an essential role in cellular integrity and barrier function in the intestine.

The integrity of TJs is vital in maintaining intestinal epithelial homeostasis both at physiological condition and in disease state. Our NEC mouse model indicates an altered expression in the claudins where there is an increase in expression of claudin-2 and with a decreased expression of claudin-3, -4 and -7. It is well known that claudin-2 creates cation selective pores and increases cation permeability in epithelia of various tissues including intestines [29–31]. We observed an increased expression of claudin-2 in our NEC intestines which is consistent with the hypothesis of leaky TJs in NEC. The function of claudin-3 and -4 in the intestine is well established as a barrier and its down-regulation observed in our NEC mouse model explains the loss of barrier function [32]. It has been reported that claudin-7 is involved in cell-matrix interactions [33, 34]. Reduced expression of claudin-7 could contribute to the loss of tissue integrity. Claudins have been studied in human subjects and increased gut permeability has been demonstrated in cases with NEC [35, 36]. Thus, our study provides the molecular basis behind the observed clinical effect. Further research could focus on modulating TJ protein expression in the preterm neonatal gut to prevent NEC.

Biotins are membrane impermeable reagents and therefore, will not diffuse through the intercellular space if TJ is intact. However, if TJ structure/function is disrupted, the biotin molecule will penetrate into the intercellular space. Biotin permeability assay has been successfully applied to many different *in vivo* systems to examine the TJ permeability barrier, such as the blood brain barrier in claudin-5-deficient mice [37], the blood brain barrier in adult zebrafish [38], and the pathogen-infected intestinal epithelia [39]. Our study also demonstrates the increased gut permeability in NEC intestines. Disruption of TJ barrier function in NEC intestines is visualized for the first time by biotin *in vivo* detection assay. Disruption of epithelial barrier has been studied in human infants using indirect markers of epithelial cells like fatty acid binding protein (I-FABP). We did not use this marker in our mouse model since intestinal injury was grossly visible in affected animals.

Leaky TJs in NEC induce inflammation in the gut as reported by other studies [11, 40–43]. Our current study also observed increased signals for inflammatory markers, NF-kB and TGF-β. Both NF-kB and TGF-β are involved in the regulation of inflammatory processes. In addition, it is worth pointing out that NEC induction not only induces inflammatory response in GI tract, but also in kidneys as we have previously reported [44]. Further studies are necessary to better understand the relationship of a disrupted TJ structure/function with inflammation and severity of the NEC and whether altered expression of TJ protein claudins can be used as a potential biomarker for NEC.

The major limitation of our current study is that it is an animal study conducted using mice subjected to feeding a hyperosmolar formula and periods of hypoxia which is not exactly the same pathology seen in human neonates where infection starts the NEC process in most cases. But, at the same time inflammation which is the end result, was witnessed in our mouse model as well. Thus, there are similarities between clinical NEC and what we witnessed in our mouse model. Our report suggests that by modulating the expression of certain TJ proteins and control of the inflammatory process could potentially change the course of NEC. However, this goal will require further basic and clinical research.

Conclusions

We have successfully induced NEC in a mouse model where there was widespread inflammation and histological changes like those seen in human neonates. Inflammation was associated with increased expression of NF-κB, TGF-β and PARP. There was increased expression of Claudin-2 along with down-regulation of Claudins-3, -4, and -7 which explains the reason for breakdown of the epithelial barrier. We have demonstrated increased leakiness through the epithelial lining using biotin tracer, that explains the clinical sepsis like features witnessed in neonates. Thus, our report provides the molecular basis behind the clinical picture of NEC and identifies molecules where future therapies could be targeted.

Abbreviations

JAM: Junction adhesion molecules; NEC: Necrotizing enterocolitis; NF-κB: Nuclear factor κB; PARP: Poly (ADP-ribose) polymerase; TGF-β: Transforming growth factor-β; TJ: Tight junction; TLR: Toll-like receptor

Acknowledgments

We thank Joani Zary Oswald and Beverly G. Jeansonne for their technical assistance.

Funding

This study is supported by the National Institutes of Health grant DK103166 (to Yan-Hua Chen).

Authors' contributions

SR performed experiments, collected and analyzed data as well as wrote the first draft of the manuscript. RT performed experiments and collected data. PG performed experiments and edited the manuscript. MH performed experiments; PS conceptualized the study, edited and revised the manuscript. YHC designed the study, interpreted data, and finalized the manuscript. All authors approved the final manuscript as submitted.

Competing interests

The authors declare that they have no competing interests.

Author details

[1]Department of Pediatrics, Brody School of Medicine, East Carolina University, Greenville, NC 27834, USA. [2]Department of Anatomy and Cell Biology, Brody School of Medicine, East Carolina University, Greenville, NC 27834, USA. [3]Department of Pediatrics, MetroHealth Medical Center, Case Western Reserve University, Cleveland, OH 44109, USA. [4]Present Address: Clinical Neonatologist, Mercy Medical Center, Cedar Rapids, IA 52403, USA. [5]Present Address: Department of Pediatrics, Division Neonatology, University of Mississippi Medical Center, Jackson, Mississippi 39216, USA.

References

1. Neu J, Walker WA. Necrotizing enterocolitis. N Engl J Med. 2011;364:255–64.
2. Pike K, Brocklehurst P, Jones D, Kenyon S, Salt A, Taylor D, et al. Outcomes at 7 years for babies who developed neonatal necrotising enterocolitis: the ORACLE Children Study. Arch Dis Child Fetal Neonatal Ed. 2012;97:F318–22.
3. Lin PW, Nasr TR, Stoll BJ. Necrotizing enterocolitis: recent scientific advances in pathophysiology and prevention. Semin Perinatol. 2008;32:70–82.
4. Gordon P, Christensen R, Weitkamp JH, Maheshwari A. Mapping the New World of Necrotizing Enterocolitis (NEC): Review and Opinion. EJ Neonatol Res. 2012;2:145–72.
5. Berseth CL. Gestational evolution of small intestine motility in preterm and term infants. J Pediatr. 1989;115:646–51.
6. Berseth CL. Neonatal small intestinal motility: motor responses to feeding in term and preterm infants. J Pediatr. 1990;117:777–82.
7. Berseth CL, Ittmann PI. Antral and duodenal motor responses to duodenal feeding in preterm and term infants. J Pediatr Gastroenterol Nutr. 1992;14: 182–6.
8. Ittmann PI, Amarnath R, Berseth CL. Maturation of antroduodenal motor activity in preterm and term infants. Dig Dis Sci. 1992;37:14–9.
9. Di Lorenzo M, Bass J, Krantis A. An intraluminal model of necrotizing enterocolitis in the developing neonatal piglet. J Pediatr Surg. 1995;30: 1138–42.
10. Santulli TV, Schullinger JN, Heird WC, Gongaware RD, Wigger J, Barlow B, et al. Acute necrotizing enterocolitis in infancy: a review of 64 cases. Pediatrics. 1975;55:376–87.
11. Gribar SC, Sodhi CP, Richardson WM, Anand RJ, Gittes GK, Branca MF, et al. Reciprocal expression and signaling of TLR4 and TLR9 in the pathogenesis and treatment of necrotizing enterocolitis. J Immunol. 2009;182:636–46.
12. Good M, Siggers RH, Sodhi CP, Afrazi A, Alkhudari F, Egan CE, et al. Amniotic fluid inhibits Toll-like receptor 4 signaling in the fetal and neonatal intestinal epithelium. Proc Natl Acad Sci U S A. 2012;109:11330–5.
13. Gonzalez-Mariscal L, Betanzos A, Nava P, Jaramillo BE. Tight junction proteins. Prog Biophys Mol Biol. 2003;81:1–44.
14. Stevenson BR, Siliciano JD, Mooseker MS, Goodenough DA. Identification of ZO-1: a high molecular weight polypeptide associated with the tight junction (zonula occludens) in a variety of epithelia. J Cell Biol. 1986;103: 755–66.
15. Furuse M, Hirase T, Itoh M, Nagafuchi A, Yonemura S, Tsukita S, et al. Occludin: a novel integral membrane protein localizing at tight junctions. J Cell Biol. 1993;123:1777–88.
16. Furuse M, Fujita K, Hiiragi T, Fujimoto K, Tsukita S. Claudin-1 and -2: novel integral membrane proteins localizing at tight junctions with no sequence similarity to occludin. J Cell Biol. 1998;141:1539–50.
17. Martin-Padura I, Lostaglio S, Schneemann M, Williams L, Romano M, Fruscella P, et al. Junctional adhesion molecule, a novel member of the immunoglobulin superfamily that distributes at intercellular junctions and modulates monocyte transmigration. J Cell Biol. 1998;142:117–27.
18. Fujita H, Chiba H, Yokozaki H, Sakai N, Sugimoto K, Wada T, et al. Differential expression and subcellular localization of claudin-7, -8, -12, -13, and -15 along the mouse intestine. J Histochem Cytochem. 2006;54:933–44.

19. Krause G, Winkler L, Mueller SL, Haseloff RF, Piontek J, Blasig IE. Structure and function of claudins. Biochim Biophys Acta. 2008;1778:631–45.
20. Schneeberger EE, Lynch RD. The tight junction: a multifunctional complex. Am J Physiol Cell Physiol. 2004;286:C1213–28.
21. Arrieta MC, Bistritz L, Meddings JB. Alterations in intestinal permeability. Gut. 2006;55:1512–20.
22. Tsukita S, Furuse M, Itoh M. Multifunctional strands in tight junctions. Nat Rev Mol Cell Biol. 2001;2:285–93.
23. Clark JA, Doelle SM, Halpern MD, Saunders TA, Holubec H, Dvorak K, et al. Intestinal barrier failure during experimental necrotizing enterocolitis: protective effect of EGF treatment. Am J Physiol Gastrointest Liver Physiol. 2006;291:G938–49.
24. Kilkenny C, Browne W, Cuthill IC, Emerson M, Altman DG, Group NCRRGW. Animal research: reporting in vivo experiments: the ARRIVE guidelines. Br J Pharmacol. 2010;160:1577–9.
25. Jilling T, Simon D, Lu J, Meng FJ, Li D, Schy R, et al. The roles of bacteria and TLR4 in rat and murine models of necrotizing enterocolitis. J Immunol. 2006;177:3273–82.
26. Caplan MS, Hedlund E, Adler L, Hsueh W. Role of asphyxia and feeding in a neonatal rat model of necrotizing enterocolitis. Pediatr Pathol. 1994;14: 1017–28.
27. Prophet E. Laboratory methods in Histotechnology. Am Reg Pathol. 1992. p. 279.
28. Ding L, Zhang Y, Tatum R, Chen YH. Detection of tight junction barrier function in vivo by biotin. Methods Mol Biol. 2011;762:91–100.
29. Weber CR, Liang GH, Wang Y, Das S, Shen L, Yu AS, et al. Claudin-2-dependent paracellular channels are dynamically gated. Elife. 2015;4:e09906.
30. Rosenthal R, Gunzel D, Krug SM, Schulzke JD, Fromm M, Yu AS. Claudin-2-mediated cation and water transport share a common pore. Acta Physiol (Oxf). 2017;219:521–36.
31. Zeissig S, Burgel N, Gunzel D, Richter J, Mankertz J, Wahnschaffe U, et al. Changes in expression and distribution of claudin 2, 5 and 8 lead to discontinuous tight junctions and barrier dysfunction in active Crohn's disease. Gut. 2007;56:61–72.
32. Lu Z, Ding L, Lu Q, Chen YH. Claudins in intestines: Distribution and functional significance in health and diseases. Tissue Barriers. 2013;1:e24978.
33. Ding L, Lu Z, Foreman O, Tatum R, Lu Q, Renegar R, et al. Inflammation and disruption of the mucosal architecture in claudin-7-deficient mice. Gastroenterology. 2012;142:305–15.
34. Lu Z, Kim DH, Fan J, Lu Q, Verbanac K, Ding L, et al. A non-tight junction function of claudin-7-Interaction with integrin signaling in suppressing lung cancer cell proliferation and detachment. Mol Cancer. 2015;14:120.
35. Grootjans J, Thuijls G, Verdam F, Derikx JP, Lenaerts K, Buurman WA. Non-invasive assessment of barrier integrity and function of the human gut. World J Gastrointest Surg. 2010;2:61–9.
36. Thuijls G, Derikx JP, van Wijck K, Zimmermann LJ, Degraeuwe PL, Mulder TL, et al. Non-invasive markers for early diagnosis and determination of the severity of necrotizing enterocolitis. Ann Surg. 2010;251:1174–80.
37. Nitta T, Hata M, Gotoh S, Seo Y, Sasaki H, Hashimoto N, et al. Size-selective loosening of the blood-brain barrier in claudin-5-deficient mice. J Cell Biol. 2003;161:653–60.
38. Jeong JY, Kwon HB, Ahn JC, Kang D, Kwon SH, Park JA, et al. Functional and developmental analysis of the blood-brain barrier in zebrafish. Brain Res Bull. 2008;75:619–28.
39. Guttman JA, Li Y, Wickham ME, Deng W, Vogl AW, Finlay BB. Attaching and effacing pathogen-induced tight junction disruption in vivo. Cell Microbiol. 2006;8:634–45.
40. Edelson MB, Bagwell CE, Rozycki HJ. Circulating pro- and counterinflammatory cytokine levels and severity in necrotizing enterocolitis. Pediatrics. 1999;103:766–71.
41. Caplan MS, Sun XM, Hseuh W, Hageman JR. Role of platelet activating factor and tumor necrosis factor-alpha in neonatal necrotizing enterocolitis. J Pediatr. 1990;116:960–4.
42. Harris MC, Costarino AT Jr, Sullivan JS, Dulkerian S, McCawley L, Corcoran L, et al. Cytokine elevations in critically ill infants with sepsis and necrotizing enterocolitis. J Pediatr. 1994;124:105–11.
43. Harris MC, D'Angio CT, Gallagher PR, Kaufman D, Evans J, Kilpatrick L. Cytokine elaboration in critically ill infants with bacterial sepsis, necrotizing entercolitis, or sepsis syndrome: correlation with clinical parameters of inflammation and mortality. J Pediatr. 2005;147:462 8.
44. Garg PM, Tatum R, Ravisankar S, Shekhawat PS, Chen YH. Necrotizing enterocolitis in a mouse model leads to widespread renal inflammation, acute kidney injury, and disruption of renal tight junction proteins. Pediatr Res. 2015;78:527–32.

24

Melatonin alleviates brain and peripheral tissue edema in a neonatal rat model of hypoxic-ischemic brain damage: the involvement of edema related proteins

Li-Xiao Xu[1†], Yuan Lv[2†], Yan-Hong Li[1], Xin Ding[3], Ying Wang[3], Xing Han[3], Ming-Hua Liu[3], Bin Sun[3*] and Xing Feng[3*]

Abstract

Background: Previous studies have indicated edema may be involved in the pathophysiology following hypoxic-ischemic encephalopathy (HIE), and melatonin may exhibit neuro-protection against brain insults. However, little is known regarding the mechanisms that involve the protective effects of melatonin in the brain and peripheral tissues after HIE. The present study aimed to examine the effects of melatonin on multiple organs, and the expression of edema related proteins in a neonatal rat model of hypoxic-ischemic brain damage (HIBD).

Methods: One hundred ninety-two neonatal rats were randomly divided into three subgroups that underwent a sham surgery or HIBD. After the HIBD or sham-injury, the rats received an intraperitoneal injection of melatonin or an equal volume vehicle, respectively. We investigated the effects of melatonin on brain, kidney, and colon edema via histological examination and the expression of edema related proteins, including AQP-4, ZO-1 and occludin, via qPCR and western blot.

Results: Our data indicated (1) Melatonin reduced the histological injury in the brain and peripheral organs induced by HIBD as assessed via H-E staining and transmission electron microscopy. (2) Melatonin alleviated the HIBD-induced cerebral edema characterized by increased brain water content. (3) HIBD induced significant changes of edema related proteins, such as AQP-4, ZO-1 and occludin, and these changes were partially reversed by melatonin treatment.

Conclusions: These findings provide substantial evidence that melatonin treatment has protective effects on the brain and peripheral organs after HIBD, and the edema related proteins, AQP4, ZO-1, and occludin, may indirectly contribute tothe mechanism of the edema protection by melatonin.

Keywords: Melatonin, Hypoxic-ischemic encephalopathy, Edema, Aquaporin-4, Zonula occludens-1, Occludin

Background

Hypoxic-ischemic encephalopathy (HIE) is a leading cause of mortality and morbidity. The most frequent etiologies of it are intrapartum or late antepartum brain hypoxia and ischemia [1, 2]. 40–60% of the HIE infants were die by 2 years of age or left severe disabilities—The majority pathological mechanism of HIE is declined cerebral blood flow which results in less oxygen delivery to the brain disabilities [3] Despite the substantial research that has been conducted regarding HIE, the therapeutic interventions remain limited. Current HIE research is focused on the identification of the underlying pathophysiology of perinatal HIE and the alleviation of these pathophysiological mechanisms, especially the reversible factors [4].

Neonatal asphyxia, or birth asphyxia is caused by deprivation of oxygen to a newborn baby that usually

* Correspondence: sunyu0628@126.com; xing_feng66@suda.edu.cn
†Equal contributors
[3]Department of Neonatology, Children's Hospital of Soochow University, Suzhou 215006, China

induce edema harm to the body, frequently to the brain to result in HIE [5]. Except brain injuries, severe neonatal asphyxia is usually accompanied with multi-organ damages (such as in heart, lungs, liver, gut, kidneys) since the preferential blood supply to the brain will aggravate peripheral tissue ischemia [6, 7]. Therefore, the management of brain and peripheral tissue edema is critical for the prognosis of HIE patients. To date, a number of theories have been proposed to explain the development of edema in the brain and peripheral tissues [5, 8] Water channel aquaporins-4 (AQP-4) is specific membrane protein that have been widely investigated, which controls the influx and efflux of transmembrane water [9]. As the constituent of the continuous intercellular barrier between epithelial cells, tight junctions (TJ) are required to separate tissue spaces and regulate the selective movement of solutes across the epithelium [10]. Because zonula occludens-1 (ZO-1) and occludin are identified within TJs, together they form a virtually impermeable barrier to fluid between closely associated cells, which is very important in the maintenance of the mucosal and vascular endothelial barrier structure [11]. However, the dynamic changes in edema related proteins, such as AQP-4, ZO-1 and occludin, in the brain and peripheral tissues following HIE and their roles in edema development in central and peripheral tissues have rarely been reported. Early inhibition of edema related proteins in the brain and peripheral tissues may represent a new treatment protocol for edema following HIE.

In recent years, melatonin has been considered a promising neuro-protective drug for various acute and chronic brain injuries [12]. Melatonin is a naturally occurring hormone that is produced by the brain and was first identified to facilitate the regulation of the sleep-wake cycle [13]. Following ischemic brain injury/stroke, melatonin treatment has demonstrated a remarkable ability to reduce the infarct volume and/or inhibit neuronal cell death in different mammalian species and experimental models [12]. Moreover, it has been reported that melatonin decreased sensorimotor asymmetry and learning deficits, which thus protected pups from the long-term consequences of neonatal asphyxia [14]. In addition, histological analysis has also demonstrated melatonin treatment can increase the number of morphologically well preserved neurons in the CA1, CA2, and CA3 areas, as well as the dentate gyrus of the hippocampus in a hypoxic-ischemic mode [12]. Melatonin can decrease the cellular damage induced by epilepsy involved activation of kainate-sensitive glutamate receptors [15]. However, to the best of our knowledge, little is known regarding the mechanisms that involve the neuroprotective effects of melatonin and its effects on peripheral tissues in a hypoxic-ischemic encephalopathy model.

In the present study, we examined the effects of melatonin on brain, kidney and colon edema, and its roles in the expression of edema related proteins, including AQP-4, ZO-1 and occludin, in a neonatal rat model of hypoxic-ischemic brain damage (HIBD). We hypothesized that melatonin treatment would reduce the edema in both the brain and peripheral tissues that was induced by HIBD, at least in part, through the modulation of edema related proteins.

Methods

Animal preparation

192 Specific pathogen Free (SPF) Sprague Dawley (SD) rats at 7 days of age and a weight of 15–20 g, regardless of gender, were obtained from the SLRC Laboratory Animal Co. Ltd., China (License Key SCXK (Hu) 2012-0002). The neonatal rats were housed in groups of 10–15 rats per cage in standard plastic cages, and they were freely fed by female rats. The animal room was maintained on a 12-h dark-light cycle, and the temperature was maintained at 25±2°C. The protocols, which include all surgical procedures and animal usage, were approved by the Animal Care and Use Committee of Soochow University and conformed to the Guide for the Care and Use of Laboratory Animals by the National Institutes of Health.

HIBD model establishment

HIBD was induced in the present study using a modified Rice-Vannucci method [16]. In brief, 7-day-old postnatal pups were anesthetized with is oflurane (3% in a mixture of medical air and oxygen, 70:30 ratio). The left common carotid artery of each pup was identified, exposed, and permanently ligated with 5-0 surgical silk via a near-midline incision. The wound was closed, and the pups were allowed to recover from the anesthesia after the procedure, which lasted approximately 5 min per pup. Following recovery with their dams for 2 h, the pups were subsequently placed in a jar perfused with a humidified and pre-warmed gas mixture (8% oxygen balanced with nitrogen) for 2.5 h. A constant temperature of 37 °C was maintained throughout all procedures. Following the hypoxia, the animals were returned to their dams, and the ambient temperature was maintained at 37 °C for 24 h. The sham animals underwent anesthesia, and the common carotid artery was exposed without ligation or hypoxia.

Experimental protocol

The animals were randomly allocated into three subgroups ($n = 64$ per group) by throwing a 9-faces dice: (A) the numbers 1, 4, 7 were in sham group (Sham group), (B) the numbers of 2, 5, 8 were in HIBD group (Mod group), and (C) the numbers of 3, 6, 9 were in HIBD + melatonin group (MT group). Immediately after the HIBD injury, the rats received an intraperitoneal injection of melatonin (10 mg/kg body weight) (Sigma, USA) in the MT group or an equal volume of vehicle in the Sham and Mod Groups.

Cerebral edema measurement

Cerebral edema was determined via brain water content (BWC) measurement using the wet weight—dry weight technique, and the results are expressed as a percentage of the water content [17].

Hematoxylin& eosin (H-E) staining of the brain, kidney and colon

The rats were sacrificed under deep anesthesia at 3, 6, 24 and 72 h after HIBD or sham-injury for H-E staining. The rats were perfused with heparinized saline and 4% neutral buffered formalin. The same cortical layer of left frontal cortex, renal cortex and colon were dissected. 5 μm thick paraffin-embedded sections were prepared for H-E staining.

Quantification of the swelling cell

For quantification analysis, the swelling cell in the H-E stained cortex, renal cortex and colon samples were defined as the cells which were abnormal enlargement of a body, transparent cytosol, light stained, and even balloon-like structures. The total number of the swelling glial cell, renal tubular epithelial cells, or colon epithelial cells were countered in 5 random fields under high magnification view. The swellingcells of cerebral glial, glomerular epithelial, colon epithelial cells were quantified by dividing to the corresponding total cells.

Transmission electron microscopy (TEM) of the brain, kidney and colon

The rats were sacrificed under deep anesthesia at 3, 6, 24 and 72 h after HIBD or sham-injury for ultrastructure examination using TEM. Slices (approximately 1 mm thick) of the same cortical layer of left frontal cortex, renal cortex and colon were placed into cold 4% glutaraldehyde solution immediately after harvest and maintained at less than 4°C. The whole process of sampling required less than 3 min. Semi-thin sections were cut from these slices, rinsed overnight in 0.1 M phosphate buffer, post-fixed for 2 h in 1% osmium tetroxide, dehydrated and then embedded in Araldite mixture. Ultrathin sections stained in uranyl acetate and lead citrate were viewed in a Philips CM 120 electron microscope (Worcester, MA, USA).

Real time-quantitative polymerase chain reaction (RT-qPCR) for AQP4, ZO-1, and occludin

The rats in the three groups were sacrificed under deep anesthesia at 3, 6, 24 and 72 h after HIBD or sham-injury for RT-qPCR [18]. The rats were transcardially perfused with 250 ml of cold heparinized 0.9% saline, and the left frontal cortex, renal cortex and colon were rapidly removed and stored in liquid nitrogen immediately until use. The AQP-4, ZO-1, and occluding mRNA levels were determined using RT-qPCR. The primer sequences and PCR conditions were as follows: AQP-4: forward, 5'- cggttcatggaaacct cact -3'; reverse, 5'- catgctggctccggtataat -3'; Zo-1: forward, 5'- gtatccgattgttgtgttcc -3'; reverse, 5'- tcacttg tagcaccatccgc -3'; occludin: forward, 5'- cacgttcgac caatgc -3'; reverse, 5'- cccgttccataggctc -3'; and β-actin: forward, 5'-cccatctatgagggttacgc -3'; reverse, 5'-tttaatgtcacgcacgatttc -3'. RT-qPCR analysis was performed using the iQ5™ Real-Time PCR System (Bio-Rad, USA), which applied real-time SYBR Green PCR technology. All samples were analyzed in triplicate. β-actin was selected as an acceptable endogenous reference "housekeeping" gene. The relative change in the target cytokine mRNA expression was determined by the following equation: fold change = 2 – [ΔΔCt], where the Ct value is the cycle number at which the fluorescence signal crosses the threshold.

Western blot

0.5–1 g of the mouse cortex, renal cortex, and colon were collected and lysed in 500 μl of homogenization buffer. Each 30 μg of the extracted protein was separated on 10% SDS-PAGE gels and transferred onto a nitrocellulose membrane. Subsequently, the membrane was reacted with mouse monoclonal AQP-4 (all antibodies are from Abcam;Cambridge,MA),mouse monoclonal ZO-1, mouse monoclonal occluding, and mouse monoclonal GAPDH. The probed membrane was then incubated with horseradish peroxidase-conjugated rabbit anti-mouse IgG. The probed proteins (AQP-4, ZO-1, occluding, and GAPDH) were visualized by enhanced chemiluminescent.

Statistical analysis

SPSS 16.0 software was used for the statistical analyses (SPSS, Inc., Chicago, IL, USA). All data are presented as the mean ± SD. The data were subjected to a one-way analysis of variance followed by a Student-Newman-Keuls test. Statistical significance was determined as $P < 0.05$.

Results

Cerebral edema measurement

Twenty-four h after HIBD, a significant increase in the BWC, which indicated cerebral edema, was identified in the cerebral cortex compared with the sham rats that received vehicle treatment ($P < 0.05$; Fig. 1). The BWC increase induced by HIBD was significantly attenuated in

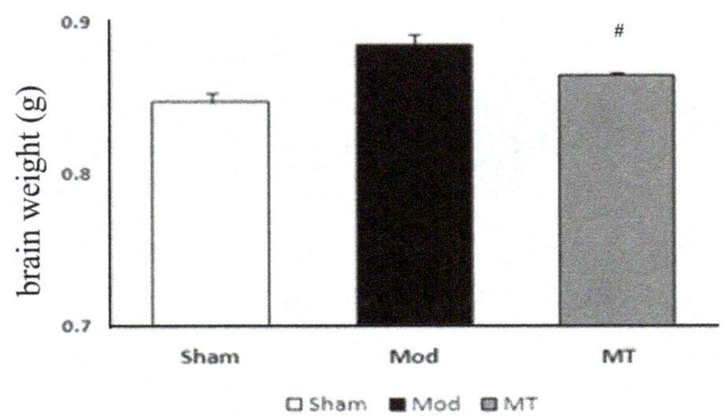

Fig. 1 Effects of melatonin treatment on the BWC ($n = 6$ per group). HIBD could result in a significant increase in the BWC in comparison with the one in the sham rats ($P < 0.05$), which was significantly attenuated following melatonin treatment ($P < 0.05$)

the HIBD rats following melatonin treatment ($P < 0.05$; Fig. 1), which indicates an improvement in cerebral edema.

Edema estimation of the brain, kidney and colon by H-E staining and edema cell quantification

In the Sham group, the cellular morphologies were normal in the brain (Fig. 2), kidney (Fig. 3) and colon (Fig. 4). In the Mod group, there was significant glial cell swelling and karyopyknosis in combination with interstitial tissue edema, capillary contracture and blank zones around the capillary (Fig. 2). And a significant swelling of the renal tubular epithelial cells was identified, as well as interstitial tissue edema (Fig. 3). Moreover, significant edema and even ballooning degeneration of the renal tubular epithelial cells were identified (Fig. 4). In the MT group, there was an improvement in the edema compared with the Mod group (Figs. 2, 3 and 4). In addition, the corresponding edema cells were quantified (Fig. 2d, 3d, and 4d) which is consistent with the observation above.

TEM of the brain, kidney and colon

In the Sham group, the cellular morphologies were normal in the brain (Fig. 5), kidney (Fig. 6) and colon (Fig. 7). In the Mod group, at 3 h after HIBD, there was a minimally dilated rough endoplasmic reticulum (ER) and edematous changes in the matrix and cristae of the mitochondria (Fig. 5). And the tubular epithelial cells were slightly swollen (Fig. 6). Moreover, the microvilli were sparse, and the rough ER was slightly dilated (Fig. 7). At 6 h after HIBD, there were more substantial edematous changes in the organelles and vacuolation of the mitochondria, as well as fusion in some intercellular junctions (Fig. 5). And the capillary lumen narrowed

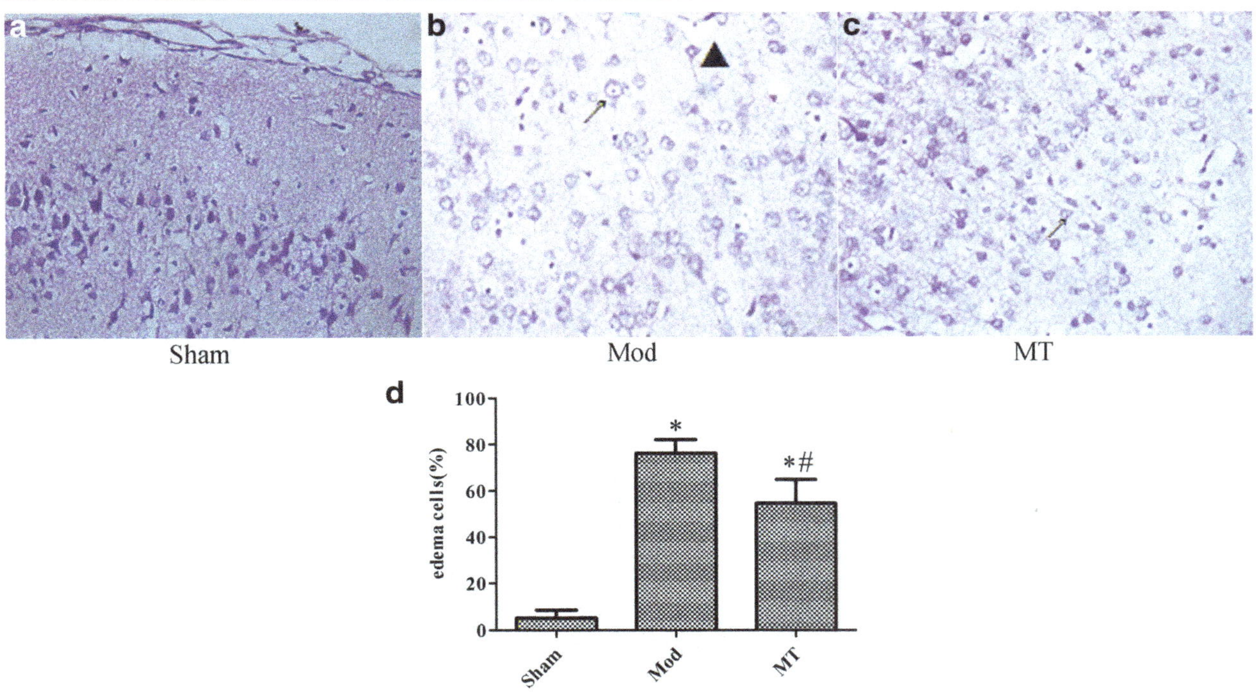

Fig. 2 Cerebral cortex under a 400 × light microscope after H-E staining. 24 h treatment of the HIBD results in insignificant glial cell swelling and karyopyknosis in combination with interstitial tissue edema, capillary contracture and blank zones around the capillary in H-E stained samples (**a** and **b**), which was improved by melatonin treatment (**c**). Furthermore, **d** showed the quantification analysis of the swollen glial cells in the total glial cells in the indicated groups.↗ represents cytotoxic edema, and ▲ represents vasogenic edema

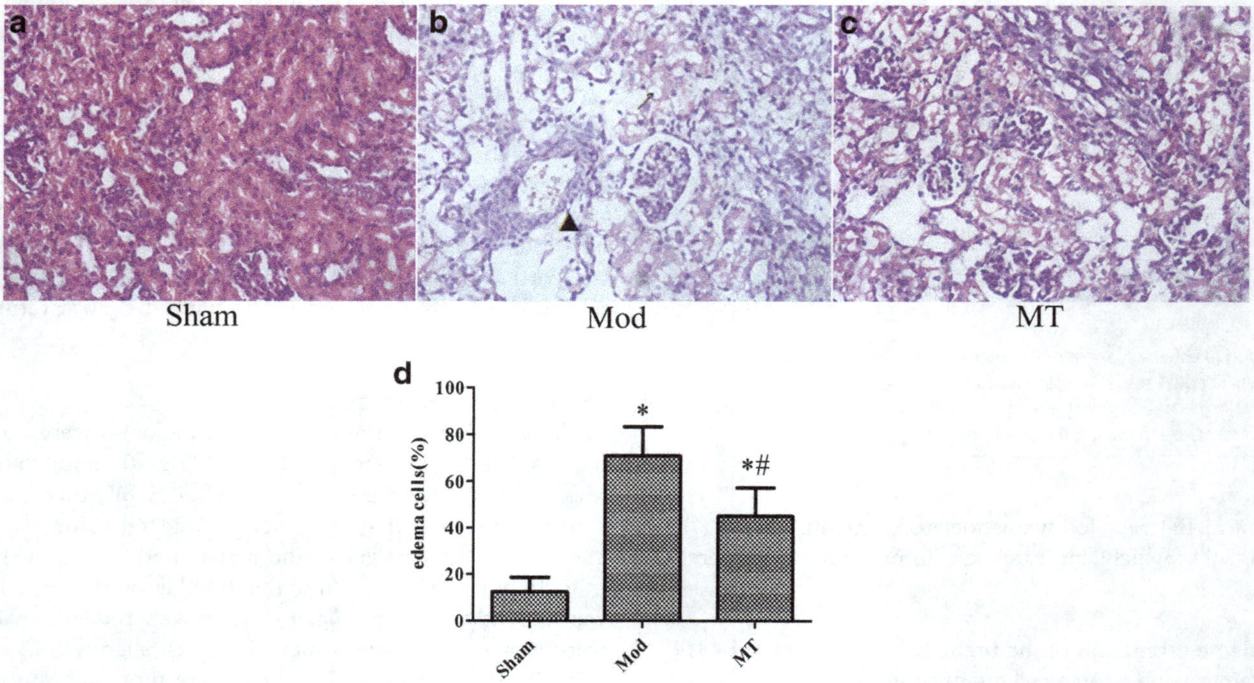

Fig. 3 Renal cortex under a 400 × light microscope after H-E staining. Similar treatment as Fig. 2 induced significant swelling of the renal tubular epithelial cells and interstitial tissue edema, which was improved by melatonin treatment in H-Estained samples (**a** and **b**). However, there were few changes regarding the glomeruli in these groups. In addition, the swollen renal tubular epithelial cells were quantified in the total renal tubular epithelial cells in the indicated groups.↗ represents cytotoxic edema, and ▲ represents vasogenic edema

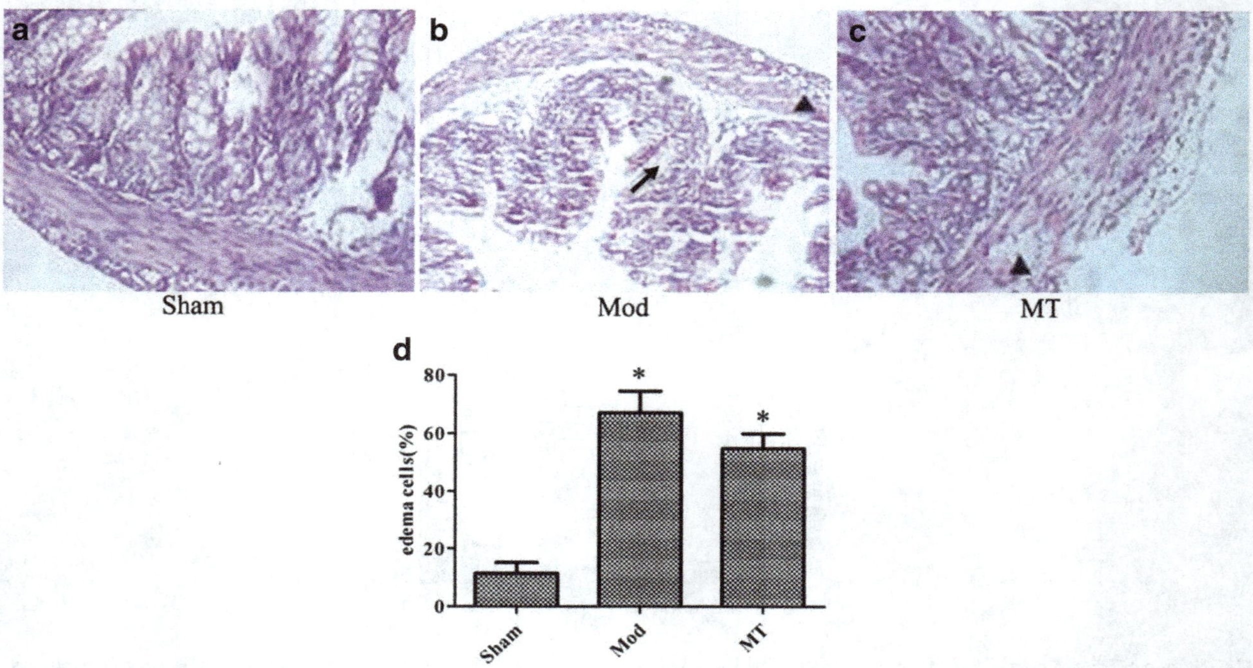

Fig. 4 Colon under a 400 × light microscope after H-E staining. 24 h-HIBD persuaded significant edema and even ballooning degeneration of the renal tubular epithelial cells (**b**) compared with sham group (**a**), and these alterations were improved by melatonin treatment (**c**). The edema colon epithelial cells were quantified as well in the total colon epithelial cells in the indicated groups (**d**). ↗ represents cytotoxic edema, and ▲ represents vasogenic edema

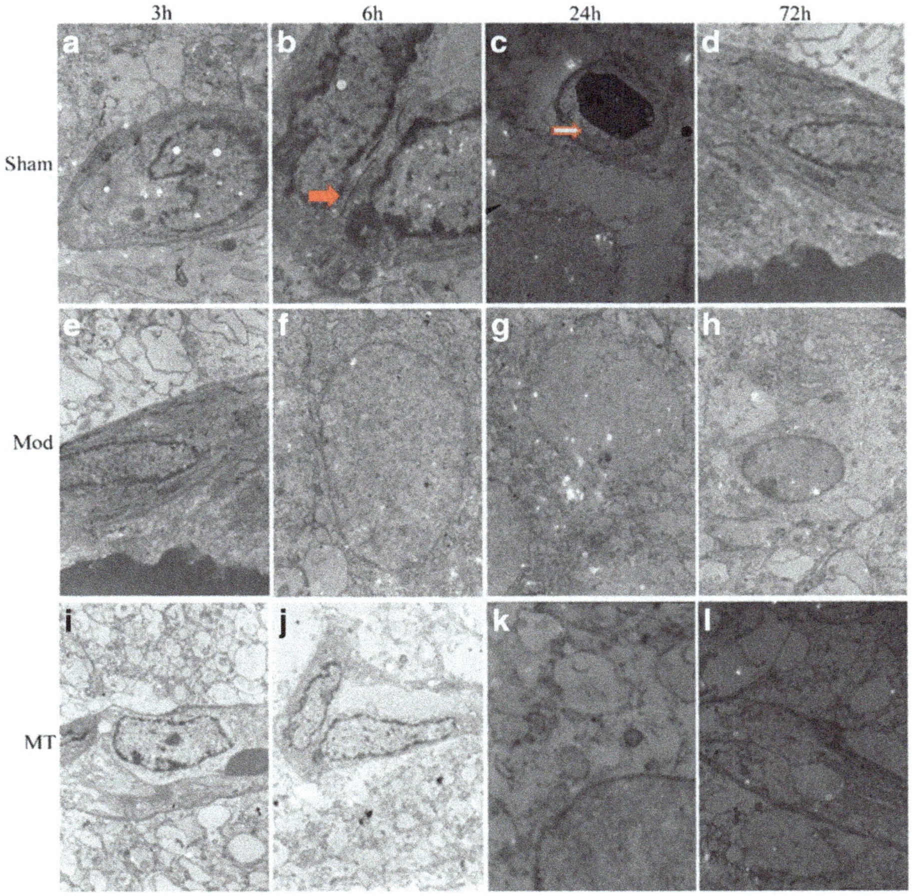

Fig. 5 Cerebral glial cells and capillaries assessed via a transmission electron microscope. HIBD could result in a remarkable pathologic change at 24 h after injury, including clearly decreased organelles and their extraordinary swelling, fused or disappeared intercellular junctions and additional stenosis and contracture of the capillary lumens (**e-h**) compared with sham group (**a-d**). Melatonin treatment could reduce the severity of pathology after injury (**i-l**). Red solid arrows represent tight junctions, red hollow arrows represent capillary lumens, and ▲ represents cell vacuoles

while the epithelial hole increased (Fig. 6). Moreover, the edematous changes in the colon cells progressed, and the junctions between the cells became somewhat vague (Fig. 7). A remarkable pathologic change occurred at 24 h after HIBD, which was characterized by clearly decreased organelles and their extraordinary swelling. Many intercellular junctions had fused or disappeared (Fig. 5). And there was a vague membrane, which made it difficult to distinguish the three layers, and the foot process was randomly arranged and further fused (Fig. 6). In the colon (Fig. 7), even the sparse distributed microvilli swelled, and the epithelial cell organelles were vague. 72 h after the operation, the situation had improved in the brain (Fig. 5), kidney(Fig. 6) and colon(Fig. 7). In the MT group, the time course of edema was similar compared with the Mod group, but the severity was reduced (Figs. 5, 6 and 7).

AQP-4 expression in the cerebral cortex, renal cortex and colon

As shown in Fig. 8a, HIBD induced a significant increase in the AQP-4 mRNA expression in the cerebral cortex compared with the sham injury at 3, 6 and 24 h after injury ($P < 0.05$). Melatonin treatment significantly decreased the AQP-4 mRNA expression in the cerebral cortex compared with the Mod Group at 3 and 24 h after the injury ($P < 0.05$). Furthermore, the data in Fig. 8b indicated that there was no significant difference in the AQP-4 mRNA expression in the renal cortex between the three groups at any time-point ($P > 0.05$). In addition, the data in Fig. 8c indicated that HIBD induced a significant increase in the AQP-4 mRNA expression in the colon compared with the sham injury only at 24 h after the injury ($P < 0.05$). The mRNA changes in the cerebral cortex and renal cortex after 24 h HIBD treatment were verified as well by western blot (Fig. 11a

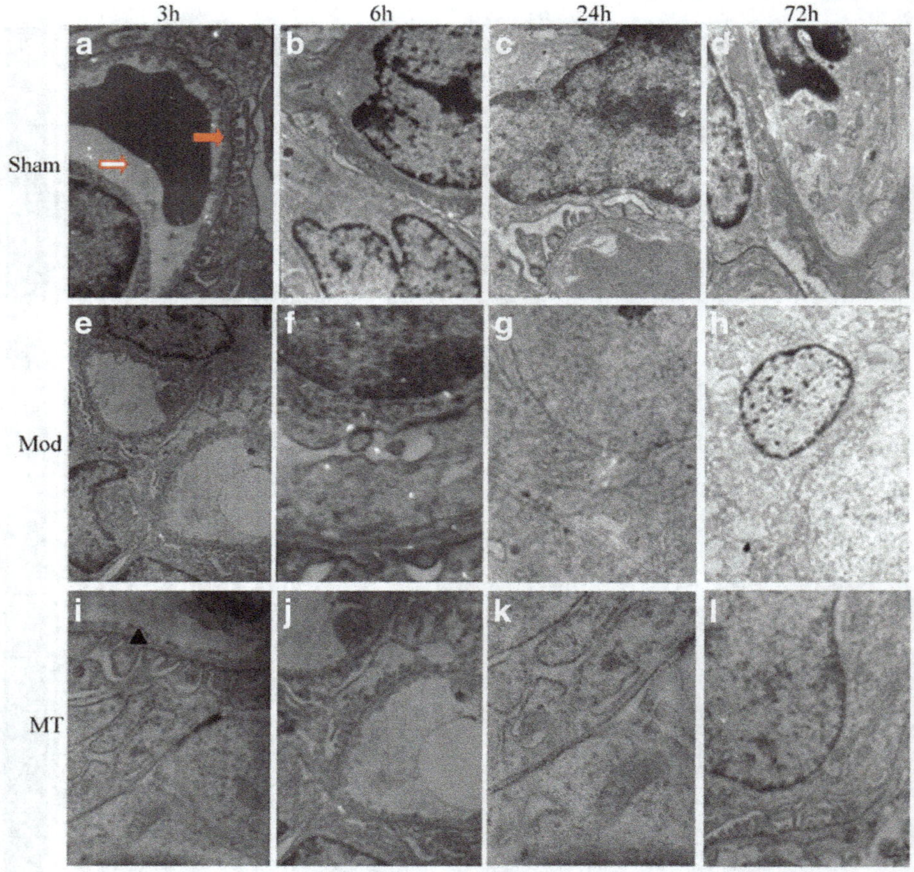

Fig. 6 Glomerular filtration barriers assessed via a transmission electron microscope. HIBD could result in a remarkable damage in the membrane and foot processes at 24h after injury, including vague membranes and randomly arranged and further fused foot process (**e-h**) compared with sham group (**a-d**). Melatonin treatment could reduce the severity of pathology after injury (**i-l**). Red solid arrows represent the foot process, red hollow arrows represent capillary lumens, and ▲ represents filtration barrier epithelial cells

and b). AQP-1 protein expression of the cerebral cortex and renal cortex were augmented significantly 24 h after HIBD and melatonin partially (cerebral cortex, Fig. 11a) or completely (renal cortex, Fig. 11b) prevented this increase. The detection of the protein expression in the colon samples did not succeed (data did not show).

ZO-1 expression in the cerebral cortex, renal cortex and colon

As shown in Fig. 9a, HIBD induced a significant decrease in the ZO-1 mRNA expression in the cerebral cortex compared with the sham injury at 6, 24 and 72 h after the injury ($P < 0.05$). There was no significant difference in the ZO-1 mRNA expression in the cerebral cortex between the Mod and MT groups at any time-point ($P > 0.05$). Furthermore, the data in Fig. 9b indicated that the ZO-1 mRNA expression in the renal cortex was significantly decreased compared with the sham injury at 6 and 24 h after the injury ($P < 0.05$). Melatonin significantly increased the ZO-1 mRNA expression in the renal cortex compared with the Mod group at 24 h after the injury ($P < 0.05$). In addition, the data in Fig. 9c indicated that HIBD induced a significant decrease in the ZO-1 mRNA expression in the colon compared with the sham injury at 6 and 24 h after the injury ($P < 0.05$), whereas melatonin treatment significantly increased the ZO-1 mRNA expression in the colon compared with the Mod group24 h after the injury ($P < 0.05$). The findings in the cerebral cortex and renal cortex at 24 h after injury were further confirmed by western blot (Fig. 11a and b). ZO-1 protein of the cerebral cortex has declined 24 h after HIBD and melatonin turn back this response significantly (Fig. 11a). Likewise, ZO-1 protein expression of the renal cortex has slightly weakened 24 h after HIBD and this decrease was prohibited considerably by melatonin treatment (Fig. 11b).

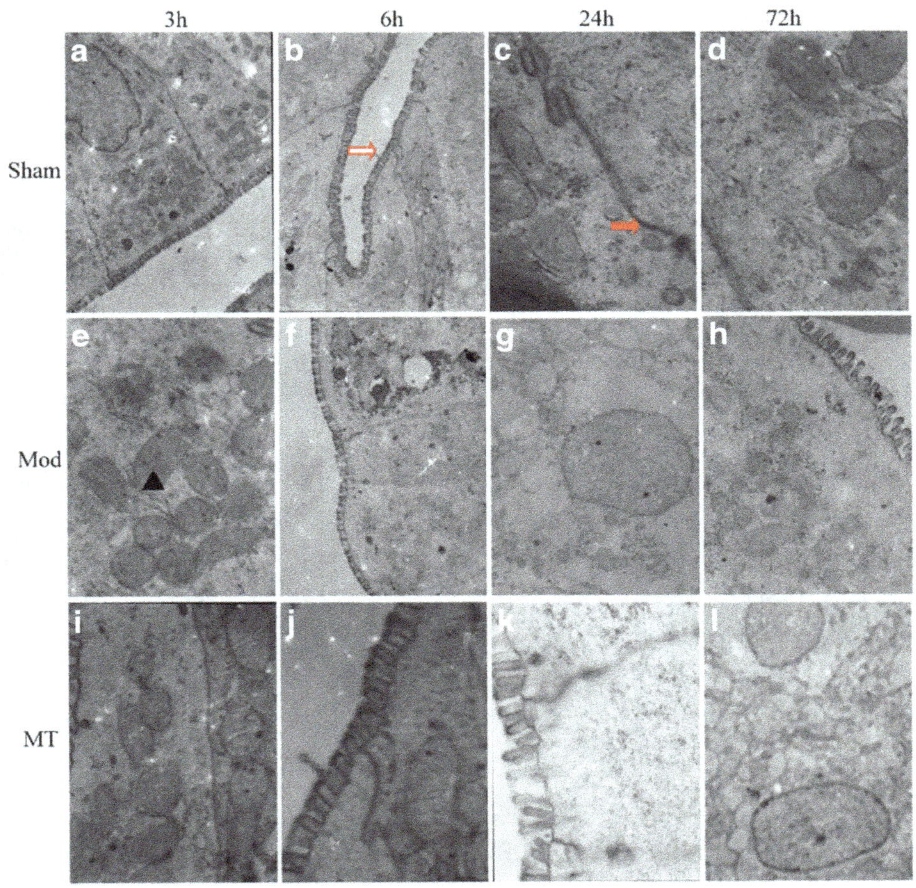

Fig. 7 Colon epithelial cells assessed via atransmission electron microscope. HIBD could result in edematous changes in the matrix, cristae in the mitochondria, the sparse distributed swelled microvilli, the vague epithelial cell organelles, remarkable decreased junctions and the loosened interstitial tissue (**e-h**) compared with sham group (**ad**). Melatonin treatment could reduce the severity of pathology after injury (**i-l**). Red solid arrows represent tight junctions, red hollow arrows represent intestinal epithelium microvilli, and ▲ represents mitochondria

Occludin expression in the cerebral cortex, renal cortex and colon

As shown in Fig. 10a, HIBD induced a significant decrease in the occluding mRNA expression in the cerebral cortex compared with the sham injury at each time-point after the injury ($P < 0.05$). Melatonin treatment significantly increased the occluding mRNA expression in the cerebral cortex compared with the Mod group at 6, 24 and 72 h after the injury ($P < 0.05$). Moreover, the data in Fig. 10b indicated that the occluding mRNA expression in the renal cortex was significantly decreased compared with the sham injury 24 h after the injury ($P < 0.05$). There was no significant difference in the occluding mRNA expression in the renal cortex between the Mod and MT groups at any time-point ($P > 0.05$). In addition, the data in Fig. 10c indicated that HIBD induced a significant decrease in the occluding mRNA expression in the colon compared with the sham injury at each time-point after the injury ($P < 0.05$), whereas there was no significant difference in the occluding mRNA expression in the colon between the Mod and MT groups at any time-point ($P > 0.05$). In addition, these results in the cerebral cortex and renal cortex after 24 h HIBD were proven by western blot (Fig. 11a and b). Theoccludin protein expression of the cerebral cortex and renal cortex have decreased significantly 24 h after HIBD and melatonin partially attenuated these changes.

Discussion

In the present study, we examined the effects of melatonin on brain, kidney and colon edema, and its roles in the expression of edema related proteins in a neonatal rat model of HIBD. The main findings are as follows: (1) Melatonin reduced the histological injuries of the brain and peripheral organs, which were induced by HIBD, as assessed via H-E staining and TEM. (2) Melatonin alleviated the HIBD-induced cerebral edema characterized by the decreased BWC. (3) HIBD induced significant

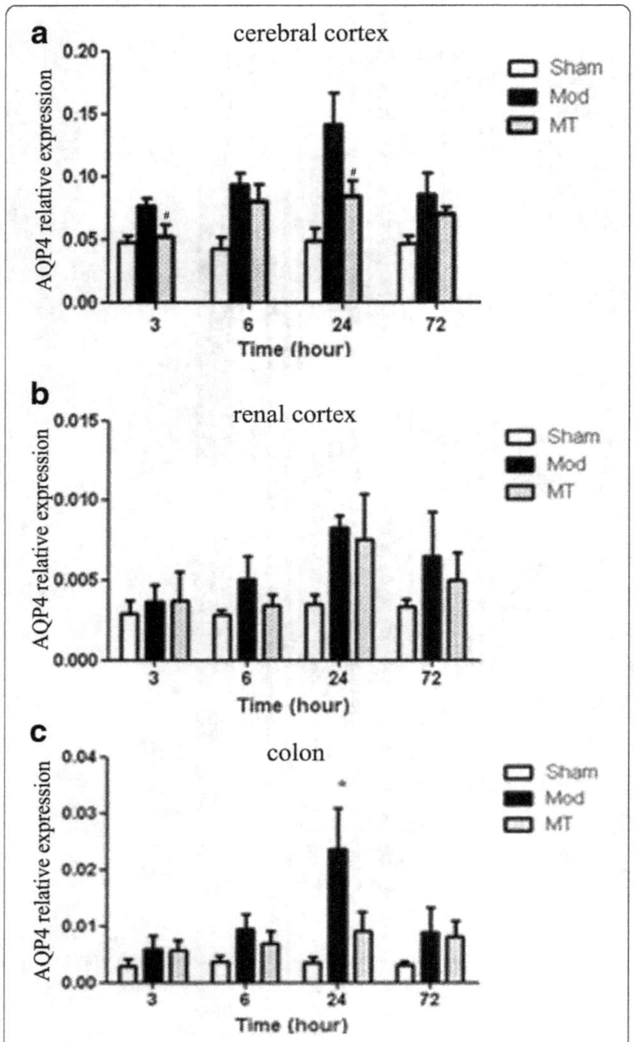

Fig. 8 Real time-qPCR for AQP-4 in the cerebral cortex (**a**), renal cortex (**b**) and colon (**c**). HIBD induced a significant increase in the AQP-4 mRNA expression in the cerebral cortex and colon. Melatonin treatment significantly decreased the AQP-4 mRNA expression in comparison with the one without melatonin treatment in HIBD group. The data represent the mean ± SD

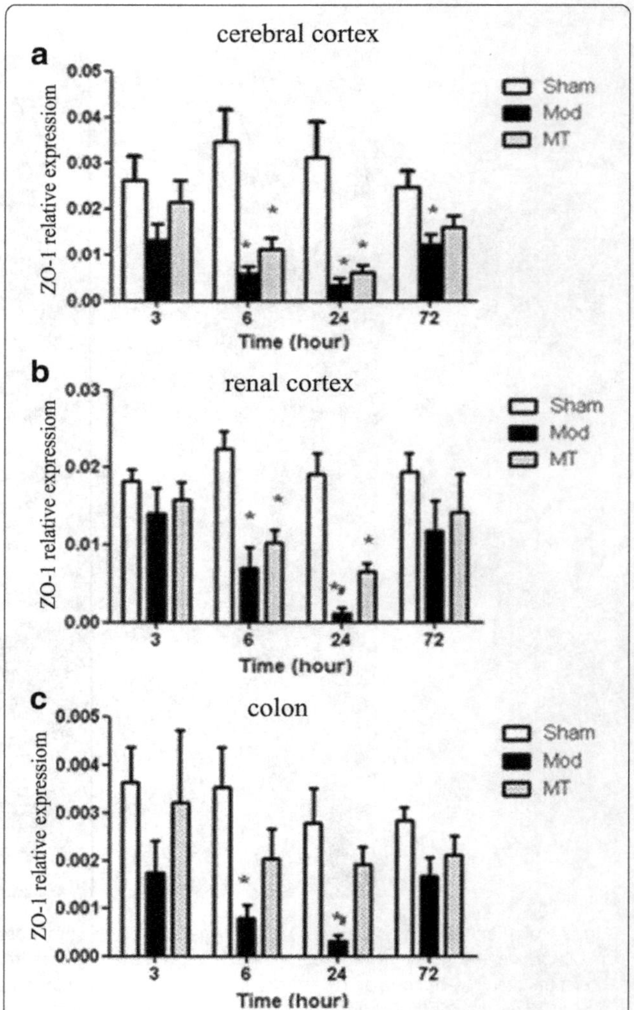

Fig. 9 Real time-qPCR for ZO-1 in the cerebral cortex (**a**), renal cortex (**b**) and colon (**c**). HIBD induced a significant decrease in the ZO-1 mRNA expression in the cerebral cortex, renal cortex and colon. Melatonin treatment could significantly increase the ZO-1 mRNA expression in the renal cortex and colon in comparison with the one without melatonin treatment in HIBD group. The data represent the mean ± SD

changes in the mRNA expression of edema related proteins, including AQP-4, ZO-1 and occludin, which were partially reversed by melatonin treatment.

AQP-4 is one of the most deeply lucubrated edema related proteins in the central nervous system, especially regarding cytotoxic cerebral edema [19]. The expression of AQP-4 is positively related to edema at an early stage after HIBD insults in rats with a genetic knockout of AQP-4 [20], which is consistent with our findings that cerebral edema characterized by increased BWC is accompanied by significantly increased AQP-4 expression in the cerebral cortex following HIBD insults. Moreover, we demonstrated that AQP-4 mRNA expression increased as early as 3 h after HIBD injury and was accompanied by the histological signs of cerebral edema, such as mitochondrial swelling, rough ER expansion, and capillary contracture surrounded by an electronic blank area, when examined by TEM, these alterations represented both cytotoxic edema and vasogenic edema. The present study demonstrated that AQP-4 mRNA expression reached its peak at 24 h after injury and subsequently decreased, which was accompanied by similar changes assessed via TEM.

Acute kidney injury typically presents with edema and necrosis, and the renal tubules exhibit an earlier and more severe manifestation [21]. In the present study, we

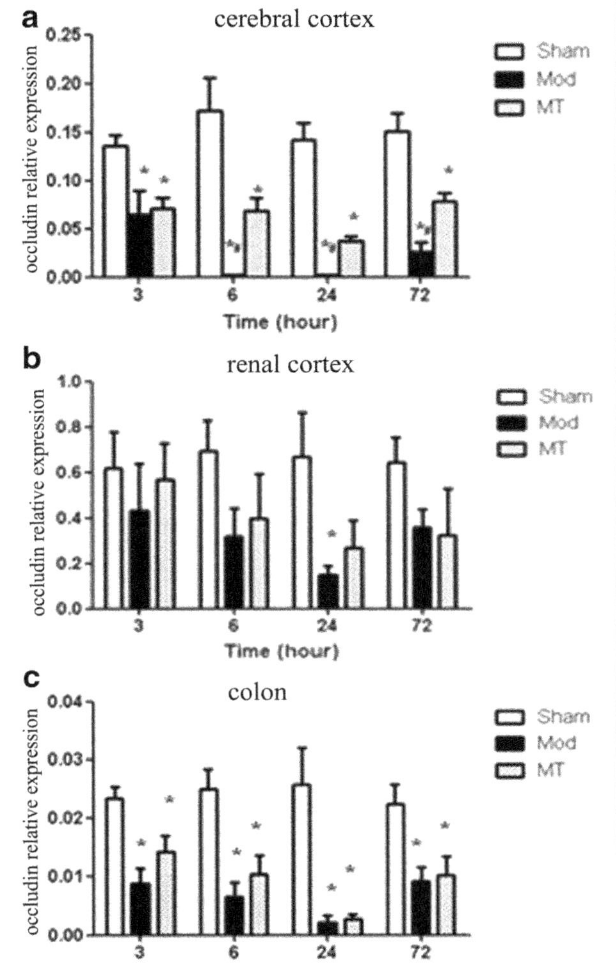

Fig. 10 Real time-qPCR for occluding in the cerebral cortex (**a**), renal cortex (**b**) and colon (**c**). HIBD induced a significant decrease in the occluding mRNA expression in the cerebral cortex, renal cortex and colon, which could be significantly increased by melatonin treatment. The data represent the mean ± SD

identified obvious edematous and necrotic changes together with interstitial edema. However, AQP-4 mRNA expression was not significantly different after hypoxic and ischemic damage, which indicates that there may be no obvious correlation between AQP4 and renal tubular epithelial cell and interstitial tissue edema. Nevertheless, based on evidence regarding the organic distribution of AQPs and the existence of more than one subtype of AQPs positioned in the kidney [22] we speculated that tubular cell edemamay be affected by other AQP subtypes; thus

Additional research is required to verify this hypothesis. Neonates with HIE typically exhibit abnormal manifestations in the digestive tract, such as gastrointestinal bleeding and feeding intolerance, and the most severe symptom is necrotizing enterocolitis. The ileum and colon are more likely to be affected because of their special blood supply characteristics and molecular basis. Previous studies have demonstrated that AQP-4 is distributed in the entire colon, mainly on the top of the villi epithelium and lumen [23]. However, little is known regarding the relationship between AQP-4 and hypoxic-ischemic intestinal damage. In our experiment, we identified colon epithelial cell edema using TEM, as well as an increased AQP-4 expression, which is consistent with the extent of edema in the colon. Thus, we could infer that AQP-4 expression may play a role in hypoxic-ischemic colon damage.

Tight junction proteins (TJPs) represent a series of proteins closely related to the blood-brain barrier (BBB) in the brain. In our experiment, we investigated two types of TJPs, including ZO-1 and occludin. The expression of ZO-1 and occluding mRNA were decreased as early as 3 h after HIBD injury, which was accompanied by signs of vasogenic edema in the brain assessed with TEM. This finding further verifies that TJPs are negatively related to edema. Tight junctions are also very important for the maintenance of epithelial homeostasis. Previous studies have indicated that TJPs are expressed on tubules [24]. Thus, the significant decrease in TJP expression, especially ZO-1 expression, may be related to the damage of tight junctions between tubules and renal interstitial, which tends to lead to vasogenic edema. In addition, the use of TEM in the present study demonstrated the existence of colon epithelial edema as early as 3 h after HIBD, and the edema peaked 24 h after injury, which was accompanied by significantly decreased ZO-1 and occluding mRNA expression in the colon. Thus, the damaged tight junction structure characterized by reduced TJP expression may be the reason for colon epithelial injury following HIBD.

To date, previous studies regarding endogenous melatonin and melatonin receptors have indicated that there is a significant decrease in both the release and function of melatonin following HIBD, which suggests melatonin may function in the pathogenesis of HIBD. Moreover, exogenous melatonin supplementation can improve the stress state, exhibit beneficial effects in the maintenance of relative homeostasis, and improve the immunological functions of HIE neonates. Thus, it is necessary to further investigate the role of melatonin in the pathophysiological mechanisms of HIBD, such as edema in the central nervous system and peripheral organs. Our study provides timely and substantial evidence for the theoretical basis of melatonin application in the clinic.

Previous studies indicate that endogenous melatonin release decreased during the hypoxic-ischemic injury in rats, which may be involved in the pathogenesis of early HIBD [10, 12]. In addition, supplement of exogenous

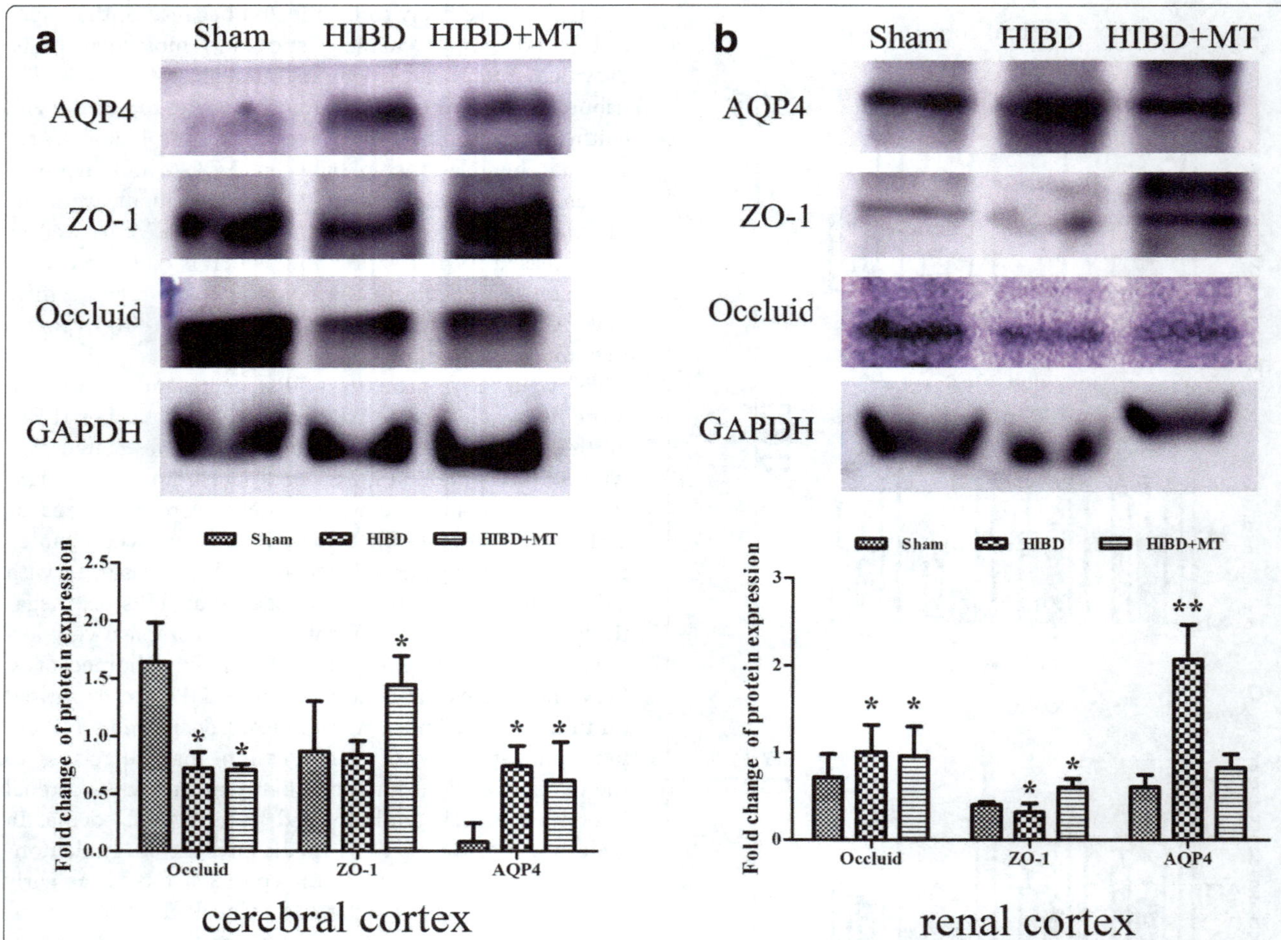

Fig. 11 Western blot of the APQ-4, ZO-1, and occludin inthe cerebral cortex, renal cortex. The protein expression of the APQ-4, ZO-1, and occluding were detected by western blot after 24 h HIBD in cerebral cortex (**a**), renal cortex (**b**). The targeted protein was indicated in the left of the images and the treatment conditions were shown on the top of the pictures. GAPDH were used as a housekeeping gene references. The shown pictures represented three other independent results. **P* < 0.05, compared with the sham operation group

melatonin after hypoxic-ischemic injury is beneficial to protect neonatal perinatal brain damage [14]. In a prospective study melatonin combining with hypothermia promoted neonatal HIE survival and health by brain magnetic resonance imaging (MRI) analysis [25]. In another preterm brain injury study, small dose (0.1 mg/kg) of melatonin demonstrated a protective activity on pregnant ewe hyopoxic/ischemia injure model [26]. On the other hand, other study of melatonin treatment in an neonatal hypoxic-ischemic damage model did not show significant improvement in (1 h) early phase [27]. These results hint that different hypoxic/ischemia model and the method of melatonin employment may affect the result, as well as more longer observation is necessary. Our results did demonstrate a significant anti-edema damage activity in longer time course observation. In addition, our result provided a possible mechanism as well that melatonin indirectly regulates the edema related factors, AQP-4, ZO-1, and occludin, to partially protect hypoxic-ischemic injures.

Several mechanisms of melatonin may be involved in its effects. For example, based on its lipophilic and partly hydrophilic dissolubility, melatonin has a high diffusing capacity, which makes it easy to enter the central nervous system and act directly on cell membranes and nuclei [28]. It was believed that metalonin acts for neuroprotection and ischemia harm protection by its anti-oxidative and anti-apoptosis properties [29–33]. Thus, regarding the edema protection property, melatonin could change the transcriptional activity of edema related molecules, such as AQP-4 and TJPs, which is important for its improvement in brain edema. Furthermore, the melatonin receptor belongs to a G-protein-coupled receptor family, and exogenous melatonin can combine with its receptors soon after HIBD, which further activates the downstream MAPK signal pathway, especially the p38 MAPK and JNK/SAPK signal pathways [34, 35], both of which are important in the regulation of HIBD pathogenesis, such as edema related proteins. Moreover, exogenous melatonin could increase endogenous melatonin release and melatonin receptor regulation via the positive feedback path, as well as enlarge their effects via a cascade reaction. In addition, vascular endothelial growth factor (VEGF) has been reported to lead to the inactivation of TJPs, such as ZO-1, by decreasing their expression and increasing phosphorylation; previous studies have indicated that melatonin can improve VEGF release [36, 37], which indirectly regulates edema related protein expression. Additional research regarding the pathways involved in the regulation of edema related proteins for melatonin is necessary.

Conclusions

In conclusion, our data indicate that melatonin treatment has protective effects on the brain and peripheral organs after HIBD. The edema related proteins, AQP-4, ZO-1, and occludin, may participate in the mechanism of edema protection by melatonin.

Abbreviations

AQPs: Aquaporins; BBB: Blood-brain barrier; BWC: Brain water content; ER: Endoplasmic reticulum; HIBD: Hypoxic-ischemic brain damage; HIE: Hypoxic-ischemic encephalopathy; MT: Melatonin; qPCR: Real-time quantitative polymerase chain reaction; SD: Sprague Dawley; SPF: Specific pathogen free; TJ: Tight junctions; TJP: Tight junction proteins; VEGF: Vascular endothelial growth factor; ZO-1: Zonula occludens-1

Acknowledgements

Not applicable.

Funding

This work was supported by grants from National Natural Science Foundation (81471488, 81502157, 81271378, 81501291), Key medical subjects of Jiangsu province (XK201120), Jiangsu Province key research and development of special funds (BE2015644), Key Laboratory of Suzhou City (SZS201108), Science and Technology Project of Suzhou (SYSD2013105, SYS201446, SYS201441), Public health technology project of Suzhou (SS201536) and the Department of Pediatrics Clinical Center of Suzhou (Szzx201504).

Authors' contributions

XLX and LY participated in project design, all the experiment processes, data analysis, and manuscript writing. LYH provided technical support in histochemical staining analysis and helped revising the manuscript. DX designed the primer of PCR, completed the real-time PCR experiments and data collecting. HX and LMH helped accomplish HIBD model, participated in western blot experiments. WY was responsible for electronic microscopy analysis. SB and FX were primarily responsible for study design and protocol development. All authors have read and approved the manuscript.

Competing interests

The authors declare that they have no competing interests.

Author details

[1]Institute of Pediatric Research, Children's Hospital of Soochow University, Suzhou 215006, China. [2]Department of Neonatology, Northern Jiangsu People's Hospital, Yangzhou 225001, China. [3]Department of Neonatology, Children's Hospital of Soochow University, Suzhou 215006, China.

References

1. Sarnat HB, Sarnat MS. Neonatal encephalopathy following fetal distress. A clinical and electroencephalographic study. Arch Neurol. 1976;33(10):696–705.
2. Volpe JJ. Neurology of the Newborn. 4. In: Hypoxic-ischemic encephalopathy: Clinical aspects. Philadelphia: WB Saunders Co; 2000. p. 331–96.
3. Allen KA, Brandon DH. Hypoxic ischemic encephalopathy: pathophysiology and experimental treatments. Newborn Infant Nurs Rev. 2011;11(3):125–33.
4. Buonocore G, Perrone S, Turrisi G, Kramer BW, Balduini W. New pharmacological approaches in infants with hypoxic-ischemic encephalopathy. Curr Pharm Des. 2012;18(21):3086–100.
5. Lupton BA, Hill A, Roland EH, Whitfield MF, Flodmark O. Brain swelling in the asphyxiated term newborn: pathogenesis and outcome. Pediatrics. 1988;82(2):139–46.
6. Wang X, Zhang J, Yang Y, Dong W, Wang F, Wang L, et al. Progesterone attenuates cerebral edema in neonatal rats with hypoxic-ischemic brain damage by inhibiting the expression of matrix metalloproteinase-9 and aquaporin-4. Exp Ther Med. 2013;6(1):263–7.
7. Barnett CP, Perlman M, Ekert PG. Clinicopathological correlations in postasphyxial organ damage: a donor organ perspective. Pediatrics. 1997;99(6):797–9.
8. Scallan J, Huxley VH, Korthuis RJ. Capillary fluid exchange: regulation, functions, and pathology[J]. Colloquium. 2010(1).
9. Liu K, Agre P. Aquaporin Water Channels. In: Lane WJLD, eidotr. Encyclopedia of Biological Chemistry. Waltham: Academic Press; 2013. p. 120-6.
10. Anderson JM, Van Itallie CM. Physiology and function of the tight junction. Cold Spring Harb Perspect Biol. 2009;1(2):a002584.
11. Günzel D, Yu AS. Claudins and the modulation of tight junction permeability. Physiol Rev. 2013;93(2):525–69.
12. Alonso-Alconada D, Alvarez A, Arteaga O, Martinez-Ibarguen A, Hilario E. Neuroprotective effect of melatonin: a novel therapy against perinatal hypoxia-ischemia. Int J Mol Sci. 2013;14(5):9379–95.
13. Brown GM. Light, melatonin and the sleep-wake cycle. J Psychiatry Neurosci. 1994;19(5):345–53.
14. Carloni S, Perrone S, Buonocore G, Longini M, Proietti F, Balduini W. Melatonin protects from the long-term consequences of a neonatal hypoxic-ischemic brain injury in rats. J Pineal Res. 2008;44(2):157–64.
15. Uz T, Giusti P, Franceschini D, Kharlamov A, Manev H. Protective effect of melatonin against hippocampal DNA damage induced by intraperitoneal administration of kainate to rats. Neuroscience. 1996;73(3):631–6.
16. Chen W, Jadhav V, Tang J, Zhang JH. HIF-1alpha inhibition ameliorates neonatal brain injury in a rat pup hypoxic-ischemic model. Neurobiol Dis. 2008;31(3):433–41.
17. Wang JW, Wang HD, Cong ZX, Zhang XS, Zhou XM, Zhang DD. Activation of metabotropic glutamate receptor 5 reduces the secondary brain injury after traumatic brain injury in rats. Biochem Biophys Res Commun. 2013;430(3):1016–21.
18. Wang JW, Wang HD, Zhong WZ. Li N, Cong ZX. Expression and cell distribution of metabotropic glutamate receptor 5 in the rat cortex following traumatic brain injury. Brain Res. 2012;1464:73–81.
19. Wang H, Wang X, Guo Q. The correlation between DTI parameters and levels of AQP-4 in the early phases of cerebral edema after hypoxic-ischemic/reperfusion injury in piglets. Pediatr Radiol. 2012;42(8):992–9.
20. Da T, Verkman AS. Aquaporin-4 gene disruption in mice protects against impaired retinal function and cell death after ischemia. Invest Ophthalmol Vis Sci. 2004;45(12):4477–83.
21. Basile DP, Anderson MD, Sutton TA. Pathophysiology of acute kidney injury. Compr Physiol. 2012;2(2):1303–53.
22. Wang W, Li C, Summer SN, Falk S, Wang W, Ljubanovic D, et al. Role of AQP1 in endotoxemia-induced acute kidney injury. Am J Physiol Renal Physiol. 2008;294(6):F1473–80.

23. Yde J, Keely S, Wu Q, et al. Characterization of AQPs in Mouse, Rat, and Human Colon and Their Selective Regulation by Bile Acids. Front Nutr. 2016;3:46.
24. Gonzalez-Mariscal L, Namorado MC, Martin D, Luna J, Alarcon L, Islas S, et al. Tight junction proteins ZO-1, ZO-2, and occludin along isolated renal tubules. Kidney Int. 2000;57(6):2386–402.
25. Aly H, Elmahdy H, El-Dib M, Rowisha M, Awny M, El-Gohary T, et al. Melatonin use for neuroprotection in perinatal asphyxia: a randomized controlled pilot study. J Perinatol. 2015;35(3):186–91.
26. Drury PP, Davidson JO, Bennet L, Booth LC, Tan S, Fraser M, et al. Partial neural protection with prophylactic low-dose melatonin after asphyxia in preterm fetal sheep. J Cereb Blood Flow Metab. 2014;34(1):126–35.
27. Berger HR, Morken TS, Vettukattil R, Brubakk AM, Sonnewald U, Wideroe M. No improvement of neuronal metabolism in the reperfusion phase with melatonin treatment after hypoxic-ischemic brain injury in the neonatal rat. J Neurochem. 2015;136(2):339–50.
28. Hardeland R. Melatonin in plants and other phototrophs: advances and gaps concerning the diversity of functions. J Exp Bot. 2015;66(3):627–46.
29. Gilad E, Cuzzocrea S, Zingarelli B, Salzman AL, Szabo C. Melatonin is a scavenger of peroxynitrite. Life Sci. 1997;60(10):L169–74.
30. Hardeland R, Tan DX, Reiter RJ. Kynuramines, metabolites of melatonin and other indoles: the resurrection of an almost forgotten class of biogenic amines. J Pineal Res. 2009;47(2):109–26.
31. Wakatsuki A, Okatani Y, Izumiya C, Ikenoue N. Melatonin protects against ischemia and reperfusion-induced oxidative lipid and DNA damage in fetal rat brain. J Pineal Res. 1999;26(3):147–52.
32. Tan DX, Manchester LC, Terron MP, Flores LJ, Reiter RJ. One molecule, many derivatives: a never-ending interaction of melatonin with reactive oxygen and nitrogen species? J Pineal Res. 2007;42(1):28–42.
33. Hassell KJ, Ezzati M, Alonso-Alconada D, Hausenloy DJ, Robertson NJ. New horizons for newborn brain protection: enhancing endogenous neuroprotection. Arch Dis Child Fetal Neonatal Ed. 2015;100(6):F541–52.
34. Xu L, Pathak PS, Fukumura D. Hypoxia-induced activation of p38 mitogen-activated protein kinase and phosphatidylinositol 3'-kinase signaling pathways contributes to expression of interleukin 8 in human ovarian carcinoma cells. Clin Cancer Res. 2004;10(2):701–7.
35. Ferreira GM, Martinez M, Camargo IC, Domeniconi RF, Martinez FE, Chuffa LG. Melatonin Attenuates Her-2, p38 MAPK, p-AKT, and mTOR Levels in Ovarian Carcinoma of Ethanol-Preferring Rats. J Cancer. 2014;5(9):728–35.
36. Fischer S, Wobben M, Marti HH, Renz D, Schaper W. Hypoxia-induced hyperpermeability in brain microvessel endothelial cells involves VEGF-mediated changes in the expression of zonula occludens-1. Microvasc Res. 2002;63(1):70–80.
37. Kaur C, Sivakumar V, Ling EA. Melatonin protects periventricular white matter from damage due to hypoxia. J Pineal Res. 2010;48(3):185–93.

25

Causes of death in very preterm infants cared for in neonatal intensive care units

Tim Schindler[1,2*], Louise Koller-Smith[1], Kei Lui[1,2], Barbara Bajuk[3], Srinivas Bolisetty[1,2]
and New South Wales and Australian Capital Territory Neonatal Intensive Care Units' Data Collection

Abstract

Background: While there are good data to describe changing trends in mortality and morbidity rates for preterm populations, there is very little information on the specific causes and pattern of death in terms of age of vulnerability. It is well established that mortality increases with decreasing gestational age but there are limited data on the specific causes that account for this increased mortality. The aim of this study was to establish the common causes of hospital mortality in a regional preterm population admitted to a neonatal intensive care unit (NICU).

Methods: Retrospective analysis of prospectively collected data of the Neonatal Intensive Care Units' (NICUS) Data Collection of all 10 NICUs in the region. Infants <32 weeks gestation without major congenital anomalies admitted from 2007 to 2011 were included. Three authors reviewed all cases to agree upon the immediate cause of death.

Results: There were 345 (7.7%) deaths out of 4454 infants. The most common cause of death across all gestational groups was major IVH (cause-specific mortality rate [CMR] 22 per 1000 infants), followed by acute respiratory illnesses [ARI] (CMR 21 per 1000 infants) and sepsis (CMR 12 per 1000 infants). The most common cause of death was different in each gestational group (22–25 weeks [ARI], 26–28 weeks [IVH] and 29–31 weeks [perinatal asphyxia]). Pregnancy induced hypertension, antenatal steroids and chorioamnionitis were all associated with changes in CMRs. Deaths due to ARI or major IVH were more likely to occur at an earlier age (median [quartiles] 1.4 [0.3–4.4] and 3.6 [1.9–6.6] days respectively) in comparison to NEC and miscellaneous causes (25.2 [15.4–37.3] and 25.8 [3.2–68.9] days respectively).

Conclusions: Major IVH and ARI were the most common causes of hospital mortality in this extreme to very preterm population. Perinatal factors have a significant impact on cause-specific mortality. The varying timing of death provides insight into the prolonged vulnerability for diseases such as necrotising enterocolitis in our preterm population.

Keywords: Preterm, Infant, Mortality, Cause of death

* Correspondence: tschindl@med.usyd.edu.au
[1]Faculty of Medicine, University of New South Wales, Sydney, Australia
[2]Department of Newborn Care, Royal Hospital for Women, Sydney, Australia

Background

For many parents, premature birth is a confronting experience whereby they are faced with a series of potentially life-changing events as their baby transitions from foetal to neonatal life. As clinicians, it is important to have a thorough understanding of preterm mortality as we counsel and prognosticate through this process. While there are good data to describe changing trends in mortality and morbidity rates for preterm populations [1–3], there is very little information on the specific causes and pattern of death in terms of age of vulnerability. It is well established that mortality increases with decreasing gestational age but there are limited data on the specific causes that account for this increased mortality.

Cause-specific mortality rates (CMR) are routinely used to describe the mortality rate from a specified cause for a population in a defined period. There are studies that addressed the cause-specific mortality in the neonatal intensive care environment and the newborn period, however, these studies generally accepted extreme prematurity or immaturity as a cause of death without specifying the immediate cause of death for this population [4–7].

We have previously published mortality data on a large cohort of preterm infants less than 32 weeks gestation admitted to a regional network of neonatal intensive care units [8]. We reported gestational age-specific mortality, including identification of perinatal risk factors that have a significant impact on overall mortality. In this study, we performed an in-depth analysis of the immediate causes of mortality in this same cohort. We investigated the CMR by gestational age at birth. We also investigated the age at death based on the cause of mortality. We also analysed the implications of the cause specific mortality on resource utilisation.

Methods

Data for this study were sourced from the prospectively collected Neonatal Intensive Care Units' (NICUS) Data Collection. NICUS Data Collection is an ongoing regional audit of neonates admitted to all 10 NICUs in New South Wales (NSW) and Australian Capital Territory (ACT). All 10 NICUs are level III or level IV facilities [9]. These units are regularly benchmarked against each other and have comparable outcomes with respect to mortality and major morbidity. Neonatal, maternal and perinatal data are prospectively collected within each NICU by a designated Clinical Audit Officer. The data undergo rigorous quality control procedures with regular audit and validation checks. All liveborn infants less than 32 weeks gestation admitted to any of these NICUs from 1st January 2007 to 31st December 2011 were identified. Infants with major congenital malformations (constituting major confounding factors for morbidity and mortality) or admitted for palliation were excluded from the analysis. The perinatal characteristics of these infants, along with gestational age-specific hospital survival rates, hospital morbidities and interventions are detailed in our earlier study [8]. This a population where the majority of women received antenatal care (97.7%), antenatal steroids (90%) and delivered at a tertiary perinatal centre (89%).

Study variables were defined according to NICUS Data Collection Manual. Definitions for other relevant major outcomes are as follows:

Cause-specific mortality rate: Number of deaths prior to hospital discharge from a specified cause for every 1000 infants admitted to a NICU. For instance, CMR for major IVH was calculated as per the formula below:

$$\frac{\text{Number of deaths due to Major IVH x 1000}}{\text{Study cohort}}$$

Ventilation days: Respiratory support with either mechanical ventilation, CPAP or high flow support (≥2 liters per minute).

Immediate cause of death: The disease, injury or complication that directly preceded death. Three authors *(TS, SB and BB)* reviewed all cases of hospital death that occurred before first discharge from hospital to home. This does not include deaths that may have occurred after hospital discharge. The cause of death recorded in the NICUS Data Collection was compared to the NICUS discharge summary for all cases. Each case was discussed in detail by all authors in each case. In cases where the immediate cause of death was unclear, further information from the case notes was sought from the individual units. For example, there were 48 cases where extreme prematurity was labelled as the immediate cause of death and these cases were further investigated to determine the complication that directly preceded death. If the immediate cause of death remained unclear at this point or if a consensus between the authors could not be reached, the individual unit was contacted directly to clarify the immediate cause of death. There were a number of cases where more than one problem could have been responsible for death. In these cases, the most significant problem, determined by the individual unit, was taken as the cause of death. In cases where intensive care was withdrawn, the antecedent problem leading to redirection of care was taken as the cause of death. In all cases, the authors were able to come to a consensus agreement on the immediate cause of death.

Deaths were categorised into the five most common groups and a miscellaneous group as defined below:

Deaths due to acute respiratory illness: Death from acute respiratory problems including hyaline membrane disease, pulmonary hypertension, pulmonary haemorrhage and pulmonary hypoplasia. Deaths attributable to chronic lung disease were not included in this group.

Deaths due to sepsis: Deaths attributed to either early or late onset sepsis. This included deaths that occurred in either the acute or subacute phase of illness. For example, an infant that progressed to subsequent organ failure as a result of sepsis would be classified as a death due to sepsis. These deaths were not differentiated by causative organism.

Deaths due to intraventricular haemorrhage: Any death attributable to Grade 3 or higher intraventricular and/or intracerebral haemorrhage. This included deaths following redirection of care because of a major haemorrhage.

Deaths due to perinatal asphyxia: Deaths that the individual unit attributed to any perinatal hypoxic insult. This included deaths that occurred in either the acute or subacute phase of illness. For example, an infant that progressed to subsequent organ failure as a result of an asphyxic event would be classified as a death due to perinatal asphyxia.

Deaths due to necrotising enterocolitis: Deaths directly attributable to the development of necrotising enterocolitis. This included deaths that occurred in either the acute or subacute phase of illness.

Deaths due to miscellaneous causes: All remaining deaths attributable to any cause not included in the five most common groups. Deaths attributable to chronic lung disease were included in this group.

These five most common groups and the remaining group of deaths due to miscellaneous causes were further analysed to identify the underlying perinatal risk factors and the pattern of death, including age at death and resource utilisation. Resource utilisation was measured by hours for respiratory support and parenteral nutrition and days for length of level 3 stay.

Statistical analyses were performed using SPSS Predictive Analytics Software (version 21, Chicago, Illinois, USA). Results were summarized as proportions, mean (±SD) and median and quartiles; Chi-square, parametric or non-parametric analyses were used where appropriate. Logistic multivariate analyses were used to determine independent significant factors associated with mortality. A Kaplan-Meier plot was created to illustrate the different chronological ages of death according to the cause of death. The study was approved by the South Eastern Sydney Illawarra Area Health Services Northern Hospital Network Human Research Ethics Committee.

Results

During the study period, there were 4501 eligible neonates registered in the NICUS database. There were 44 neonates with major congenital malformations, two born at 22 weeks gestation and one at 24 weeks gestation admitted to NICU for palliation and they were excluded from the study. Of 4454 infants included, there were 345 deaths during the study period.

Table 1 shows the results of the univariate and multivariate analyses on perinatal characteristics between infants who survived and those who died prior to discharge. Extreme prematurity was strongly associated with increased mortality. Using 29–31 weeks gestation as referent, 26–28 week infants and 22–25 week infants had adjusted odds ratios (95% CI) of 3.46 (2.24–5.35) and 16.34 (10.23–25.97) respectively. Other perinatal factors associated with increased mortality were male gender, small for gestation and low Apgar score. Neonatal factors associated with increased mortality were early onset sepsis, persistent pulmonary hypertension, pulmonary haemorrhage, major IVH, moderate-severe hypoxic ischaemic encephalopathy and NEC. Breech delivery was associated with mortality but this was not significant after adjustment for risk factors. Similarly, the increased mortality associated with surfactant treated hyaline membrane disease was not significant after multivariate analysis.

The cause-specific mortality patterns based on individual perinatal factors are represented in Table 2. In comparison to infants who survived, infants who died from sepsis were more likely to have a history of chorioamnionitis. Infants who died from NEC were more likely to be small for gestational age, had younger mothers, were more likely to have a history of hypertensive disease during pregnancy and less likely to have a history of chorioamnionitis. Infants who died due to major IVH were less likely to have a history of hypertensive disease during pregnancy, more likely to have a history of antepartum haemorrhage, less likely to have received antenatal steroids and more likely to be outborn. With respect to ARI, infants were less likely to have received antenatal steroids and more likely to have a history of antepartum haemorrhage. Infants who died due to asphyxia had older mothers, were less likely to have had antenatal care or receive antenatal steroids and were more likely to have a history of antepartum haemorrhage. The gestational ages and birthweights of infants who died due to asphyxia were higher than those who died from other causes.

Table 3 shows the distribution of the common causes of death stratified by gestation. The most common cause of death across all gestational groups was major IVH (CMR 22 per 1000 infants), followed by an acute respiratory illness [ARI] (CMR 21 per 1000 infants) and sepsis (CMR 12 per 1000 infants). In infants born at 22–25 weeks gestation, the commonest cause of death was ARI (CMR 119 per 1000 infants), followed by IVH (CMR 117 per 1000 infants) and sepsis (CMR 54 per 1000 infants). Chronic lung disease had a CMR of 13 per 1000 infants in this group. In infants born at 26–28 weeks gestation,

Table 1 Perinatal and clinical characteristics of infants who died

Variable	Survived	Died	Univariate analysis	P	Multivariate analysis
	n = *4109*	*n* = *345*	OR (95% CI)		Adjusted OR (95% CI)
Maternal age(mean ± SD)	30 ± 6	30 ± 6	—	0.978	—
Maternal indigenous status	229 (6%)	22 (6%)	1.15 (0.73–1.81)	0.301	—
Attended antenatal care	4021 (98%)	330 (96%)	0.48 (0.27–0.84)	0.009	0.83 (0.39–1.77)
Assisted conception	512 (13%)	41 (12%)	0.94 (0.67–1.33)	0.761	—
Multiple Births	1210 (29%)	82 (24%)	0.75 (0.58–0.97)	0.026	1.03 (0.72–1.47)
Hypertensive Disease of Pregnancy	802 (20%)	46 (13%)	0.63 (0.46–0.87)	0.005	0.93 (0.59–1.45)
Antepartum Haemorrhage	985 (24%)	123 (36%)	1.76 (1.39–2.21)	0.000	1.23 (0.90–1.68)
Chorioamnionitis	838 (20%)	94 (27%)	1.46 (1.14–1.87)	0.003	0.89 (0.76–1.04)
Antenatal Steroids	3724 (91%)	288 (84%)	0.52 (0.38–0.71)	0.000	0.84 (0.53–1.32)
Out born	452 (11%)	52 (15%)	1.44 (1.05–1.96)	0.022	0.98 (0.62–1.56)
Vaginal Breech Delivery	210 (5%)	62 (18%)	4.07 (2.99–5.54)	0.000	1.33 (0.87–2.04)
Gestation, weeks	29 ± 2	26 ± 2	—	0.000	—
Gestation					
22–25 weeks	344	178	—	0.000	16.34 (10.23–25.97)
4026–28 weeks	1248	118			3.46 (2.24–5.35)
4029–31 weeks	2517	49			1.00 (referent)
Male gender	2134 (52%)	223 (65%)	1.69 (1.34–2.13)	0.000	1.47 (1.10–1.96)
Birth weight, g	1285 ± 377	895 ± 362	—	0.000	—
Small for Gestational Age	286 (7%)	37 (11%)	1.61 (1.12–2.31)	0.009	2.14 (1.28–3.56)
APGAR <7 at 5 mins	697 (17%)	186 (56%)	5.73 (4.56–7.18)	0.000	2.41 (1.79–3.23)
Early Onset Sepsis	66 (2%)	28 (8%)	5.41 (3.43–8.54)	0.000	4.21 (2.34–7.56)
Late Onset Sepsis	742 (18%)	75 (22%)	1.26 (0.96–1.65)	0.054	—
Surfactant treated HMD	2371 (58%)	294 (85%)	4.23 (3.12–5.73)	0.000	0.84 (0.55–1.27)
PPHN	143 (3%)	62 (18%)	6.08 (4.41–8.38)	0.000	3.06 (2.02–4.64)
Pulmonary haemorrhage	69 (2%)	58 (17%)	11.8 (8.18–17.1)	0.000	4.26 (2.65–6.87)
IVH Grade III/IV	96 (2%)	112 (32%)	20.1 (14.8–27.2)	0.000	9.27 (6.30–13.64)
HIE Stage 2	8 (0.2%)	24 (7%)	38.3 (17.0–86.0)	0.000	4.52 (3.18–6.43)
NEC Stage 2	92 (2%)	40 (12%)	5.73 (3.88–8.45)	0.000	2.02 (1.59–2.57)

The number of infants n (%), mean ± SD and median (quartiles) are shown. Significant variables defined by univariate analysis are entered into a multivariate analysis. Odds ratio and adjusted odds ratios are shown

the commonest cause of death was IVH (CMR 24 per 1000 infants), while infants born at 29–31 weeks gestation, it was perinatal asphyxia (CMR 5 per 1000 infants).

A Kaplan-Meier curve (Fig. 1) was created to illustrate the age of death based on the most common causes of death. The overall survival curve shows that 80% of infants who die, die within the first three weeks and 90% die within the first five weeks of life. Cause-specific curves demonstrate that infants who die due to ARI or major IVH are more likely to die early (median age [quartiles] at death 1.4 [0.3–4.4] and 3.6 [1.9–6.6] days respectively). Infants who die from NEC and miscellaneous causes are more likely to die later (median age at death 25.2 [15.4–37.3] and 25.8 [3.2–68.9] days respectively).

Resource utilisation from birth is compared for each of the most common causes of death in Fig. 2. Length of level 3 stay in days, hours of respiratory support and hours of parenteral nutrition have been used as surrogate markers for resource utilisation. Resource utilisation is highest in infants who die of NEC for length of level 3 stay, duration of respiratory support and duration of parenteral nutrition and lowest in infants who die from respiratory problems.

Discussion

To our knowledge, this is the largest population based study describing CMR for an extreme to very preterm population. Compared with published data from other preterm populations over a shorter review period, the

Table 2 Perinatal characteristics based on the cause-specific mortality

		Causes of death									
Variable	Survived	Sepsis		Necrotizing enterocolitis		Major IVH		Respiratory		Perinatal asphyxia	
Total	*4109*	*55*	P	*39*	P	*99*	P	*95*	P	*25*	P
Maternal Age	30 ± 6	31 ± 5	0.326	28 ± 6	0.049	30 ± 6	0.719	30 ± 7	0.413	33 ± 5	0.029
Caucasian	3218 (78%)	44 (80%)	0.763	33 (85%)	0.342	77 (78%)	0.898	77 (81%)	0.522	22 (88%)	0.241
Antenatal Care	4021 (98%)	52 (95%)	0.095	37 (95%)	0.203	95 (96%)	0.202	92 (97%)	0.501	23 (92%)	0.045
Assisted Conception	512 (13%)	10 (18%)	0.203	7 (18%)	0.303	11 (11%)	0.688	11 (12%)	0.797	1 (4%)	0.201
Multiple											
Twins	1084 (26%)	14 (26%)	0.877	9 (23%)	0.641	19 (19%)	0.108	21 (22%)	0.349	3 (12%)	0.103
Triplets	115 (3%)	2 (4%)	0.709	2 (5%)	0.382	2 (2%)	0.642	3 (3%)	0.834	2 (8%)	0.118
Hypertensive Disease of Pregnancy	802 (20%)	10 (18.2%)	0.804	12 (30.8%)	0.078	6 (6.1%)	0.001	11 (11.6%)	0.053	5 (20%)	0.952
Antepartum Haemorrhage	985 (24%)	15 (27.3%)	0.569	13 (33.3%)	0.173	33 (33.3%)	0.032	36 (37.9%)	0.002	14 (56%)	0.000
Chorioamnionitis	838 (20%)	28 (51%)	0.000	3 (8%)	0.050	21 (21%)	0.842	26 (27%)	0.096	6 (24%)	0.656
No Antenatal Steroids	385 (9%)	2 (4%)	0.146	3 (8%)	0.720	23 (23%)	0.000	22 (23%)	0.000	7 (28%)	0.002
Out born	452 (11%)	5 (9%)	0.653	2 (5%)	0.242	28 (28%)	0.000	12 (13%)	0.616	1 (4%)	0.264
Mode of Delivery											
Normal Vaginal	1253 (31%)	13 (24%)	0.272	10 (26%)	0.512	35 (35%)	0.300	25 (26%)	0.381	3 (12%)	0.045
Vaginal Breech	210 (5%)	12 (22%)	0.000	1 (3%)	0.471	19 (19%)	0.000	21 (22%)	0.000	4 (16%)	0.014
Instrumental	79 (2%)	1 (1.8%)	0.955	0 (0%)	0.382	2 (2%)	0.944	0 (0%)	0.172	0 (0%)	0.484
LSCS	2562 (62%)	29 (53%)	0.144	28 (72%)	0.225	43 (43%)	0.000	49 (52%)	0.032	18 (72%)	0.321
Gestation, weeks	29 ± 2	26 ± 2	0.000	27 ± 2	0.000	25 ± 2	0.000	25 ± 2	0.000	29 ± 2	0.456
Male gender	2134 (52%)	28 (51%)	0.880	27 (69%)	0.031	69 (70%)	0.000	61 (64%)	0.018	18 (72%)	0.045
Birth weight, g	1285 ± 377	865 ± 289	0.000	895 ± 243	0.000	836 ± 225	0.000	807 ± 280	0.000	1343 ± 478	0.446
Birth weight <10th percentile	508 (12%)	9 (16%)	0.371	9 (23%)	0.044	9 (9%)	0.327	10 (11%)	0.590	4 (16%)	0.582
APGAR <7 at 5 mins	697 (17%)	26 (47%)	0.000	8 (21%)	0.566	58 (59%)	0.000	63 (69%)	0.000	22 (88%)	0.000
Resources utilisation											
Length of NICU Stay, days	56.8 (41.9–78.7)	7.3 (1.0–18.1)	0.000	25.2 (15.4–37.3)	0.000	3.6 (1.9–6.6)	0.000	1.4 (0.3–4.4)	0.000	2.5 (0.5–3.5)	0.000
Duration of Resp Support, hours	194 (40–853)	173 (13–421)	0.020	457 (267–785)	0.002	86 (44–145)	0.000	31 (7–104)	0.000	57 (12–84)	0.001
Duration of TPN, hours	231 (134–387)	143 (5–417)	0.004	374 (247–635)	0.000	42 (0–109)	0.000	0 (0–60)	0.000	0 (0–48)	0.000

n (%), (mean ± SD) and median (quartiles) are shown, Chi-square, *t*-test and Mann–Whitney U tests are used where appropriate. Perinatal characteristics for each cause of death are compared characteristics of survivors

most common causes of death in this population were similar [9, 10]. The most significant difference in this population was a relative higher incidence of major IVH as the principal cause of death [11, 12]. This is an interesting finding as the overall incidence of major IVH in our preterm population is comparable with other preterm populations [13]. As survival rates in extreme prematurity continue to improve, neonatologists are increasingly focused on neurological outcomes in surviving infants. There is an increasing tendency to redirect care in the setting of major IVH within this network, which is very likely to have impacted on cause-specific mortality in the extremely preterm groups. There is likely to be practice variation with respect to redirection of care between NICUs, however, these differences are difficult to objectively assess. Cause-specific mortality was not calculated for each individual unit, which may have allowed analysis of the effects of practice variation on cause-specific mortality.

Death due to ARI was expectedly the leading cause of mortality in the extreme preterm population however infants in older gestational age groups were more likely to die from other causes such as IVH and asphyxia. It is not surprising that perinatal asphyxia becomes the most common cause of death with increasing gestation as the infants in these groups are less likely to die from problems that are more prevalent in the extreme preterm population such as respiratory problems.

As expected, the most significant predictor of death in our preterm population was gestational age regardless of the cause of death. Other perinatal factors that were associated with a higher mortality were male gender, low

Table 3 Causes of death stratified by gestational age

	Gestational age group			
Cause of death	22–25 weeks	26–28 weeks	29–31 weeks	All GA groups
Total number of neonates	*n* = *522*	*n* = *1366*	*n* = *2566*	*n* = *4454*
Total deaths	178 (341/1000)	118 (86/1000)	49 (19/1000)	345 (77/1000)
Sepsis	28 (54/1000)	22 (16/1000)	5 (2/1000)	55 (12/1000)
NEC	9 (17/1000)	23 (17/1000)	7 (3/1000)	39 (9/1000)
Major IVH	61 (117/1000)	33 (24/1000)	5 (2/1000)	99 (22/1000)
Respiratory	62 (119/1000)	23 (17/1000)	10 (4/1000)	95 (21/1000)
HMD	47 (90/1000)	8 (6/1000)	0 (0/1000)	55 (12/1000)
Pulm HTN	2 (4/1000)	4 (3/1000)	2 (1/1000)	8 (2/1000)
Pulm Haem	6 (11/1000)	4 (3/1000)	2 (1/1000)	12 (3/1000)
Pulm Hypopl	7 (13/1000)	6 (4/1000)	6 (2/1000)	19 (4/1000)
PTX	0 (0/1000)	1 (1/1000)	0 (0/1000)	1 (0/1000)
Perinatal Asphyxia	2 (4/1000)	9 (7/1000)	14 (5/1000)	25 (6/1000)
Miscellaneous	16 (31/1000)	8 (6/1000)	8 (3/1000)	32 (7/1000)
CLD	7 (13/1000)	1 (1/1000)	1 (<1/1000)	9 (2/1000)

The number in parenthesis represents the cause-specific mortality rate (CMR) per 1000 infants

birth weight, small for gestational age and low Apgar score at five minutes. All of these results are consistent with previously published data [6–8, 14–17].

There were a number of perinatal factors that influenced the cause-specific mortality in this population. Hypertensive disease during pregnancy was associated with a decreased number of deaths due to major IVH. This is consistent with findings from other studies, which show that hypertensive disease is protective for major IVH [18, 19]. Chorioamnionitis was found more prevalently in infants who died from sepsis, which was also consistent with other studies that show an association between maternal chorioamnionitis and neonatal sepsis [19, 20]. It was not surprising to find that infants who die due to respiratory problems, IVH and asphyxia are less likely to have received steroids antenatally. Other expected findings included associations between being outborn and death

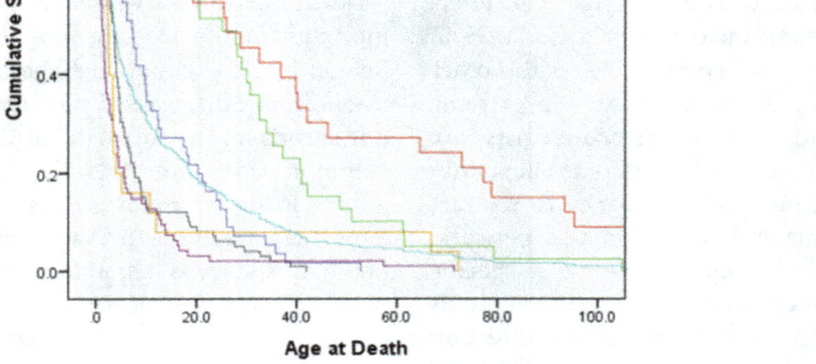

Fig. 1 Kaplan-Meier plot illustrating the cause specific mortality according to the age of death

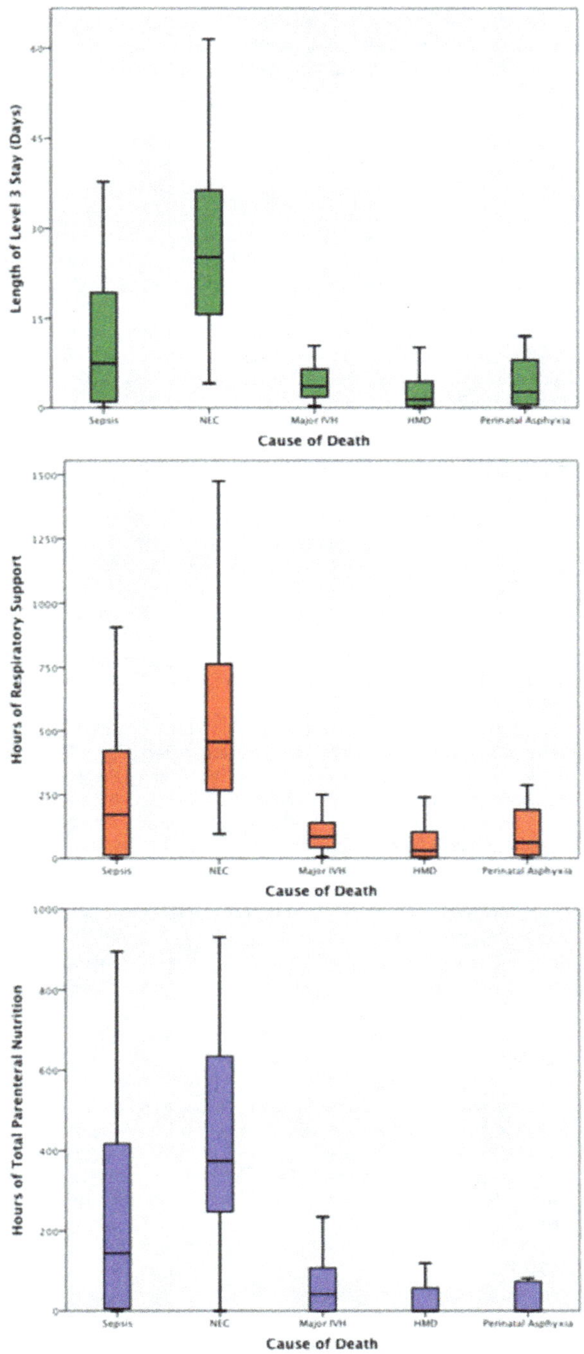

Fig. 2 Comparison of resource utilisation from birth in relation to cause of death category: Top – length of level 3 stay (days); Middle – hours of respiratory support; Bottom – hours of parenteral nutrition. Median (*bar*), quartiles (*box*) and 95% CI (error bars) are shown

due to IVH [21] and having no antenatal care and death due to perinatal asphyxia [22].

It is interesting to note that although maternal age was not different among infants who died and infants who survived, the average maternal age varied with the cause of death. Mothers of infants who died due to necrotising enterocolitis had a lower average age, which is consistent with published data from large preterm populations that show that the incidence of necrotising enterocolitis is lower in infants born to older mothers [23]. Mothers of infants who died due to perinatal asphyxia had a higher average age, which is consistent with literature that suggests that advanced maternal age is associated with neonatal encephalopathy in term infants [22].

The period of vulnerability of death varied significantly with each cause of death. Infants who die from ARI and IVH usually die within the first two to three weeks of life, which is an expected result. The majority of deaths relating to sepsis died early reflecting early onset sepsis. The survival curve decreases relatively steadily after this reflecting variability in the onset of late sepsis. Very premature infants continue to be vulnerable to NEC [24, 25] and thus deaths due to NEC behaved very differently to the other common causes of death. There are very few early deaths attributable to NEC followed by a steady decrease in the survival curve due to the onset of NEC after two to three weeks of age.

Analysis of our surrogate markers of resource consumption consistently showed that there are significant differences depending on the cause of death. It is clear that infants who die from ARI and IVH consumed the least resources during their hospital stay. Infants who died from sepsis consumed more resources than infants who died in the immediate postnatal period but less than those who died from NEC. This is unsurprising and is consistent with the mean age at death and survival curves for these causes of death.

This study represents the largest analysis of causes of death in preterm infants, including data from multiple NICUs across a large area. Although analysed retrospectively, all NICUS data are collected prospectively. One of the major strengths of this study compared with previous similar studies is that there was a detailed investigation to ascertain the exact cause of death for every infant. An accurate immediate cause of death was determined and agreed upon for all infants who died during the study period.

The most significant limitation of this study is that to be eligible for inclusion, infants must have been admitted to a NICU. The study provides no information on the foetal mortality associated with important prenatal risk factors, which potentially biases the associations between these risk factors and cause of death. Infants who were born alive at the threshold of viability but not actively resuscitated are also not included in the analysis, which may bias the distribution of cause of death in the extreme preterm population.

It is important to note that the NICUS Data Collection is a regional audit from 10 different NICUs. These data were not separated by NICUS and we were therefore not able to analyse the cause-specific mortality for each unit individually. Although these NICUs have comparable outcomes and all participate in regular meetings to discuss management of the preterm infant, practice variation between units is difficult to assess and may have an effect on cause-specific mortality.

Conclusions

In performing a detailed analysis of the causes of death in this population, this study provides insight into the specific reasons that preterm infants die and demonstrates that perinatal factors have a significant impact on cause-specific mortality. The varied timing of death, depending on the primary cause of death, highlights that preterm infants who survive the immediate newborn period remain vulnerable to life-threatening conditions such as sepsis and necrotising enterocolitis.

Abbreviations

ACT: Australian Capital Territory; ARI: Acute repiratory illness; CMR: Cause-specific mortality rate; IVH: Intraventricular haemorrhage; NEC: Necrotising enterocolitis; NICU: Neonatal intensive care unit; NICUS: Neonatal intensive care units' data collection; NSW: New South Wales

Acknowledgements

The authors would like to thank Running for Premature Babies for supporting the conduct of this study by funding a research fellowship for one of the authors (TS) and for their contributions to the Royal Hospital for Women NICU.

Funding

Not applicable.

Authors' contributions

TS assisted with the study design, reviewed the cases, performed the statistical analysis and drafted the manuscript. LKS assisted with the statistical analysis. KL assisted with the statistical analysis and assisted with the manuscript. BB extracted the data and reviewed the cases. SB conceived the concept of the study and its design, reviewed the cases and assisted with the manuscript. All authors read and approved the final manuscript.

Competing interests

The authors declare that they have no competing interests.

Author details

[1]Faculty of Medicine, University of New South Wales, Sydney, Australia. [2]Department of Newborn Care, Royal Hospital for Women, Sydney, Australia. [3]New South Wales Pregnancy and Newborn Services Network (PSN), Sydney, Australia.

References

1. Moore T, Hennessy EM, Myles J, Johnson SJ, Draper ES, Costeloe KL, et al. Neurological and developmental outcome in extremely preterm children born in England in 1995 and 2006: the EPICure studies. BMJ. 2012;345:e7961.
2. Shah PS, Sankaran K, Aziz K, Allen AC, Seshia M, Ohlsson A, et al. Outcomes of preterm infants <29 weeks gestation over 10-year period in Canada: a cause for concern? J Perinat Med. 2012;32(2):132–8.
3. Kusuda S, Fujimura M, Uchiyama A, Totsu S, Matsunami K. Trends in morbidity and mortality among very-low-birth-weight infants from 2003 to 2008 in Japan. Pediatr Res. 2012;72:531–8.
4. Barria-Pailaquilen RM, Mendoza-Maldonado Y, Urrutia-Toro Y, Castro-Mora C, Santander-Manriquez G. Trends in infant mortality rate and mortality for neonates born at less than 32 weeks and with very low birth weight. Rev Lat-Am Enferm. 2011;19:977–84.
5. Battin MR, Knight DB, Kuschel CA, Howie RN. Improvement in mortality of very low birthweight infants and the changing pattern of neonatal mortality: the 50-year experience of one perinatal centre. J Paediatr Child H. 2012;48:596–9.
6. Feng Y, Abdel-Latif ME, Bajuk B, Lui K, Oei JL. Causes of death in infants admitted to Australian neonatal intensive care units between 1995 and 2006. Acta Paediatr. 2013;102:e17–23.
7. Patel RM, Kandefer S, Walsh MC, Bell EF, Carlo WA, Laptook AR, et al. Causes and Timing of Death in Extremely Premature Infants from 2000 through 2011. New Engl J Med. 2015;372:331–40.
8. Bolisetty S, Legge N, Bajuk B, Lui K. Preterm infant outcomes in New South Wales and the Australian Capital Territory. J Paediatr Child H. 2015;51:713–21.
9. Papile LA, American Academy of Pediatrics Committee on Fetus And Newborn. Levels of neonatal care. Pediatrics 2012;130:587–97.Simpson CD, Ye XY, Hellmann J, Tomlinson C. Trends in cause-specific mortality at a Canadian outborn NICU. Pediatrics. 2010;126:e1538–44.
10. Stichtenoth G, Demmert M, Bohnhorst B, Stein A, Ehlers S, Heitmann F, et al. Major contributors to hospital mortality in very-low-birth-weight infants: data of the birth year 2010 cohort of the German Neonatal Network. Klin Padiatr. 2012;224:276–81.
11. Corchia C, Ferrante P, Da Fre M, Di Lallo D, Gagliardi L, Carnielli V, et al. Cause-specific mortality of very preterm infants and antenatal events. J Pediatr. 2013;162:1125–32.
12. Batton DG, DeWitte DB, Pryce CJ. One hundred consecutive infants born at 23 weeks and resuscitated. Am J Perinat. 2011;28:299–304.
13. Lui K, Modi N, Sjors G, Reichman B, Darlow B, San Feliciano L et al. Variability in rates of major intraventricular hemorrhage (IVH) and its impact on mortality in very preterm between 8 national neonatal databases: The International Network for Evaluation of Outcomes (iNeo) experience. San Diego: Poster session presented at: Pediatric Academic Societies; 2015.
14. Evans N, Hutchinson J, Simpson JM, Donoghue D, Henderson-Smart D. Prenatal predictors of mortality in very preterm infants cared for in the Australian and New Zealand Neonatal Network. Arch Dis Child-Fetal. 2007;92:F34–40.
15. Behrman RE, Stith Butler A. Institute of Medicine Committee on Understanding Premature Birth and Assuring Healthy Outcomes Board on Health Sciences Outcomes. Preterm Birth: Causes, Consequences, and Prevention. Washington: The National Academies Press; 2007.
16. Doyle LW, Victorian Infant Collaborative Study Group. Evaluation of neonatal intensive care for extremely low birth weight infants in Victoria over two decades: II. Efficiency. Pediatrics. 2004;113:510.
17. Stoll BJ, Hansen NI, Bell EF, Shankaran S, Laptook AR, Walsh MC, et al. Neonatal outcomes of extremely preterm infants from the NICHD Neonatal Research Network. Pediatrics. 2010;126:443.
18. Perlman JM, Risser RC, Gee JB. Pregnancy-induced hypertension and reduced intraventricular hemorrhage in preterm infants. Pediatric Neurol. 1997;17:29–33.

19. Gagliardi L, Rusconi F, Bellu R, Zanini R. Association of maternal hypertension and chorioamnionitis with preterm outcomes. Pediatrics. 2014;134:e154–61.
20. Cornette L. Fetal and neonatal inflammatory response and adverse outcome. Semin Fetal Neonatal Med. 2004;9:459–70.
21. Palmer KG, Kronsberg SS, Barton BA, Hobbs CA, Hall RW, Anand KJ. Effect of inborn versus outborn delivery on clinical outcomes in ventilated preterm neonates: secondary results from the NEOPAIN trial. J Perinat Med. 2005;25(4):270–5.
22. Kurinczuk JJ, White-Koning M, Badawi N. Epidemiology of neonatal encephalopathy and hypoxic-ischaemic encephalopathy. Early Hum Dev. 2010;86(6):329–38.
23. Kanungo J, James A, McMillan D, Lodha A, Faucher D, Lee SK, et al. Advanced maternal age and the outcomes of preterm neonates: a social paradox? Obstet Gynecol. 2011;118(4):872–7.
24. Neu J, Walker WA. Necrotizing enterocolitis. New Engl J Med. 2011;364:255–64.
25. Mohamed A, Shah PS. Transfusion associated necrotizing enterocolitis: a meta-analysis of observational data. Pediatrics. 2012;129:529–40.

26

The association between vancomycin trough concentrations and acute kidney injury in the neonatal intensive care unit

Vidit Bhargava[1*], Michael Malloy[2] and Rafael Fonseca[2]

Abstract

Background: Vancomycin has recently gained popularity as an empiric therapy for late onset sepsis in the NICU. Changes in resistance patterns in common organisms has resulted in targeting higher trough concentrations of vancomycin. Consequently, an increase in vancomycin associated nephrotoxicity has been speculated. The objective of this study is to compare the incidence of acute kidney injury (AKI) in neonates with serum vancomycin trough concentrations less than 10 mg/L, 10–15 mg/L, or greater than 15 mg/L.

Methods: A retrospective chart review of patients in the neonatal intensive care unit (NICU) was conducted to determine the incidence of AKI in neonates receiving vancomycin.

Results: The overall incidence of AKI was 2.7%. Comparison of the incidence of AKI in the three groups using Mantel-Haenszel Chi-Square test showed a statistically significant association between increasing vancomycin trough concentration and incidence of AKI.

Conclusion: There is a low incidence of AKI in neonates receiving vancomycin. However, there is a positive correlation between increasing vancomycin trough concentrations and an increasing serum creatinine.

Keywords: AKI, Nephrotoxicity, Prematurity, Vancomycin

Background

Vancomycin is a glycopeptide antibiotic which gained popularity in 1980's for treatment of coagulase negative Staphylococcus (CONS) and Methicillin resistant staphylococcus aureus (MRSA). Late onset sepsis is a common concern in premature infants in neonatal intensive care unit (NICU). Vancomycin is widely used as an empiric therapy for late onset sepsis, and in confirmed infections with CONS and MRSA. [1, 2] Consequently, vancomycin is used in the NICU even though limited information is available concerning the dosing, monitoring, and adverse effects of this medication in neonates. Additionally, increasing antibiotic resistance among familiar pathogens in the NICU, as evidenced by higher minimum inhibitory concentrations (MICs), has resulted in targeting higher vancomycin trough concentrations. [3, 4] Vancomycin associated nephrotoxicity has not been well studied in the neonatal population and limited data exists on the association between higher vancomycin trough and incidence of acute kidney injury (AKI).

This study aims to measure the association between increasing trough concentrations and AKI in neonates receiving vancomycin therapy. We also look at the effect of co-administration of other nephrotoxic agents on the incidence of AKI.

Methods

A retrospective chart review was performed for patients in NICU at University of Texas Medical Branch (UTMB) at Galveston. The electronic medical record was reviewed between January 2008 and December 2012 to determine the incidence of AKI in neonates receiving vancomycin. The patient population consisted of premature neonates admitted to NICU at UTMB and received at least one course of vancomycin. Each patient may have received several courses of vancomycin during this

* Correspondence: vibharga@utmb.edu
[1]Department of Pediatrics, University of Texas Medical Branch, 301 UNIVERSITY BLVD, GALVESTON 77555, TEXAS, USA

period. Courses of vancomycin were included in the study group if they met the following inclusion criteria: a) Duration of treatment at least 5 days b) Availability of serum creatinine (SCr) values both prior to and after completing the vancomycin therapy and c) at least one vancomycin trough collected during the duration of treatment. Courses of vancomycin therapy were excluded if: a) evidence of pre-existing renal insufficiency or congenital anomalies including renal agenesis, renal hypoplasia, polycystic kidney disease, or renal dysplasia were present b) extracorporeal membrane oxygenation was required or c) there was incomplete data in the UTMB electronic medical record, Epic. Baseline serum creatinine was defined as the serum creatinine obtained prior to starting vancomycin therapy. Post vancomycin creatinine was defined as the serum creatinine value obtained at the end of vancomycin therapy or after a suspected episode of AKI.

Courses of vancomycin therapy were divided into three groups based on highest achieved vancomycin trough concentrations; less than 10 mg/L, 10–15 mg/L, or greater than 15 mg/L. Standardized vancomycin dosage proposed by Capparelli et al., based on gestational age was used for each patient.[5] The trough was obtained prior to the fourth dose. If the trough was found sub-therapeutic or toxic, changes in dose or frequency of vancomycin administration were accordingly made. The change in dose was subsequently followed by a repeat trough measurement prior to the 4th dose. For each course of vancomycin therapy, multiple vancomycin trough concentrations may have been measured, but the highest achieved trough concentration was used to classify courses of vancomycin therapy into the three study groups. The incidence of AKI was determined in each group. AKI was defined as an increase in SCr of at least 0.5 mg/L or an increase of at least 100% from lowest trough previously available. This definition is based on pRIFLE criteria for renal injury proposed by Akcan-Arikan et al. and the increase in serum creatinine proposed by moghal et al. [6–8] A decrease in urine output was not used as a defining criteria due to lack of this being a universal finding.

Data collected included gestational age; postnatal age; gender; birth weight; APGAR scores; vancomycin dose, frequency, duration, and trough concentrations; date and time of vancomycin doses and trough concentrations; concurrent nephrotoxic medications administered including amphotericin B, acyclovir, amikacin, captopril, dobutamine, dopamine, enalapril, epinephrine, ganciclovir, gentamicin, indomethacin, ibuprofen, naficillin, and tobramycin; blood culture results; type of infection; presence of a patent ductus arteriosus; and final discharge status. Maternal history was also collected and included the presence of pregnancy-induced hypertension, chorioamnionitis, diabetes, renal dysfunction, or urinary tract infection.

Mantel-Haenszel Chi-Square test was used to compare the incidence of AKI between the three groups. A p-value of < 0.05 was considered to be statistically significant. Regression analysis was used to examine the relationship between vancomycin trough concentrations and serum creatinine. All statistical analyses were done using SAS 9.3©. The study was approved by the institutional review board (IRB) at UTMB, Galveston.

Results

Nine hundred and sixty-two patients receiving vancomycin therapy administered between January 2008 and December 2012 were evaluated for study inclusion. Eight hundred and fifty-two patients were excluded due to inability to meet one or more inclusion criteria. The majority of patients were excluded due to vancomycin being administered for less than five days. The second most common reason for exclusion was incomplete data in the electronic medical record. Therefore, 110 patients were included in the analysis. The majority of patients were male. The mean birth weight was 1200 g, and the mean gestational age was 29 weeks. (Table 1) Central line associated blood stream infection (CLABSI), sepsis and necrotizing enterocolitis (NEC) were the most common suspected diagnoses for which patients were started on vancomycin therapy. The most common organism was Coagulase Negative Staphylococcus aureus (32 patients) followed by Enterococcus faecalis (5 patients) and Staphylococcus aureus.

One hundred ten patients were further studied to determine an association with AKI. There were 72 patients with a highest vancomycin trough concentration less than 10 mg/L, 27 patients with a highest vancomycin trough concentration of 10–15 mg/L, and 11 patients with a highest vancomycin trough concentration greater than 15 mg/L. The incidence of AKI was 1.39% (1/72 patients) in the group achieving vancomycin trough concentrations less than 10 mg/L, 0% (0/27 patients) in the group achieving vancomycin trough concentrations between 10–15 mg/L, and 18.18% (2/11 patients) in the group achieving vancomycin trough concentrations greater than 15 mg/L (Table 2). There was a statistically significant association between AKI and vancomycin trough groups ($p = 0.04$). Regression analysis between

Table 1 Baseline characteristics of patients

N = 110	
Male/Female	58/52
Birth weight (grams) ± SD	1200 ± 734
Gestational age (weeks) ± SD	29 ± 5
Postnatal age at time of first vancomycin course (days) ± SD	23 ± 27

Table 2 Incidence of acute kidney injury

Group	Total number of patients	Patients with AKI	Incidence of AKI
Vancomycin trough < 10 mg/L	72	1	1.38%
Vancomycin trough 10–15 mg/L	27	0	0%
Vancomycin trough > 15 mg/L	11	2	18.18%
TOTAL	110	3	2.7%

increasing vancomycin trough concentrations and post vancomycin serum creatinine values demonstrated a positive correlation value of 0.32 ($p < 0.05$) (Fig.1).

Each of the patients with AKI were also receiving at least one concurrent nephrotoxic medication including dobutamine, dopamine, and/or gentamicin (Table 3). Gentamicin was the only nephrotoxic drug that a large percentage of the 87 patients received during vancomycin therapy (79%). There was no significant correlation between post vancomycin creatinine values and the total number of days' gentamicin was received ($p = 0.10$) or of a change in creatinine of greater than or equal to 0.5 mg/dl from pre- to post-vancomycin administration ($p = 0.13$). In an ANOVA regression equation with gentamicin days run as a covariate with vancomycin trough group, however, gentamicin days were significantly associated with post vancomycin creatinine values ($p = 0.04$). The vancomycin trough groups remained significantly associated with post vancomycin creatinine values independent of gentamicin days ($p < 0.01$).

Discussion

There has been an on-going debate on the dosage, frequency of administration and the most appropriate monitoring of vancomycin therapy. This is the result of multiple factors responsible for clearance of vancomycin including gestational age, post-natal age, weight, renal tubular function and creatinine levels. [9] Historically, area-under-the-curve concentration versus time to the minimum inhibitory concentration (AUC:MIC), was accepted as the pharmacokinetic and pharmacodynamic predictor of adequate treatment with vancomycin. AUC: MIC > 400 has been recommended to achieve desired anti-microbial effect in both adult and pediatric populations. [10] A consensus statement released by the American Society of Health-System Pharmacists, the Infectious Diseases Society of America, and the Society of Infectious Diseases Pharmacists in 2009 recommended vancomycin as the first choice drug for MRSA with MIC < 2. [10] The consensus statement also recommends assessment of vancomycin clinical effectiveness through serum vancomycin trough concentrations at steady state. Studies have demonstrated that trough between 7–10 mg/L corresponds to AUC:MIC > 400 if the MIC of MRSA is < 1. [11] However, with increasing MIC's higher trough concentrations are recommended. In serious clinical infections such as endocarditis, meningitis, hospital-acquired pneumonia, bacteremia, and osteomyelitis trough concentrations between 15–20 are recommended.[12] These higher troughs allow for greater vancomycin exposure, a higher AUC and the ability to reach the goal AUC:MIC ≥ 400, or a trough concentration approximately four to five times the MIC

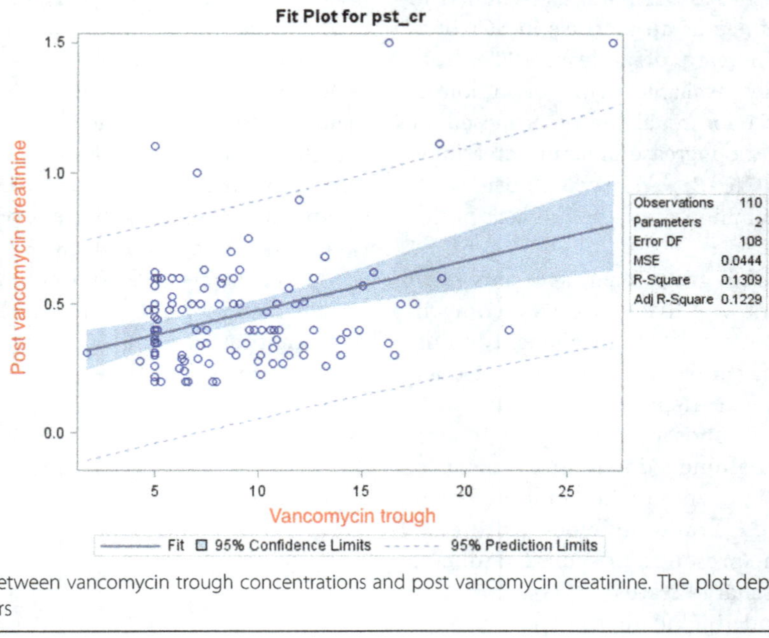

Fig. 1 Showing a Fit plot between vancomycin trough concentrations and post vancomycin creatinine. The plot depicts a positive co-relation between the two parameters

Table 3 Cases of acute kidney injury

Case	Trough (mg/L)	Timing of trough	Dose of vancomycin	Frequency	Duration of treatment	Total vancomycin days
1	<5.0	Prior to 4th dose	20 mg/kg 20 mg/kg	Q18H Q12H	4 days 5 days	9 days
2	18.8	Prior to 4th dose	20 mg/kg	Q24H	6 days	6 days
3	27.2	Prior to 4th dose	20 mg/kg 15 mg/kg	Q24H Q24H	5 days 6 days	11 days

of the infecting organism. [12] Concerns for increased nephrotoxicity, an adverse effect traditionally associated with vancomycin, has accompanied the recommendation for more aggressive dosing.

In adults, increasing serum vancomycin trough concentrations have been associated with increasing incidence of AKI. In a study done to evaluate vancomycin-associated nephrotoxicity incidence in adults with MRSA infections with serum trough concentrations of 15–20 mg/L and receiving concomitant nephrotoxic medications, a significantly higher incidence of AKI was noted.[3] A 2011 prospective study also showed similar results. Adults with MRSA infections had a greater risk of AKI with serum vancomycin trough concentration greater than 15 mg/L.[13] Similarly, adults with MRSA pneumonia were shown to be at a 3–5 times greater risk for developing AKI with vancomycin serum trough concentrations of 15 mg/L.[14] On the other hand, there are other studies in adults which did not show increased risk of AKI with elevated serum vancomycin trough > 15 mg/L. In study done by Prabaker et al., an overall incidence of 2.1% was noticed with vancomycin serum trough concentration between 15–20 mg/L [15].

Nephrotoxicity in the neonatal population is poorly defined. Several definitions of acute kidney injury (AKI) exist in the literature; however, there are no standard criteria for diagnosing AKI in neonates. Commonly used definitions of AKI in neonates include oliguria of less than 1 mL/kg/h of urine output that develops 24 h after birth and persists for at least 24 h, an increase in serum creatinine (SCr) to greater than 1.5 mg/L 72 h after birth, or an increase in SCr between 0.5 and 1 mg/L per day.[8, 16] Nephrotoxicity attributed to vancomycin use is not clearly defined in neonates; however, the mechanism of injury to the kidney is believed to be the result of proximal tubule damage. [17, 18] Although causality has not been proven, a higher risk of vancomycin-induced nephrotoxicity in the pediatric population with higher vancomycin trough concentrations has been speculated.

Due to pharmacokinetic differences between adults and neonates, and since neonates have immature renal function compared to adults, the applicability and adverse effects of increased target troughs in premature neonates remain unknown. Lastly, it has been documented in adult populations that concurrent treatment using other known nephrotoxic agents, such as aminoglycosides, is associated with an increased risk for nephrotoxicity with vancomycin. [19] Again, it is unclear whether this is true in the neonatal population.

Previously done studies in children receiving vancomycin alone have reported incidence of AKI from 9%–14%. Linder et al. and Nahata et al. found the incidence of AKI in neonatal population to be low. Their studies did not show statistically significant difference in the incidence of AKI with concomitant administration of gentamicin.[20, 21] However, McKamy and Knoderer et al. reported slightly higher overall incidence of AKI at 14% in children between the ages 1 month and 17 years.[17, 22] Both the studies also reported significantly higher incidence of AKI with vancomycin trough > 15 mg/L at 28% and 18% respectively.

In our study, the overall incidence of AKI was low at 2.71%. A statistically significant association between AKI and vancomycin trough groups was found ($p = 0.04$). There was also a positive correlation between vancomycin trough concentrations and post vancomycin creatinine values, indicating that vancomycin may have some role in AKI in predisposed individuals. It also indicates that higher vancomycin troughs are associated with rising creatinine values post treatment. Additionally, we looked at several covariates using a linear regression model to assess whether these were significantly associated with higher post vancomycin creatinine values. Highest vancomycin trough value ($p < 0.001$), total vancomycin days ($p \sim 0.0021$) and gestational age (p value < 0.001) were found to have an independent association. Gender and APGAR scores were also looked at and were not found to be significantly associated with vancomycin trough and rising creatinine values. Even after controlling for these independent variables, the highest trough value and post vancomycin creatinine values showed a significant association.

Also of interest is the observation that vancomycin trough groups continued to be positively associated with increasing post vancomycin creatinine values independent of the number of days of gentamicin the infants had received. In addition, independent of vancomycin trough groups there was a positive association between the number of days that gentamicin was received and post vancomycin creatinine values. Thus, gentamicin, another potentially nephrotoxic had its effect on post vancomycin creatinine values obscured by the effect of vancomycin. Only after having the effect of vancomycin controlled for in the regression equation was gentamicin's effect revealed. Because of the small number of courses associated with our definition of acute kidney failure whether or not vancomycin and gentamicin were additive in their nephrotoxic effects cannot be determined in this analysis. Larger studies are needed to confirm these findings.

Our study has limitations. The study was retrospective in nature and had a small sample size. Due to the lack of a standardized definition a hybrid definition of AKI was used in this study. Another limitation is that patients may have received multiple courses of vancomycin therapy during the same admission. However, courses of vancomycin therapy were often separated by weeks. Further, for each course of vancomycin therapy, multiple vancomycin trough concentrations may have been measured, but the highest achieved trough concentration was used to divide the vancomycin courses into the three study groups. Finally, despite the fact that patients were often on concurrent nephrotoxic medications, only three cases of AKI were identified in this study which is different from the previously reported studies.

Conclusion

Based on our study, vancomycin troughs greater than 20 mg/dl may be associated with increased incidence of AKI. We recommend close monitoring of vancomycin trough concentrations during therapy and appropriate alteration in dosage/frequency should be made based on serum trough concentrations. However, this was a single-center retrospective study, and larger prospective studies are required to validate this finding.

Abbreviations

AKI: Acute kidney injury; AUC: MIC: Area-under-the-curve concentration versus time to the minimum inhibitory concentration; CONS: Coagulase negative staphylococcus aureus; MRSA: Methicillin resistant staphylococcus aureus; NICU: Neonatal intensive care unit; SCr: Serum creatinine; UTMB: University of Texas Medical Branch

Acknowledgements

Not applicable

Funding

Not applicable.

Authors' contributions

VB was involved in writing the manuscript and collection of data. MM was involved in data interpretation and statistical analysis of the data. He was also involved in critical review of the article and multiple corrections prior to submission. RF is the chief investigator in the study. He was involved in designing the study, reviewing the results and reviewing the manuscript and the whole project at each stage. All authors read and approved the final manuscript.

Competing interests

The authors declare that they have no competing interests.

Author details

[1]Department of Pediatrics, University of Texas Medical Branch, 301 UNIVERSITY BLVD, GALVESTON 77555, TEXAS, USA. [2]Department of Pediatrics, Division of Neonatology, University of Texas Medical Branch, 301 UNIVERSITY BLVD, GALVESTON 77555, TEXAS, USA.

References

1. Klingenberg C, Aarag E, Ronnestad A, Sollid JE, Abrahamsen TG, Kjeldsen G, Flaegstad T. Coagulase-negative staphylococcal sepsis in neonates. Association between antibiotic resistance, biofilm formation and the host inflammatory response. Pediatr Infect Dis J. 2005;24(9):817–22.
2. Healy CM, Palazzi DL, Edwards MS, Campbell JR, Baker CJ. Features of invasive staphylococcal disease in neonates. Pediatrics. 2004;114(4):953–61.
3. Hidayat LK, Hsu DI, Quist R, Shriner KA, Wong-Beringer A. High-dose vancomycin therapy for methicillin-resistant Staphylococcus aureus infections: efficacy and toxicity. Arch Intern Med. 2006;166(19):2138–44.
4. Sakoulas G, Moise-Broder PA, Schentag J, Forrest A, Moellering Jr RC, Eliopoulos GM. Relationship of MIC and bactericidal activity to efficacy of vancomycin for treatment of methicillin-resistant Staphylococcus aureus bacteremia. J Clin Microbiol. 2004;42(6):2398–402.
5. Capparelli EV, Lane JR, Romanowski GL, McFeely EJ, Murray W, Sousa P, Kildoo C, Connor JD. The influences of renal function and maturation on vancomycin elimination in newborns and infants. J Clin Pharmacol. 2001;41(9):927–34.
6. Akcan-Arikan A, Zappitelli M, Loftis LL, Washburn KK, Jefferson LS, Goldstein SL. Modified RIFLE criteria in critically ill children with acute kidney injury. Kidney Int. 2007;71(10):1028–35.
7. Moghal NE, Brocklebank JT, Meadow SR. A review of acute renal failure in children: incidence, etiology and outcome. Clin Nephrol. 1998;49(2):91–5.
8. Viswanathan S, Manyam B, Azhibekov T, Mhanna MJ. Risk factors associated with acute kidney injury in extremely low birth weight (ELBW) infants. Pediatr Nephrol. 2012;27(2):303–11.
9. Pacifici GM, Allegaert K. Clinical pharmacokinetics of vancomycin in the neonate: a review. In: Clinics (Sao Paulo). 67th ed. 2012. p. 831–7.
10. Rybak MJ, Lomaestro BM, Rotschafer JC, Moellering Jr RC, Craig WA, Billeter M, Dalovisio JR, Levine DP. Therapeutic monitoring of vancomycin in adults summary of consensus recommendations from the American Society of Health-System Pharmacists, the Infectious Diseases Society of America, and the Society of Infectious Diseases Pharmacists. Pharmacotherapy. 2009;29(11):1275–9.
11. Frymoyer A, Guglielmo BJ, Hersh AL. Desired vancomycin trough serum concentration for treating invasive methicillin-resistant Staphylococcal infections. Pediatr Infect Dis J. 2013;32(10):1077–9.
12. Liu C, Bayer A, Cosgrove SE, Daum RS, Fridkin SK, Gorwitz RJ, Kaplan SL, Karchmer AW, Levine DP, Murray BE, et al. Clinical practice guidelines by the infectious diseases society of america for the treatment of methicillin-resistant Staphylococcus aureus infections in adults and children. Clin Infect Dis. 2011;52(3):e18–55.
13. Bosso JA, Nappi J, Rudisill C, Wellein M, Bookstaver PB, Swindler J, Mauldin PD. Relationship between vancomycin trough concentrations and nephrotoxicity: a prospective multicenter trial. Antimicrob Agents Chemother. 2011;55(12):5475–9.
14. Jeffres MN, Isakow W, Doherty JA, Micek ST, Kollef MH. A retrospective analysis of possible renal toxicity associated with vancomycin in patients with health care-associated methicillin-resistant Staphylococcus aureus pneumonia. Clin Ther. 2007;29(6):1107–15.
15. Prabaker KK, Tran TP, Pratummas T, Goetz MB, Graber CJ. Elevated vancomycin trough is not associated with nephrotoxicity among inpatient veterans. J Hosp Med. 2012;7(2):91–7.

16. Ringer SA. Acute Renal Failure in the Neonate. 2010.
17. McKamy S, Hernandez E, Jahng M, Moriwaki T, Deveikis A, Le J. Incidence and risk factors influencing the development of vancomycin nephrotoxicity in children. J Pediatr. 2011;158(3):422–6.
18. Zappitelli M, Selewski DT, Askenazi DJ. Nephrotoxic Medication Exposure and Acute Kidney Injury in Neonates. 2012.
19. Fauconneau B, Favreliere S, Pariat C, Genevrier A, Courtois P, Piriou A, Bouquet S. Nephrotoxicity of gentamicin and vancomycin given alone and in combination as determined by enzymuria and cortical antibiotic levels in rats. Ren Fail. 1997;19(1):15–22.
20. Linder N, Edwards R, MeClead R, Mortensen ME, Walson P, Koren G. Safety of vancomycin with or without gentamicin in neonates. Neonatal Netw. 1993;12(8):27–30.
21. Nahata MC. Lack of nephrotoxicity in pediatric patients receiving concurrent vancomycin and aminoglycoside therapy. Chemotherapy. 1987;33(4):302–4.
22. Knoderer CA, Nichols KR, Lyon KC, Veverka MM, Wilson AC. Are Elevated Vancomycin Serum Trough Concentrations Achieved Within the First 7 Days of Therapy Associated With Acute Kidney Injury in Children? J Pediatric Infect Dis Soc. 2014;3(2):127–31.

Urinary Neutrophil Gelatinase-associated Lipocalin in the evaluation of Patent Ductus Arteriosus and AKI in Very Preterm Neonates

Anna Sellmer[1,2*], Bodil H. Bech[3], Jesper V. Bjerre[1], Michael R. Schmidt[4], Vibeke E. Hjortdal[5], Gitte Esberg[1], Søren Rittig[1] and Tine B. Henriksen[1,2]

Abstract

Background: A patent ductus arteriosus (PDA) is frequently found in very preterm neonates and is associated with increased risk of morbidity and mortality. A shunt across a PDA can result in an unfavorable distribution of the cardiac output and may in turn result in poor renal perfusion. Urinary Neutrophil Gelatinase-associated Lipocalin (U-NGAL) is a marker of renal ischemia and may add to the evaluation of PDA. Our primary aim was to investigate if U-NGAL is associated with PDA in very preterm neonates. Secondary, to investigate whether U-NGAL and PDA are associated with AKI and renal dysfunction evaluated by fractional excretion of sodium (FENa) and urine albumin in a cohort of very preterm neonates.

Methods: A cohort of 146 neonates born at a gestational age less than 32 weeks were consecutively examined with echocardiography for PDA and serum sodium, and urine albumin and sodium were measured on postnatal day 3 and U-NGAL and serum creatinine day 3 and 6. AKI was defined according to modified neonatal Acute Kidney Injury Network (AKIN) criteria. The association between U-NGAL and PDA was investigated. And secondly we investigated if PDA and U-NGAL was associated with AKI and renal dysfunction.

Results: U-NGAL was not associated with a PDA day 3 when adjusted for gestational age and gender. A PDA day 3 was not associated with AKI when adjusted for gestational age and gender; however, it was associated with urine albumin. U-NGAL was not associated with AKI, but was found to be associated with urine albumin and FENa.

Conclusions: Based on our study U-NGAL is not considered useful as a diagnostic marker to identify very preterm neonates with a PDA causing hemodynamic changes resulting in early renal morbidity. The interpretation of NGAL in preterm neonates remains to be fully elucidated.

Keywords: Acute kidney injury, Neutrophil gelatinase-associated lipocalin, Patent ductus arteriosus, Very preterm neonates

* Correspondence: anna.sellmer@clin.au.dk
[1]Department of Pediatrics, Aarhus University Hospital, Palle Juul-Jensens Boulevard 99, DK 8200 Aarhus, Denmark
[2]Perinatal Epidemiology Research Unit, Department of Pediatrics, Aarhus University Hospital, Palle Juul-Jensens Boulevard 99, DK 8200 Aarhus, Denmark

Background

A patent ductus arteriosus (PDA) in preterm neonates is associated with an increased risk of morbidity and mortality [1, 2]. On day 3 of life, up to 50% of neonates born before 32 weeks of gestation have a PDA [1, 3]. However, not every PDA challenges the preterm neonate. We have previously demonstrated that a PDA diameter above 1.5 mm on postnatal day 3 can be used to identify a clinically significant PDA [1]. However, further diagnostic tools are needed in order to understand the potential impact of PDA presence and optimize handling of PDA in very preterm neonates.

Neutrophil gelatinase-associated lipocalin (NGAL) is expressed in low concentrations in many organs and the expression is up-regulated during infection, inflammation, and ischemia [4, 5]. Furthermore, NGAL is believed to be involved in renal development [6]. Urinary NGAL is produced in the renal tubule of the thick ascending limb of Henle and the collecting ducts [7]. In preterm neonates, NGAL has been suggested to be associated with Acute Kidney Injury (AKI) [8, 9].

U-NGAL has been hypothesized to be increased in the presence of a PDA [10]. A shunt across a PDA may result in an unfavorable distribution of the cardiac output between the pulmonary and the systemic circulation. This may in turn result in poor renal perfusion. This could cause AKI or renal dysfunction due to ischemia which could increase U-NGAL [11].

The aim of this study was to evaluate if U-NGAL can be used as a diagnostic marker to identity very preterm neonates with a PDA causing hemodynamic changes resulting in renal morbidity within the first week of life. To do this we investigated if U-NGAL is associated with PDA in very preterm neonates. Secondly we investigated whether U-NGAL and PDA were associated with AKI and renal dysfunction evaluated by fractional excretion of sodium and urine albumin in a cohort of very preterm neonates.

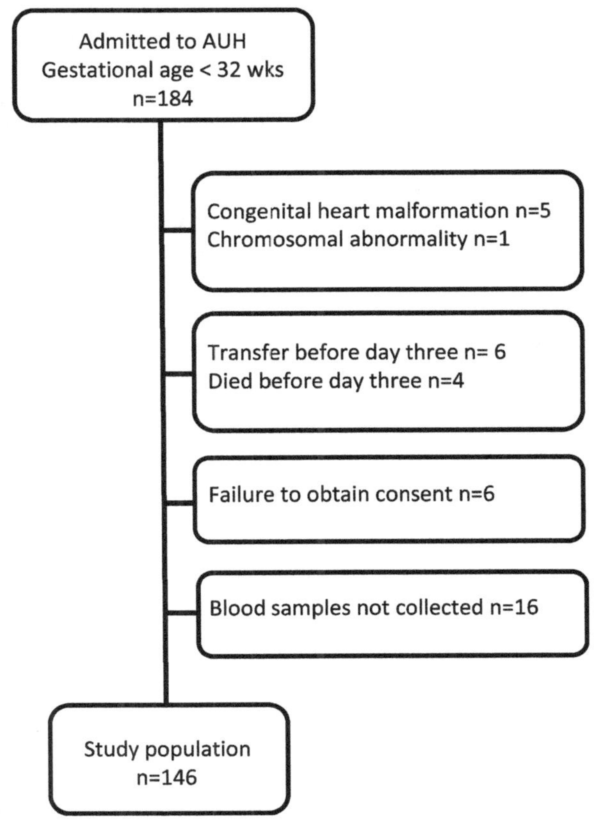

Fig. 1 Study population from 184 very preterm neonates admitted to Aarhus University Hospital (AUH)

Methods

Study population

The study population has previously been described [1], in brief, newborns born at gestational age below 32 weeks admitted to Aarhus University Hospital were eligible. We excluded neonates with chromosomal abnormalities or congenital heart malformations other than atrial septum defects from the study (Fig. 1).

Data collection and definitions

Irrespective of clinical symptoms, all very preterm neonates had an echocardiography on day 3 (equal to 72 h). Urine samples and blood samples were collected day 3 and 6. Urine was collected with a cotton ball placed at the perineum [8, 9, 12]. The diaper was checked at least every 4 h and the cotton transferred to a refrigerator. Cotton was centrifuged at 1000 rpm for 1 min and the urine was stored at −80 °C within 24 h after collection.

From the patient medical records we collected the following clinical details: gestational age at birth (determined by ultrasound), birth weight, multiple births, Apgar score, early onset sepsis (defined as seven days of antibiotics initiated within the first 3 days after birth) [13, 14], surfactant administration, packed red blood cell transfusion (within the first 3 days), use of inotropes (within the first 3 days), maternal preeclampsia, antenatal steroid administration, and mode of delivery.

Clinical guidelines

Management of the PDA was in accordance with institutional clinical guideline. Treatment with Ibuprofen (Pedea, Orphan Europe SARL Puteaux, France) was initiated based on detection by echocardiography alone if the gestational age at birth was less than 28 weeks; otherwise treatment was initiated based on a combination of specific echocardiographic findings and clinical symptoms. Ibuprofen was never administered before day 3.

Echocardiographic measurements

A complete diagnostic echocardiography was performed by two senior pediatric echocardiographers (J Bjerre and MR Schmidt) by use of standard neonatal windows. A Philips IE33 Ultrasound machine with a 12-MHz cardiology probe (Philips Healthcare, Andover, Massachusetts, USA) was used. A PDA was defined as present if flow could be visualized on colour Doppler. The PDA diameter was measured in two-dimensional mode at the most narrow point. A mean value of three cardiac cycles was calculated. A large PDA was defined as a PDA with a diameter of 1.5 mm or more and a small PDA as a PDA with a diameter below 1.5 mm.

U-NGAL measurement

The U-NGAL test Reagent Kit from BioPorto was used (BioPorto, Copenhagen, Denmark) as routine analysis on the Cobas 6000 analyzer system (Roche, Basel, Switzerland) at the Department of Biochemistry, Aarhus University Hospital. Also, serum creatinine (SCr), serum sodium, urinary albumin and sodium were measured as routine analyses at the Department. AKI was defined according to the definition proposed by Jetton et Askenazi based on the neonatal acute kidney injury (AKIN) classification [15–17]. AKI Stage 0: no change or rise SCr < 0.3 mg/dl; Stage 1: increase SCr 0.3 mg/dl or increase SCr 150–200% from previous trough value; Stage2: increase SCr 200–300% from previous trough value; Stage 3: increase SCr 200% from previous trough value or 2.5 mg/dl or recipient of dialysis [15]. Six stable neonates only had one SCr measured, this was within normal range and they were categorized as not having AKI. To evaluate renal dysfunction we measured urine albumin and calculated fractional excretion of sodium (FENa). Fractional excretion of sodium was calculated using the following formula: FENa (%) = (UNa/ PNa) * (SCr/ UCr) * 100, where UNa = urine sodium (mmol/l); PNa = plasma sodium (mmol/l); SCr serum creatine (μmol/l); and UCr = urine creatinine (μmol/l).

Statistical analysis

U-NGAL, urine albumin, SCr, and FENa were transformed by the natural logarithm (ln) to normalize the distribution of residuals. Geometric means were compared using the Student's t-test and proportions using Fisher's exact test. Univariate and multivariate log-linear regression was performed in order to examine the association between U-NGAL and PDA day 3, PDA size, perinatal characteristics, and sepsis. We consequently exponentiated the differences estimated on the natural log scale to obtain ratios of the medians. The formula ($\exp^{beta}$ -1) * 100% was used to express the percent change. These ratios are presented as crude and adjusted percent change per unit of explanatory variable or difference from reference group with 95% confidence interval (CI). Univariate and multivariate log-log regression was performed to examine the association between U-NGAL and parameters of renal dysfunction. The formula (1.01^{beta}-1)* 100% was used to express the percent change in U-NGAL per 1% change in urine albumin, SCr or FENa with 95% CI. Univariate and multivariate logistic regression was performed to examine the association between AKI and PDA. Odds ratio (OR) was presented with 95% CI. Estimates were adjusted for gestational age as a continuous variable (weeks) and gender and sepsis as dichotomized variables. Robust cluster standard errors were used in order to take into account the correlation between twins. Data were analyzed with STATA special edition version 11 (College Station, Texas, USA). All tests were two-sided. *P*-values of less than 0.05 were considered statistically significant.

Results

Patient characteristics

A total of 146 neonates were included in the study (Fig. 1). A PDA day 3 was found in 67 (46%) neonates on day 3 and 41 (61%) of neonates with PDA had a large PDA. Characteristics of the 146 very preterm neonates in the study are found in Table 1. Neonates with large and small PDA had comparable characteristics (data not shown).

U-NGAL in neonates with PDA

U-NGAL levels day 3 in neonates with PDA and no PDA on day 3 in four gestational age groups are found in Fig. 2. The highest level of U-NGAL day 3 was found in neonates with a small PDA compared to neonates with no PDA or a large PDA day 3 (Table 2). Median U-NGAL day 3 was 53% higher in neonates with a PDA compared to neonates without a PDA (Table 3). However, after adjusting for gender, gestational age, and sepsis by multivariate linear regression the association was no longer present. And no association was found between PDA or PDA size day 3 and U-NGAL.

AKI in neonates with PDA

A total of seven neonates were found to have AKI. AKI was found more frequently in neonates with PDA compared to neonates with no PDA and especially in neonates with a large PDA compared to no PDA day 3 (Table 2). However, when adjusted for gestational age no association between PDA day 3 and AKI was found. The odds of AKI decreased some 40% for every 1 week increase in gestational age at birth (OR = 0.64; 95% CI 0.4–0.96).

Mean SCr, urinary albumin, and FENa are described in Table 2. No difference in SCr was found between PDA groups. We found that urine albumin and FENa was higher in neonates with PDA day 3 compared to neonates

Table 1 Characteristics of 146 very preterm neonates postnatal day 3

	no PDA ($n = 79$)	PDA ($n = 67$)	*P* value
Gestational age weeks, median (range)	29 (24; 31)	27 (23; 31)	<0.01
Birth weight grams, median (range)	1190 (470;2160)	940 (570;1840)	<0.05
Singleton, number (%)	59 (75)	32 (48)	<0.01
SGA, number (%)	28 (35)	14 (21)	0.07
Sex (female:male)	27:52	28:39	0.39
Apgar score at 1 min, median (IQR)	8 (5;10)	7 (5;8)	<0.05
Apgar score at 5 min, median (IQR)	9 (7;10)	10 (9;10)	0.30
Sepsis, number (%)	9 (11)	13 (20)	0.25
Surfactant, number (%)	29 (37)	37 (55)	<0.05
PRBC transfusion, number (%)	8 (10)	16 (24)	<0.05
Inotropes, number (%)	5 (6)	7 (11)	0.39
Preeclampsia, number (%)	27 (34)	7 (11)	<0.01
Antenatal steroids, number (%)	75 (97)	61 (95)	0.66
Cesarean delivery, number (%)	56 (71)	44 (66)	0.59

SGA small-for-gestational-age (birth weight below 3rd percentile for gestational age); Sepsis defined as 7 days of antibiotics initiated before day 3; *PRBC* packed red blood cell transfusion within first 3 days of life; Inotropes used within the first 3 days of life

with no PDA. On regression we found PDA and PDA size to be associated with urine albumin also when adjusted for adjusting for gender, gestational age, and sepsis. No association between PDA or PDA size and FENa was found when adjusted for gestational age.

U-NGAL in neonates with AKI

We found no association between U-NGAL measured day 3 and AKI (Table 3). In 126 neonates we measured U-NGAL day 6. However, also on day 6 we found no association between U-NGAL and AKI. No association between U-NAGL day 3 and SCr was found. We did find an association between U-NGAL day 3 and both urine albumin and FENa also when adjusting for gender, gestational age, and sepsis.

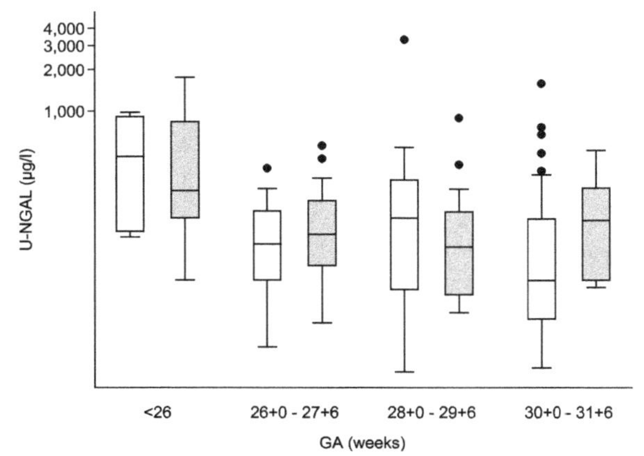

Fig. 2 Urine neutrophil gelatinase-associated lipocalin (U-NGAL) in 146 very preterm neonates with no PDA (*white*) and PDA (*grey*) assessed at postnatal day 3

Discussion

In 146 consecutively examined very preterm neonates, we found that the mere presence of a PDA and the PDA size day 3 was not associated with U-NGAL after adjusting for gestational age and gender. AKI was found more often in neonates with PDA, but after adjusting for gestational age there was no association between PDA day 3 and AKI. We found that neonates with PDA day 3 had higher urine albumin compared to neonates with no PDA. PDA and PDA size was associated with urine albumin also when adjusted for gestational age, gender, and sepsis. U-NGAL was not associated with AKI, it was however found to be associated with both urine albumin and FENa.

Tosse et al. found that U-NGAL in neonates with a birth weight below 1,500 g was higher if a PDA that needed either medical or surgical intervention was present than in neonates with no PDA or a PDA with no need for intervention [10]. They diagnosed the PDA by echocardiography on day 1–3 but the need for medical or surgical intervention was based on respiratory setback, oliguria or failure to thrive. Recently PDA diameter has been recognized as an important marker to evaluate the magnitude and clinical significance of the PDA [1, 18–20]. We used a PDA diameter above 1.5 mm on day 3 to identify the clinically significant PDA as we have previously shown that it is associated with severe morbidity and mortality [1]. Markers of organ dysfunction prior to clinical morbidity are needed in order to evaluate the PDA. The hemodynamic effects of a PDA may cause renal hypoperfusion and renal ischemia leading

Table 2 U-NGAL, SCr, FENa, urine albumin, and AKI in 146 very preterm neonates postnatal day 3

	no PDA	PDA	small PDA	large PDA
	n = 79	*n* = 67	*n* = 26	*n* = 41
U-NGAL day 3 (μg/l)	104 (79; 136)	158 (125; 201)*	177 (117; 266)*	148 (110; 200)*
U-NGAL day 6 (μg/l)	87 (63; 118)	139 (103; 190)*	166 (103; 267)*	126 (83; 190)
SCr (μmol/l)	78 (75; 82)	78 (75; 82)	78 (73; 84)	78 (74; 83)
Urinary albumin (mg/l)	29 (24; 36)	62 (51; 77)*	56 (41; 76)*	67 (51; 90)*
FENa (%)	2.6 (2.3; 2.9)	3.6 (3.2; 4.2)*	3.8 (3.0; 4.8)*	3.6 (3.0; 4.2)*
AKI, number (%)	1 (1)	6 (9)*	2 (8)	4 (10)*

NGAL urine neutrophil gelatinase-associated lipocalin, *SCr* serum creatinine, *AKI* acute kidney injury, *FENa* fractional excretion of sodium, *PDA diameter <1.5 mm* small PDA, *PDA diameter ≥1.5 mm* large PDA. Values are geometric mean (95% confidence interval) or number (percentage). *$p < 0.05$ compared to neonates with no PDA. U-NGAL day 6 was only measured in 126 neonates

to AKI [21, 22]. Also management of the PDA including Indomethacin, Ibuprofen or fluid restrictions may alter renal function or cause AKI [23, 24]. Neonates in this study were not subjected to any of these treatment strategies prior to the first echocardiography and collection of urine day 3.

In concordance with previous studies we found that U-NGAL decrease with higher gestational age at birth or birth weight and also that U-NAGL is higher in girls than in boys in preterm neonates [8, 9, 25]. Gestational age could therefore partly explain why Tosse et al. report higher U-NGAL levels in neonates with PDA needing intervention compared to neonates with no PDA or a PDA with no need for intervention. Neonates who required intervention in the study by Tosse et al. had a lower gestational age at birth than the neonates with PDA in our study, whereas the non-intervention group and the neonates with no PDA had similar gestational ages as ours. Tosse et al. did not adjust for gestational age in their analysis. When adjusted for gestational age and gender we found no association between PDA and U-NGAL which is in also in agreement with Laundry et al. [9].

AKI is defined as a sudden decline in kidney function resulting in derangements in fluid balance, electrolytes, and waste products. Currently a modified neonatal Kidney Injury: Improving Global Outcomes (KIDGO) classification of AKI accepted at the National Institute of Diabetes and Kidney Disease (NIDDK) workshop 2013 is used [26]. The applicability of these criteria for AKI in neonates is problematic because they include SCr and urinary output. Neonates often have non-oliguric renal failure [27]. SCr is difficult to interpret in preterm neonates due to incomplete nephrogenesis and the potential

Table 3 Influence of perinatal characteristics, sepsis, renal parameters, AKI, and PDA on U-NGAL in 146 very preterm neonates

	Percent change in U-NGAL Day 3		
	Crude	Adjusted GA, gender	Adjusted GA, gender, sepsis
Per gestational week	−17 (−23; −10)		
Girls only	−12 (−22; −0.2)		
Boys only	−20 (−27; −12)		
Male gender vs. female	−58 (−70; −40)		
Sepsis vs. no sepsis	329	240 (103; 466)	
Per percent increase SCr	0.4	0.3 (−0.6; 1.2)	0.7 (−0.2; 1.5)
Per percent increase urine albumin	0.6	0.5 (0.3; 0.7)	0.5 (0.3; 0.6)
Per percent increase FENa	0.7	0.5 (0.2; 0.8)	0.3 (0.0; 0.6)
PDA vs. no PDA day 3	53	0.3 (−30; 40)	0.4 (−27; 35)
Small PDA vs. no PDA	70	14 (−27; 76)	0.0 (−32; 47)
Large PDA vs. no PDA	42	−5 (−34; 38)	2.3 (−32; 41)
AKI vs. no AKI	−15	−18 (−63; 80)	−25 (−63; 52)
AKI vs. no AKI	34[a]	24 (−60; 295)	19 (−60; 269)

Percent change in U-NGAL (95% CI) concentration by one unit increase in gestational age, by 1% increase in SCr, urinary albumin, and FENa and difference in concentration between groups (male vs. female, sepsis vs. no sepsis, PDA vs. no PDA, AKI vs. no AKI). [a]U-NGAL measured day 6 in 126 neonates all other U-NGAL was measured day 3

U-NGAL urine neutrophil gelatinase-associated lipocalin, *GA* gestational age, *SCr* serum creatinine, *FENa* fractional excretion of sodium, *AKI* acute kidney injury, *PDA diameter < 1.5 mm* small PDA, *PDA diameter ≥ 1.5 mm* large PDA

impact of bilirubin on the measure of SCr. In the first days of life maternal renal function also plays a significant role in the magnitude of newborn SCr due to placental transfer [27]. Previous studies using a plethora of AKI definitions have found an association between AKI or altered renal function and PDA [28, 29]. At the time our study was designed and performed the modified neonatal AKIN classification as proposed by Jetton et Askenazi was used [15]. This definition does not include urinary output. In a cohort of very preterm neonates that all had an echocardiography day 3 to diagnose PDA we found that seven neonates (5%) had AKI within the first week of life. We found that AKI was associated with gestational age, but not PDA.

The renal function in premature neonates is affected by both immaturity with a decreased ability to reabsorb electrolytes and protein and to concentrate urine and by an increased risk of injury during the early postnatal period due to multifactorial morbidity, medication, umbilical artery catheter, and hemodynamic instability [26, 30, 31]. Urinary albumin is inversely related to gestational age, which may reflect tubular immaturity, tubular damage and glomerular dysfunction [12, 30, 32]. We found urine albumin to be associated with PDA and PDA size also when adjusted for gestational age, gender, and sepsis. A recent study found urinary albumin to be increased in preterm neonates treated with indomethacin compared to neonates that did not receive indomethacin. No information on the PDA was given in that study [33]. Urinary albumin has been found to be increased in preterm neonates with asphyxia and respiratory distress and has been suggested as a possible biomarker of AKI in newborns [32, 34] and preterm neonates [35]. In concordance with our findings FENa is known to be very high in preterm neonates and inversely related to gestational age [36]. Several mechanisms may cause this including immature tubular function, low density of sodium transporters in the tubular epithelium, and a physiological response to redistribution of extracellular fluids. After adjusting for gestational age, gender and sepsis we found no association between FENa and PDA.

Due to the difficulties in diagnosing AKI in preterm neonates, studies have investigated different biomarkers in order to allow also for earlier identification of neonates with AKI [26, 37]. An association between AKI and U-NGAL has been described in preterm neonates [8, 9, 38–40]. The definition of AKI differed in these studies, but they all included SCr. We found that U-NGAL was not an early marker of AKI in our population as we found no association between U-NGAL day 3 and AKI. Furthermore U-NGAL day 6 was not associated with AKI. In concordance with our findings Gubhaju et al. found no association between AKI and U-NGAL [30]. Gubhaju et al. recently described an association between U-NGAL and urine total protein, but contrary to us they did not find a positive association between U-NGAL and urine albumin [30]. Increased U-NGAL in extremely preterm neonates may be associated with infection, inflammation or indicate differentiation and growth of renal epithelium caused by immature nephrons stimulating glomerulogenesis [38, 41, 42]. We found U-NGAL to be associated with sepsis in very preterm neonates.

In our analyses we adjusted for gestational age, gender, and sepsis as previous studies found that they may influence U-NGAL levels. We included a total of 146 very preterm neonates in this study. Despite this being the largest cohort evaluating U-NGAL in preterm neonates, a larger cohort would be needed to allow control for more covariates and to facilitate subanalyses by gestational-age. Day-to-day variation has been described in both U-NGAL and SCr. Unfortunately; we could not collect all samples at the exact same time after birth. However, the variation in time of collection was similar in neonates with and without PDA. Renal complications in neonates with PDA may be due to hemodynamic effects of the PDA or to treatment strategies used. We were able to measure U-NGAL (day 3) before Ibuprofen was administered. However, all but one of the six neonates with PDA that were diagnosed with AKI received Ibuprofen in the interval between the two measurements of SCr used to define AKI.

Conclusion

In this cohort of 146 very preterm neonates we found no association between U-NGAL and PDA day 3 after adjusting for gestational age and gender. We found that PDA day 3 was associated with urine albumin; however PDA was not associated with AKI and FENa when adjusted for gestational age and gender. No association between U-NGAL and AKI was found. U-NGAL day 3 was associated with both urine albumin and FENa. Non-renal disease may constitute important confounders in the interpretation of NGAL and highlight the need for an enhanced understanding of the interactions between cardiovascular function, inflammation, AKI, and the risk of adverse outcome. At the present time U-NGAL is not useful as a diagnostic marker to identity very preterm neonates with a PDA causing hemodynamic changes resulting in renal morbidity within the first week of life.

Abbreviations

AKI: Acute kidney injury; FENa: Fractional excretion of sodium; GA: Gestational age; PDA: Patent ductus arteriosus; SCr: Serum creatinine; U-NGAL: Urinary neutrophil gelatinase-associated lipocalin

Acknowledgements
The authors would like to thank the parents of the infants enrolled, the staff at the neonatal intensive care unit at Aarhus University Hospital, Aarhus, and a special thanks to laboratory technician Jane Knudsen for handling plasma and urine samples.

Funding
Funding for this study was obtained from Aarhus University Faculty of Health and The Institute of Clinical Medicine, Aase and Ejnar Danielsen Foundation, Sophus Jacobsen and Astrid Jacobsen Foundation, Kurt Bønnelycke and Grethe Bønnelycke Foundation, Helga and Peter Korning Foundation, and Karl G. Andersons Foundation. The funders had no role in the study design, data collection and analysis, decision to publish, or preparation of the manuscript.

Authors' contributions
AS designed the study, collected data, performed data analysis and wrote the first draft of the paper and edited the following versions. BHB designed the study, assisted data analysis and edited the manuscript. JVB designed the study, performed echocardiography and contributed to the final manuscript. MRS designed the study, performed echocardiography and contributed to the final manuscript. VEH designed the study, assisted data analysis and edited the manuscript. GE took part in collection of data and contributed to the final manuscript. SR assisted data analysis and edited the manuscript. TBH designed the study, took part in collection of data, assisted data analysis and edited the manuscript. All authors read and approved the final manuscript.

Competing interests
The authors declare that they have no competing interests.

Author details
[1]Department of Pediatrics, Aarhus University Hospital, Palle Juul-Jensens Boulevard 99, DK 8200 Aarhus, Denmark. [2]Perinatal Epidemiology Research Unit, Department of Pediatrics, Aarhus University Hospital, Palle Juul-Jensens Boulevard 99, DK 8200 Aarhus, Denmark. [3]Department of Public Health, Section for Epidemiology, Aarhus University, Bartholins Allé 2, DK-8000 Aarhus, Denmark. [4]Department of Cardiology, Aarhus University Hospital, Palle Juul-Jensens Boulevard 99, DK 8200 Aarhus, Denmark. [5]Department of Cardiothoracic surgery, Aarhus University Hospital, Palle Juul-Jensens Boulevard 99, DK 8200 Aarhus, Denmark.

References

1. Sellmer A, Bjerre JV, Schmidt MR, McNamara PJ, Hjortdal VE, Host B, et al. Morbidity and mortality in preterm neonates with patent ductus arteriosus on day 3. Arch Dis Child Fetal Neonatal Ed. 2013;98(6):F505–10.
2. Noori S, McCoy M, Friedlich P, Bright B, Gottipati V, Seri I, et al. Failure of ductus arteriosus closure is associated with increased mortality in preterm infants. Pediatrics. 2009;123(1):e138–44.
3. Schneider DJ. The patent ductus arteriosus in term infants, children, and adults. Semin Perinatol. 2012;36(2):146–53.
4. Borregaard N, Cowland JB. Neutrophil gelatinase-associated lipocalin, a siderophore-binding eukaryotic protein. Biometals. 2006;19(2):211–5.
5. Mussap M, Degrandi R, Fravega M, Fanos V. Acute kidney injury in critically ill infants: the role of urine Neutrophil Gelatinase-Associated Lipocalin (NGAL). J Matern Fetal Neonatal Med. 2010;23 Suppl 3:70–2.
6. Mori K, Nakao K. Neutrophil gelatinase-associated lipocalin as the real-time indicator of active kidney damage. Kidney Int. 2007;71(10):967–70.
7. Mori K, Lee HT, Rapoport D, Drexler IR, Foster K, Yang J, et al. Endocytic delivery of lipocalin-siderophore-iron complex rescues the kidney from ischemia-reperfusion injury. J Clin Invest. 2005;115(3):610–21.
8. Askenazi DJ, Montesanti A, Hunley H, Koralkar R, Pawar P, Shuaib F, et al. Urine biomarkers predict acute kidney injury and mortality in very low birth weight infants. J Pediatr. 2011;159(6):907–12.
9. Lavery AP, Meinzen-Derr JK, Anderson E, Ma Q, Bennett MR, Devarajan P, et al. Urinary NGAL in premature infants. Pediatr Res. 2008;64(4):423–8.
10. Tosse V, Pillekamp F, Verde P, Hadzik B, Sabir H, Mayatepek E, et al. Urinary NT-proBNP, NGAL, and H-FABP May predict hemodynamic relevance of patent ductus arteriosus in very low birth weight infants. Neonatology. 2012;101(4):260–6.
11. Mishra J, Ma Q, Prada A, Mitsnefes M, Zahedi K, Yang J, et al. Identification of neutrophil gelatinase-associated lipocalin as a novel early urinary biomarker for ischemic renal injury. J Am Soc Nephrol. 2003;14(10):2534–43.
12. Fell JM, Thakkar H, Newman DJ, Price CP. Measurement of albumin and low molecular weight proteins in the urine of newborn infants using a cotton wool ball collection method. Acta Paediatr. 1997;86(5):518–22.
13. Stoll BJ, Gordon T, Korones SB, Shankaran S, Tyson JE, Bauer CR, et al. Early-onset sepsis in very low birth weight neonates: a report from the National Institute of Child Health and Human Development Neonatal Research Network. J Pediatr. 1996;129(1):72–80.
14. Simonsen KA, Anderson-Berry AL, Delair SF, Davies HD. Early-onset neonatal sepsis. Clin Microbiol Rev. 2014;27(1):21–47.
15. Jetton JG, Askenazi DJ. Update on acute kidney injury in the neonate. Curr Opin Pediatr. 2012;24(2):191–6.
16. Askenazi DJ, Griffin R, McGwin G, Carlo W, Ambalavanan N. Acute kidney injury is independently associated with mortality in very low birthweight infants: a matched case-control analysis. Pediatr Nephrol. 2009;24(5):991–7.
17. Mehta RL, Kellum JA, Shah SV, Molitoris BA, Ronco C, Warnock DG, et al. Acute kidney injury network: report of an initiative to improve outcomes in acute kidney injury. Crit Care. 2007;11(2):R31.
18. Kluckow M, Evans N. Early echocardiographic prediction of symptomatic patent ductus arteriosus in preterm infants undergoing mechanical ventilation. J Pediatr. 1995;127(5):774–9.
19. Evans N, Iyer P. Assessment of ductus arteriosus shunt in preterm infants supported by mechanical ventilation: effect of interatrial shunting. J Pediatr. 1994;125(5 Pt 1):778–85.
20. Kluckow M, Jeffery M, Gill A, Evans N. A randomised placebo-controlled trial of early treatment of the patent ductus arteriosus. Arch Dis Child Fetal Neonatal Ed. 2014;99(2):F99–104.
21. Shimada S, Kasai T, Hoshi A, Murata A, Chida S. Cardiocirculatory effects of patent ductus arteriosus in extremely low-birth-weight infants with respiratory distress syndrome. Pediatr Int. 2003;45(3):255–62.
22. Bomelburg T, Jorch G. Abnormal blood flow patterns in renal arteries of small preterm infants with patent ductus arteriosus detected by Doppler ultrasonography. Eur J Pediatr. 1989;148(7):660–4.
23. Gersony WM, Peckham GJ, Ellison RC, Miettinen OS, Nadas AS. Effects of indomethacin in premature infants with patent ductus arteriosus: results of a national collaborative study. J Pediatr. 1983;102(6):895–906.
24. Ohlsson A, Shah SS. Ibuprofen for the prevention of patent ductus arteriosus in preterm and/or low birth weight infants. Cochrane Database Syst Rev. 2011;7:CD004213.
25. Askenazi DJ, Koralkar R, Levitan EB, Goldstein SL, Devarajan P, Khandrika S, et al. Baseline values of candidate urine acute kidney injury biomarkers vary by gestational age in premature infants. Pediatr Res. 2011;70(3):302–6.
26. Selewski DT, Charlton JR, Jetton JG, Guillet R, Mhanna MJ, Askenazi DJ, et al. Neonatal acute kidney injury. Pediatrics. 2015;136(2):e463–73.
27. Askenazi DJ, Ambalavanan N, Goldstein SL. Acute kidney injury in critically ill newborns: what do we know? What do we need to learn? Pediatr Nephrol. 2009;24(2):265–74.
28. Walker MW, Clark RH, Spitzer AR. Elevation in plasma creatinine and renal failure in premature neonates without major anomalies: terminology, occurrence and factors associated with increased risk. J Perinatol. 2011;31(3):199–205.
29. Iacobelli S, Bonsante F, Ferdinus C, Labenne M, Gouyon JB. Factors affecting postnatal changes in serum creatinine in preterm infants with gestational age <32 weeks. J Perinatol. 2009;29(3):232–6.
30. Gubhaju L, Sutherland MR, Horne RS, Medhurst A, Kent AL, Ramsden A, et al. Assessment of renal functional maturation and injury in preterm neonates during the first month of life. Am J Physiol Renal Physiol. 2014;307(2):F149–58.
31. Koralkar R, Ambalavanan N, Levitan EB, McGwin G, Goldstein S, Askenazi D. Acute kidney injury reduces survival in very low birth weight infants. Pediatr Res. 2011;69(4):354–8.

32. Tsukahara H, Fujii Y, Tsuchida S, Hiraoka M, Morikawa K, Haruki S, et al. Renal handling of albumin and beta-2-microglobulin in neonates. Nephron. 1994; 68(2):212–6.
33. Kent AL, Brown L, Broom M, Broomfield A, Dahlstrom JE. Increased urinary podocytes following indomethacin suggests drug-induced glomerular injury. Pediatr Nephrol. 2012;27(7):1111–7.
34. Askenazi DJ, Koralkar R, Hundley HE, Montesanti A, Parwar P, Sonjara S, et al. Urine biomarkers predict acute kidney injury in newborns. J Pediatr. 2012; 161(2):270–5.
35. DeFreitas MJ, Seeherunvong W, Katsoufis CP, RamachandraRao S, Duara S, Yasin S, et al. Longitudinal patterns of urine biomarkers in infants across gestational ages. Pediatr Nephrol. 2016;31(7):1179–88.
36. Gallini F, Maggio L, Romagnoli C, Marrocco G, Tortorolo G. Progression of renal function in preterm neonates with gestational age < or = 32 weeks. Pediatr Nephrol. 2000;15(1-2):119–24.
37. Zaffanello M, Antonucci R, Cuzzolin L, Cataldi L, Fanos V. Early diagnosis of acute kidney injury with urinary biomarkers in the newborn. J Matern Fetal Neonatal Med. 2009;22 Suppl 3:62–6.
38. Genc G, Avci B, Aygun C, Ozkaya O, Kucukoduk S. Urinary neutrophil gelatinase-associated lipocalin in septic preterm babies: a preliminary study. Am J Perinatol. 2013;30(8):655–60.
39. Sarafidis K, Tsepkentzi E, Diamanti E, Agakidou E, Taparkou A, Soubasi V, et al. Urine neutrophil gelatinase-associated lipocalin to predict acute kidney injury in preterm neonates. A pilot study. Pediatr Nephrol. 2014;29(2):305–10.
40. Tabel Y, Elmas A, Ipek S, Karadag A, Elmas O, Ozyalin F. Urinary neutrophil gelatinase-associated lipocalin as an early biomarker for prediction of acute kidney injury in preterm infants. Am J Perinatol. 2014;31(2):167–74.
41. La MG, Galletti S, Capelli I, Vandini S, Nisi K, Aquilano G, et al. Urinary neutrophil gelatinase-associated lipocalin at birth predicts early renal function in very low birth weight infants. Pediatr Res. 2011;70(4):379–83.
42. Parravicini E, Nemerofsky SL, Michelson KA, Huynh TK, Sise ME, Bateman DA, et al. Urinary neutrophil gelatinase-associated lipocalin is a promising biomarker for late onset culture-positive sepsis in very low birth weight infants. Pediatr Res. 2010;67(6):636–40.

Permissions

All chapters in this book were first published in PEDIATRICS, by BioMed Central; hereby published with permission under the Creative Commons Attribution License or equivalent. Every chapter published in this book has been scrutinized by our experts. Their significance has been extensively debated. The topics covered herein carry significant findings which will fuel the growth of the discipline. They may even be implemented as practical applications or may be referred to as a beginning point for another development.

The contributors of this book come from diverse backgrounds, making this book a truly international effort. This book will bring forth new frontiers with its revolutionizing research information and detailed analysis of the nascent developments around the world.

We would like to thank all the contributing authors for lending their expertise to make the book truly unique. They have played a crucial role in the development of this book. Without their invaluable contributions this book wouldn't have been possible. They have made vital efforts to compile up to date information on the varied aspects of this subject to make this book a valuable addition to the collection of many professionals and students.

This book was conceptualized with the vision of imparting up-to-date information and advanced data in this field. To ensure the same, a matchless editorial board was set up. Every individual on the board went through rigorous rounds of assessment to prove their worth. After which they invested a large part of their time researching and compiling the most relevant data for our readers.

The editorial board has been involved in producing this book since its inception. They have spent rigorous hours researching and exploring the diverse topics which have resulted in the successful publishing of this book. They have passed on their knowledge of decades through this book. To expedite this challenging task, the publisher supported the team at every step. A small team of assistant editors was also appointed to further simplify the editing procedure and attain best results for the readers.

Apart from the editorial board, the designing team has also invested a significant amount of their time in understanding the subject and creating the most relevant covers. They scrutinized every image to scout for the most suitable representation of the subject and create an appropriate cover for the book.

The publishing team has been an ardent support to the editorial, designing and production team. Their endless efforts to recruit the best for this project, has resulted in the accomplishment of this book. They are a veteran in the field of academics and their pool of knowledge is as vast as their experience in printing. Their expertise and guidance has proved useful at every step. Their uncompromising quality standards have made this book an exceptional effort. Their encouragement from time to time has been an inspiration for everyone.

The publisher and the editorial board hope that this book will prove to be a valuable piece of knowledge for researchers, students, practitioners and scholars across the globe.

List of Contributors

Jie Qiu, Fang Li, Qian-hong Tong, Hui Rong and Rui Cheng
Department of Newborn Infants, Children's Hospital of Nanjing Medical University, Nanjing 210008, China

Yun-fei Jiang
Department of Pediatrics, Yixing People's Hospital Affiliated to Jiangsu University, Yixing 214200, China

A. E. Lange, H. Bahlmann and M. Heckmann
Departments of Paediatrics and Neonatology and Paediatric Intensive Care Medicine, University of Greifswald, Greifswald, Germany

M. Napp and J. Lange
Department of Trauma Surgery, University of Greifswald, Greifswald, Germany

Till Ittermann
Institute for Community Medicine, Div. SHIP - Clinical Epidemiological Research, University Medicine Greifswald, Greifswald, Germany

Paul-Christian Krueger
Department of Radiology, University of Greifswald, Greifswald, Germany

R. Kasch
Department of Orthopaedics and Orthopaedic Surgery, University of Greifswald, Greifswald, Germany

A. E. Lange
Klinik und Poliklinik für Kinder- und Jugendmedizin, F.-Sauerbruch-tr., 17487 Greifswald, Germany

Ashish KC, Johan Wrammert, Viktoria Nelin, Uwe Ewald, Stefan Peterson and Mats Målqvist
International Maternal and Child Health, Department of Women's and Children's Health, Uppsala University, Uppsala, Sweden

Ashish KC
United Nation's Children's Fund (UNICEF), Nepal Country Officer, UN House, Lalitpur, Nepal

Robert B. Clark
Latter-day Saint Charities, Salt Lake City, UT, USA

Stefan Peterson
Global Health, Public Health Services, Karolinska Institute, Stockholm, Sweden
School of Public Health, Makerere University, Kamala, Uganda
Health Section, Programme Division, United Nations Children Fund (UNICEF), United Nations Plaza, New York, NY 10017, USA

Mark Adams, Hans Ulrich Bucher and Dirk Bassler
Division of Neonatology, University Hospital Zurich and University of Zurich, Wagistrasse 14, 8952 Schlieren, Switzerland

Mark Adams, Julia Braun, Milo Alan Puhan and Viktor Von Wyl
Epidemiology, Biostatistics and Prevention Institute, University of Zurich, Zurich, Switzerland

Irene N. Simiyu, Deborah N. Mchaile and Kahindo Katsongeri
Kilimanjaro Christian Medical University College (KCMUCo), Moshi, Tanzania

Deborah N. Mchaile and Rune N. Philemon
Department of Paediatrics, Kilimanjaro Christian Medical Centre (KCMC), Moshi, Tanzania

Kahindo Katsongeri
Department of Obstetrics and Gynaecology, Kilimanjaro Christian Medical Centre, Moshi, Tanzania

Rune N. Philemon
Department of Community Health, KCMUCo, Institute of Public Health, Moshi, Tanzania

Sia E. Msuya
Community Health Department, Kilimanjaro Christian Medical Centre, Moshi, Tanzania
Department of Epidemiology and Biostatistics, KCMUCo, Institute of Public Health, Moshi, Tanzania

Deborah N. Mchaile
KCMC Hospital, Moshi, Tanzania

Amy Metcalfe
Department of Obstetrics and Gynecology, University of Calgary, Foothills Medical Centre, 4th Floor North Tower, 1403 29th St NW, Calgary, AB T2N 2T9, Canada

Sarka Lisonkova, Yasser Sabr and KS Joseph
Department of Obstetrics and Gynecology, University of British Columbia, Vancouver, BC, Canada

Yasser Sabr
Department of Obstetrics and Gynecology, King Saud University and King Khalid University Hospital, Riyadh, Saudi Arabia

Amelie Stritzke
Department of Pediatrics, Section of Neonatology, University of Calgary, Calgary, AB, Canada

KS Joseph
School of Population and Public Health, University of British Columbia, Vancouver, BC, Canada

Shilpa Vyas-Read, Usama Kanaan, Prabhu Shankar, David P. Carlton and Anne Fitzpatrick
Pediatrics, Emory University School of Medicine, Atlanta, GA, USA

Usama Kanaan
Sibley Heart Center, Pulmonary Hypertension Program, Atlanta, GA, USA

Jane Stremming
Department of Pediatrics, University of Colorado, Denver, CO, USA

Curtis Travers
Biostatistics, Pediatric Research Alliance, Atlanta, GA, USA

Shilpa Vyas-Read
Division of Neonatology, Emory University School of Medicine, 2015 Uppergate Dr. NE, 3rd floor, 30322 Atlanta, GA, USA

Jillian A. Patterson and Jane B. Ford
Clinical and Population Perinatal Health Research, Kolling Institute, Northern Sydney Local Health District, St Leonards, NSW 2065, Australia

Jillian A. Patterson, Jennifer R. Bowen and Jane B. Ford
Sydney Medical School Northern, University of Sydney, Sydney, Australia

Jennifer R. Bowen
Royal North Shore Hospital, Northern Sydney Local Health District, St Leonards, NSW 2065, Australia

Sally Francis
Blood Watch Program, NSW Clinical Excellence Commission, Sydney, NSW 2000, Australia

Stacey C. Dusing and Emily C. Marcinowski
Department of Physical Therapy, Motor Development Lab, Virginia Commonwealth University, Office: 1200 E Broad St. B106, Richmond, VA 23298, USA

Tanya Tripathi
Rehabilitation and Movement Sciences Program, Virginia Commonwealth University, Richmond, USA

Leroy R. Thacker
Schools of Nursing and Medicine, Virginia Commonwealth University, Richmond, USA

Lisa F. Brown
School of Nursing, Virginia Commonwealth University, Richmond, USA

Karen D. Hendricks-Muñoz
Children's Hospital of Richmond, Virginia Commonwealth University, Richmond, USA

Hans Jørgen Timm Guthe and Ansgar Berg
Department of Pediatrics and Adolescent Medicine, Haukeland University Hospital, Bergen, Norway
Department of Clinical Science, University of Bergen, Bergen, Norway

Torbjørn Nedrebø
Surgical Department, Haraldsplass Deaconess Hospital, Bergen, Norway

Jan Kristian Damås
Centre of Molecular Inflammation Research, Department of Cancer Research and Molecular Medicine, Norwegian University of Science and Technology, Trondheim, Norway
Department of Infectious Diseases, St. Olav's Hospital, Trondheim, Norway

Torbjørn Nedrebø and Helge Wiig
Department of Biomedicine, University of Bergen, Bergen, Norway

Bonnie Stevens
The Hospital for Sick Children, Lawrence S. Bloomberg Faculty of Nursing, University of Toronto, 686 Bay Street, Toronto, Ontario M5G 0A4, Canada

Janet Yamada
Daphne Cockwell School of Nursing, Ryerson University, 350 Victoria Street, Toronto, Ontario M5B 2K3, Canada

Marsha Campbell-Yeo
School of Nursing and Departments of Pediatrics, Psychology, and Neuroscience, Dalhousie University, IWK Health Centre, Forrest Building, Halifax, Nova Scotia B3H 4R2, Canada

Sharyn Gibbins
Trillium Health Partners, 100 Queensway West, Mississauga, Ontario L5B 1B8, Canada

Denise Harrison
Faculty of Health Sciences, School of Nursing, University of Ottawa, Children's Hospital of Eastern Ontario, Research Institute, 451 Smyth Road, Ottawa, Ontario K1H 8M5, Canada

Kimberley Dionne
The Hospital for Sik Children, 686 Bay Street, Toronto, Ontario M5G 0A4, Canada

Anna Taddio
The Hospital for Sick Children, Leslie Dan Faculty of Pharmacy, University of Toronto, 686 Bay Street, Toronto, Ontario M5G 0A4, Canada

Carol McNair
The Hospital for Sick Children, 686 Bay Street, Toronto, Ontario M5G 0A4, Canada

Andrew Willan
The Hospital for Sick Children, Dalla Lana School of Public Health, University of Toronto, 686 Bay Street, Toronto, Ontario M5G 0A4, Canada

Marilyn Ballantyne
Holland Bloorview Kids Rehabilitation Hospital, Lawrence S. Bloomberg Faculty of Nursing, University of Toronto, 150 Kilgour Road, Toronto, Ontario M4G 1R8, Canada

Kimberley Widger
The Hospital for Sick Children, Lawrence S. Bloomberg Faculty of Nursing, University of Toronto, 155 College Street, Suite 130, Toronto, Ontario M5T 1P8, Canada

Souraya Sidani
Daphne Cockwell School of Nursing, Ryerson University, 350 Victoria Street, Toronto, Ontario M5B 2K3, Canada

Carole Estabrooks
Faculty of Nursing, University of Alberta, 3-141 Edmonton Clinic Health Academy, 11405 87 Avenue, Edmonton, Alberta T6G 1C9, Canada

Anne Synnes
Division of Neonatology, Department of Pediatrics, University of British Columbia, 2D19-4480 Oak Street, Vancouver, British Columbia V6H 4V4, Canada

Janet Squires
Faculty of Health Sciences, School of Nursing, University of Ottawa, Ottawa Hospital Research Institute, 451 Smyth Road, Ottawa, Ontario K1H 8M5, Canada

Charles Victor
Institute for Clinical Evaluative Sciences (ICES), The Institute of Health Policy, Management and Evaluation, University of Toronto, Veterans Hill Trail, 2075 Bayview Avenue G1 06, Toronto, Ontario M4N 3M5, Canada

Shirine Riahi
The Hospital for Sick Children, 686 Bay Street, Toronto, Ontario M5G 0A4, Canada

Amala James Alenchery, Joanne Thoppil and Carl Denis Britto
Undergraduates, St. John's Medical College Hospital, Bangalore, India

Lavina Fernandez
Social Scientist, St. John's Medical College Hospital, Bangalore, India

P. N. Suman Rao
Department of Neonatology, St. John's Medical College Hospital, Sarjapur Road, Koramangala, Bangalore 560034, India

Jimena Villar de Onis
Maternal Health Research Coordinator, Compañeros En Salud, Chiapas, Mexico

Kenichi Tanaka, Hiroko Mori, Hiroshi Mitsubuchi and Masanori Iwai
Division of Neonatology, Kumamoto University Hospital, 1-1-1 Honjo, Chuo-ku, Kumamoto 860-8556, Japan

Rieko Sakamoto, Shirou Matsumoto and Kimitoshi Nakamura
Department of Pediatrics, Graduate School of Life Science, Kumamoto University, 1-1-1 Honjo, Chuo-ku, Kumamoto 860-8556, Japan

Eungu Kang
Department of Pediatrics, Hanyang University Guri Hospital, Hanyang University College of Medicine, Guri, Korea

Yoon-Myung Kim, Jin-Ho Choi, Han-Wook Yoo and Beom Hee Lee
Department of Pediatrics, Asan Medical Center Children's Hospital, University of Ulsan College of Medicine 88, Olympic-ro 43-Gil, Songpa-Gu, Seoul 05505, Korea

Minji Kang and Sun-Hee Heo
Asan Insitute for Life Sciences, Asan Medical Center Children's Hospital, 88, Olympic-ro 43-Gil, Songpa-Gu, Seoul 05505, Korea

Gu-Hwan Kim, In-Hee Choi, Han-Wook Yoo and Beom Hee Lee
Medical Genetics Center, Asan Medical Center Children's Hospital, University of Ulsan College of Medicine, 88, Olympic-ro 43-Gil, Songpa-Gu, Seoul 05505, Korea

Chi-Ju Yang, Ming Li and Xi-Gui Chen
Center of Neonatal Disease Screening, Maternal and Child Health Care Hospital, Number 12, Gongxiao Road, Jining, Shandong Province, People's Republic of China

Na Wei
Clinical Laboratory of Linyi People's Hospital, Linyi, Shandong Province, People's Republic of China

Kun Xie, Jian-Qiu Li, Cheng-Gang Huang, Yong-Sheng Xiao and Wen-Hua Liu
Zhejiang Biosan Biochemical Technologies Co., Ltd., Hangzhou, Zhejiang Province, People's Republic of China

Ji Yoon Han, Chung Joon Moon, Young Ah Youn, In Kyung Sung and In Goo Lee
Department of Pediatrics, College of Medicine, Seoul St. Mary's Hospital, The Catholic University of Korea, 222 Banpodaero, Seochogu, Seoul 137-701, South Korea

Andrea Green Hines and Alison Freifeld
Adult Infectious Diseases, University of Nebraska Medical Center, Omaha, NE, USA

Andrea Green Hines, Xing Zhao and Kari A. Simonsen
Pediatric Infectious Diseases, University of Nebraska Medical Center, Omaha, NE, USA

Ann Anderson Berry and Lynne Willett
Neonatology, University of Nebraska Medical Center, Omaha, NE, USA

Peter C. Iwen
Pathology and Microbiology, University of Nebraska Medical Center, Omaha, NE, USA

Shigeo Iijima, Daizo Ueno, Toru Baba and Akira Ohishi
Department of Pediatrics, Hamamatsu University School of Medicine, 1 - 20 - 1 Handayama, Hamamatsu, Shizuoka 431 - 3192, Japan

Silvia Maya-Enero, Francesc Botet-Mussons and Josep Figueras-Aloy
Neonatology Service, Hospital Clínic, seu Maternitat, ICGON (Institut Clínic de Ginecologia, Obstetrícia i Neonatologia), Barcelona University, Sabino de Arana, 1, 08028 Barcelona, Spain

Montserrat Izquierdo-Renau, Marta Thió and Martin Iriondo-Sanz
Neonatology Service, Hospital Sant Joan de Déu, BCNatal (Centre de Medicina Maternofetal i Neonatal de Barcelona, Hospital Sant Joan de Déu, Hospital Clínic), Barcelona University, Passeig de Sant Joan de Déu, 2, 08950 Esplugues de Llobregat, Barcelona, Spain

Manuela Capozza, Antonio Di Mauro and Nicola Laforgia
Neonatology and Neonatal Intensive Care Unit, Department of Biomedical Science ad Human Oncology, University of Bari "Aldo Moro", Bari, Italy

Iolanda Chinellato
S.C. Pediatria, P.O.C. SS. Annunziata Hospital, Taranto, Italy

Vito Guarnieri and Maria Accadia
Medical Genetics, IRCCS Casa Sollievo della Sofferenza Hospital, San Giovanni Rotondo, Foggia, Italy

Natascia Di Iorgi
Department of Pediatrics, Endocrine, Diabetes and Metabolic Unit, Istituto Giannina Gaslini, University of Genova, Genoa, Italy

Cristina Traggiai
Neonatology and Neonatal Intensive Care Unit, Istituto Giannina Gaslini, Genoa, Italy

Girolamo Mattioli
Pediatric Surgery Unit, Istituto Giannina Gaslini, University of Genoa, Genoa, Italy

Manuela Capozza
Policlinico Hospital, Piazza Giulio Cesare n. 11, 70124 Bari, Italy

Merab Nyishime, Ryan Borg, Willy Ingabire, Bethany Hedt-Gauthier, Evrard Nahimana, Neil Gupta, Christine Mutaganzwa, Francois Biziyaremye and Hema Magge
Partners In Health/Inshuti Mu Buzima (PIH/IMB), Kigali, Rwanda

Fulgence Nkikabahizi, Claudine Mukayiranga and Francine Mwamini
Ministry of Health, Kigali, Rwanda

Bethany Hedt-Gauthier
Department of Global Health and Social Medicine, Harvard Medical School, Boston, USA

Neil Gupta and Hema Magge
Brigham and Women's Hospital, Boston, USA

Anne Hansen, Michelle Labrecque and Hema Magge
Boston Children's Hospital, Boston, USA

Hema Magge
Institute for Healthcare Improvement, Addis Ababa, Ethiopia

Miyuki Kondo, Akira Ohishi, Toru Baba, Tomoka Fujita and Shigeo Iijima
Department of Pediatrics, Hamamatsu University School of Medicine, 1 - 20 - 1 Handayama, Hamamatsu, Shizuoka 431 - 3192, Japan

Srikanth Ravisankar and Parvesh M. Garg
Department of Pediatrics, Brody School of Medicine, East Carolina University, Greenville, NC 27834, USA

Rodney Tatum, Maja Herco and Yan-Hua Chen
Department of Anatomy and Cell Biology, Brody School of Medicine, East Carolina University, Greenville, NC 27834, USA

Prem S. Shekhawat
Department of Pediatrics, MetroHealth Medical Center, Case Western Reserve University, Cleveland, OH 44109, USA

Srikanth Ravisankar
Clinical Neonatologist, Mercy Medical Center, Cedar Rapids, IA 52403, USA

Parvesh M. Garg
Department of Pediatrics, Division Neonatology, University of Mississippi Medical Center, Jackson, Mississippi 39216, USA

Li-Xiao Xu and Yan-Hong Li
Institute of Pediatric Research, Children's Hospital of Soochow University, Suzhou 215006, China

Yuan Lv
Department of Neonatology, Northern Jiangsu People's Hospital, Yangzhou 225001, China

Xin Ding, Ying Wang, Xing Han, Ming-Hua Liu, Bin Sun and Xing Feng
Department of Neonatology, Children's Hospital of Soochow University, Suzhou 215006, China

Tim Schindler, Louise Koller-Smith, Kei Lui and Srinivas Bolisetty
Faculty of Medicine, University of New South Wales, Sydney, Australia

Tim Schindler, Kei Lui and Srinivas Bolisetty
Department of Newborn Care, Royal Hospital for Women, Sydney, Australia

Barbara Bajuk
New South Wales Pregnancy and Newborn Services Network (PSN), Sydney, Australia

Vidit Bhargava
Department of Pediatrics, University of Texas Medical Branch, 301 UNIVERSITY BLVD, GALVESTON 77555, TEXAS, USA

Michael Malloy and Rafael Fonseca
Department of Pediatrics, Division of Neonatology, University of Texas Medical Branch, 301 UNIVERSITY BLVD, GALVESTON 77555, TEXAS, USA

Anna Sellmer, Jesper V. Bjerre, Gitte Esberg, Søren Rittig and Tine B. Henriksen
Department of Pediatrics, Aarhus University Hospital, Palle Juul-Jensens Boulevard 99, DK 8200 Aarhus, Denmark

Anna Sellmer and Tine B. Henriksen
Perinatal Epidemiology Research Unit, Department of Pediatrics, Aarhus University Hospital, Palle Juul-Jensens Boulevard 99, DK 8200 Aarhus, Denmark

Bodil H. Bech
Department of Public Health, Section for Epidemiology, Aarhus University, Bartholins Allé 2, DK-8000 Aarhus, Denmark

Michael R. Schmidt
Department of Cardiology, Aarhus University Hospital, Palle Juul-Jensens Boulevard 99, DK 8200 Aarhus, Denmark

Vibeke E. Hjortdal
Department of Cardiothoracic surgery, Aarhus University Hospital, Palle Juul-Jensens Boulevard 99, DK 8200 Aarhus, Denmark

Index

P

R

S

T

V

Z

information can be obtained
CGtesting.com
he USA
53020123
0004B/80

9 781639 274222

CPSIA information can be obtained
at www.ICGtesting.com
Printed in the USA
LVHW061753020123
736284LV00004B/80

9 781639 274222